Cranial Intelligence

by the same author

Body Intelligence
Creating a New Environment
Second Edition
Ged Sumner
ISBN 978 1 84819 026 9
eISBN 978 0 85701 011 7

You Are How You Move
Experiential Chi Kung
Ged Sumner
ISBN 978 1 84819 014 6
eISBN 978 0 85701 002 5

of related interest

The Insightful Body
Healing with SomaCentric Dialoguing
Julie McKay
ISBN 978 1 84819 030 6
eISBN 978 0 85701 026 1

A Practical Guide to Biodynamic Craniosacral Therapy

Cranial Intelligence

GED SUMNER and STEVE HAINES

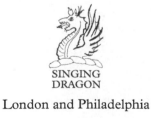

SINGING
DRAGON

London and Philadelphia

First published in 2010
by Singing Dragon
an imprint of Jessica Kingsley Publishers
73 Collier Street
London N1 9BE, UK
and
400 Market Street, Suite 400
Philadelphia, PA 19106, USA

www.singingdragon.com

Library of Congress Cataloging in Publication Data
A CIP catalog record for this book is available from the Library of Congress

British Library Cataloguing in Publication Data
A CIP catalogue record for this book is available from the British Library

ISBN 978 1 84819 028 3
eISBN 978 0 85701 012 4

Printed and bound in Great Britain

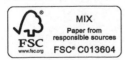

Contents

List of figures

Acknowledgements

The authors would like to acknowledge the significant contributions made by Franklyn Sills in the development of biodynamic craniosacral therapy. He has been a major influence and inspiration for both authors. He has originated many key parts of the biodynamic paradigm and created definitions of the work that have been adopted within the field. We have tried our best to acknowledge the historical roots of the work. Any errors in interpretation are our own. The authors would also like to acknowledge the ground-breaking work of the cranial osteopaths, especially Sutherland and Becker, both of whose bodies of work this book draws upon.

The artwork was by Helena Lee and Steve Haines. A huge thanks to Helena for her essential input to the drawings and the style. A big thanks also to Viola Sampson for her clear and extensive feedback and editing suggestions on the whole of the first draft. We are grateful for the comments on chapters of the first draft from Silvia Neira, Liz Garner, Katherine Ukleja and Michael Kern.

Ged Sumner: I would like to acknowledge the key influences of Michael Kern and Paul Vick, both of whom have inspired and confirmed many discoveries along with creating opportunities to teach and support me while evolving as a teacher, plus the many conversations about the theory and teaching of the work with other senior tutors who have helped to formulate a personal clarity.

Steve Haines: I would like to say additional thanks to Francoise Wright Brown, an amazing practitioner, Katherine Ukleja, an essential source of support, inspiration and clear thinking, and Michael Kern, for the many opportunities and encouragement he has given me to develop my skills. My dad died during the writing of this book. He nicknamed it 'Ouch'; I could never quite convince him I do more than work with pain. He would have been very happy and proud it got finished. Finally, thanks to Kate, obviously.

Foreword

It seems like a long time since we started to develop a biodynamic approach to craniosacral therapy. It started back in 1986 when a colleague, Claire Dolby DO, suggested that I develop a cranial course outside of osteopathic practice that was more directly influenced by Sr Sutherland's later work. We had both met while in osteopathic college. Claire was afraid that the cranial approach was not reaching enough people and that there was a real opportunity to create a new profession. So, with some trepidation, we started the first training group at the Karuna Institute in 1987. It was only 36 days long and geared for people already practising some sort of orthodox or complementary healing form. We took a mixed approach where there was a predominantly biomechanical mental-set oriented to analysis, motion testing and various techniques geared to resolve resistance and compressive forms in the body. This was supplemented by some orientation to the fluid tide and potency, and an introduction to dynamic stillness. It also had a cathartic edge with unwinding techniques and emotional releases without a real grounding in, or understanding of, trauma skills.

At a tutor's meeting in 1992 we all agreed that we were not really teaching what we were practising, which was much more oriented to primary respiration and a biodynamic approach to the work. We decided to change the curriculum at that point. It took another ten years to develop new teaching approaches and slowly change the curriculum. In this period I had to develop both new perceptual exercises and a new language for the work. This included perceptual processes that oriented students to the various levels of expression of primary respiration, new terms like mid tide, state of balance, relational field, primal midline and holistic shift and a real reorientation of student mentorship in the trainings. We also increased the course length to 50 days spread over two years. We clearly saw that it takes at least two years for students to deepen into the work and to develop the perceptual skills needed in the work. A number of us (initially myself, Claire Dolby, Michael Kern, Colin Perrow, Katherine Ukleja and Paul Vick) also taught outside England: in America, Canada, Germany, Italy and Switzerland, to name just a few places. Along with Michael Kern DO, I also helped start the

Craniosacral Educational Trust in London. The various people who have taken the work out into the world have developed it in different ways, and biodynamics is a growing, developing and diverse field of work.

A biodynamic approach to craniosacral therapy entails a real perceptual shift from the patterns and conditions present within the system, to the inherent forces that organize them. The student learns to perceive primary respiration, the inherent health within the human system, and orients to conditional patterns and their organizing fulcrums within this context. Thus the practitioner orients to formative forces, not just to their effects (like strain patterns, compressions, pathologies, etc.). The most important components of a biodynamic approach includes the development of a state of presence, the ability to establish a clear and negotiated relational field, the ability to orient to primary respiration both in yourself and in another person, and the perceptual skills to orient to what is called the inherent treatment plan and to be able to track to its unfoldment with appropriate clinical skills.

I started to write new texts for the field in 1995, which were published in 2000. They were out of date from the moment they were available! I am in the process of framing new texts, but it was to my delight that Ged Sumner and Steve Haines contacted me about the new book they were producing. Both were originally trained at the CTET in London and Steve has been a tutor both on the CTET course and at the Karuna Institute, while Ged, who originally taught at the CTET, has developed trainings in Australasia. Their book provides a practical approach to the work based upon their clinical experience, with lots of exercises, a focus on embodiment and a clear orientation to the simplicity and power of a biodynamic approach. I hope their new text becomes a real resource both for trainings and in professional life. May we all continue to learn, deepen and continually clarify our relationship both to this wonderful work and to the nature of life itself.

Franklyn Sills
Co-Director
The Karuna Institute

Preface

This book emerged from our experience of teaching biodynamic craniosacral therapy around the world. The goal is for it to be an intensely practical book directly relevant to clinical experience as a bodyworker. Primarily it is written for people interested in craniosacral therapy; however, we hope that there is much that is useful for all sorts of bodyworkers. The first five chapters have debates on boundaries, perception, working safely with trauma, birth and how stories are held in the body that are relevant to many therapeutic approaches. The final chapter on practice development covers issues pertinent to all practitioners struggling to set up a successful practice. The authors have studied and been around many forms of natural medicine; however, the biodynamic craniosacral approach offers something very profound and inspires a whole way of meeting the world and living your life that is sensitive and connected.

There are a number of key ideas that are fundamental to biodynamics: the breath of life and its expressions, how patterns of experience shape the body, meeting overwhelm with resources, being in a relational field, being in stillness, embryology, birth and ignition processes. These will be explored in Chapters 1 to 7.

Alongside the key concepts are a number of key skills essential to the practice of biodynamic craniosacral therapy. These are: the power of presence, developing perception, recognizing the holistic shift, working with the inherent treatment plan, facilitating states of balance, orienting to tides, relating to Becker's three-stage process, working with augmentation or conversation skills and skills to orient to the deeper forces of health. All of these key skills will be introduced in Chapters 1 and 2, and are referred to throughout the book.

Anatomy is the language of the body. If you do not speak the language when you go to a new country then you can still have a great time. If you can speak the language, things will happen much more quickly and there are far more possibilities. Knowing the anatomy and physiology of the human system allows a practitioner to ask much more interesting questions of the body and to respond to the puzzles and challenges of disorder in much more effective ways. An intelligent system will know that you know; it will respond to your ability to bear witness to what you are feeling. As such, certain pieces of anatomy are explored more fully: the nervous system, the spine, the cranium, the organs, the connective tissue matrix, the fluid systems of the body, the facial complex including the jaw and throat and the major joints. Some of these subjects are assigned to whole chapters in the latter half of the book; others, fluids and tissues especially, are woven into the whole text.

Throughout the book are experiential awareness exercises that lead you through explorations of your anatomy and biodynamic health expressions. These are a key part of the book and when practised start to reveal a new relationship through touch and perception. From teaching experience, the authors strongly recommend these as powerful ways to increase your sensitivity.

1

Relational Touch

1.1 THE RELATIONAL FIELD
The phenomenon of contact

Words are powerful things in the modern world. We read them and listen to them and the concepts and ideas behind them deeply influence us. However, words are learnt things and before words came touch. This was our first experience of life. The embryo is fully tactile in its orientation to its environment – movement of tissues and fluids are its sensate world, it is growing in the mother's body and later attached to the mother through the umbilical cord. Imagine what that must be like, growing in utero, and receiving blood into your body. The baby's world is completely engaged in movements and sensations within and without its body. The experience of growing and forming a body can only be guessed at, but these early enfoldments of fluids and tissues are a powerful movement into form.

Birth itself is a pushing and squeezing of the baby's body and is a unique, whole-body, sensory experience. The new baby craves touch, its survival depends on contact. It seeks contact with the mother's breast for assurance – the power of touch is etched into our brain and every cell in our body seeks relationship. In a healthy environment, touch means safety, assurance, nutrition and familiarity. These are our first communications with the world. Our first attachments are primarily based around touch.

It's no wonder that touch continues to be a huge force in our lives. So much of our expression and communication is conditioned on how we touch and how others touch us. Our needs in life often revolve around the kind of touch we are receiving or not receiving. Touch can elicit a gamut of emotions. Modern society has had a tendency to move away from strong expressions of touch. Children are often touched much less than they need; adults can hold back from touch as they feel too vulnerable or exposed. Therefore, to offer touch as a therapist can evoke an array of feelings. The nature of biodynamic touch is that it is non-imposing, without desire, open and unpressured. This is a rare kind of touch. Often people have never been touched in this way. Often the touch we are used to is qualified with another's needs. Biodynamic touch comes from a place of originality within us, it's a state of creative presence that is not caught up with the conditioned mind. The kind of touch offered in biodynamic craniosacral therapy brings people back to a more primal cellular experience that they had when they were in utero. It takes us back to the first moments of growth before experience changes us and creates patterned behaviour. It's an undifferentiated touch.

Attachment, neuroscience and relational touch

As we grow we attach. Attachment is necessary for our survival. Our first attachment is to our mother's uterus. The fertilized egg implants deeply into the wall of the uterus and this starts the process of development of the body. The growing embryo attaches even more strongly through the umbilicus and shares blood with the mother. The baby attaches to the breast and then forms powerful attachments to its caregivers.[1] These relationships are vital to life. As the baby grows it's clear that it's the relationships themselves that are the most important thing. The baby is driven to form relationships; this is instinctively its prime directive.

If it forms stable and secure relationships then it continues to develop healthily. If these relationships are not secure, the baby's development is affected. The baby's brain grows rapidly during the first few years of its life and neural pathways are being laid down that will determine how it responds to its environment later on.

There are key moments and windows of development that require the right external environment, feedbacks and emotions to be present for optimal growth. When there isn't ideal development then there are levels of dysfunction in the body and mind.[2] Key developments in the brain's hard-wiring and functioning can be affected by the lack of a secure and healthy caregiving environment.

A biodynamic craniosacral therapist offers a relational touch that duplicates these ideal early states. By offering this original space you mimic the security our brain is looking for. You mimic a field of relationships that is creative and non-judgemental. There is no imposition; clients are offered a place to grow again. When you become adept at creating this space you will notice that primary forces in the body start to move and reveal themselves throughout the body's tissues, leading to reorganizations that can go down to the neural and cellular level. The brain and body can reprogramme themselves.

The influence of another presence

Just being there is no small thing. When we are present with someone's expressions of their life force, there's a profound effect created that brings about healing. How relieving it is to be heard. Just to be heard. Not having someone qualify the hearing by providing a solution, intervening, or trying to offer something else. Rare indeed it is that someone will just listen intelligently without intervening with their own life story, opinions, solutions or ideas/concepts/fantasies of what is happening.

When you experience this, a wonderful healing takes place and there is a natural relief of your suffering. This can be so profound that you have physical sensations and changes as well as emotional expressions. Someone has acknowledged who you are. It might only be for a short time or just a moment but that's all it needs. It's the deepest form of communication, being to being. There are no words in this connection and it feels timeless. As a craniosacral therapist you bring into the therapeutic space your beingness. The more deeply you can manifest this, the more powerfully people respond to your touch and presence.

Sit for a moment and see if you can be with your state of beingness. When you reside in it you can truly be the witness. Its qualities are presence, clarity, simplicity and non-doing. It's a state of repose and acuity, it's not a sleepy state. You are actually bringing together a balance of internal and external awareness into harmony. From this place you can begin to see what is happening. Let go of ideas of what you might find, or formats for making sense of things. Try to observe what is, unfettered by your own fantasies or anxieties. Only then will you be able to have any sense of what is happening in yourself or in another person.

At the heart of the craniosacral touch there is this state of being present. Practice will make you more skilful at being able to manifest this. Eventually this starts to become part of you in a more apparent way. What you will notice too is a burgeoning sense of spaciousness, both gross and subtle. You will feel bigger and fuller as if you not only occupy your body but the space around it too. Also you will notice a mental and emotional spaciousness that allows you a deeper and richer contact with your thoughts and feelings. The spaciousness allows a disengagement, so that a natural state of non-attachment comes about.

You can engender this state through a practice of opening into this spaciousness. The wider the space, the deeper and more energetic the manifestation of health. As you widen out there is an expression of energetic forces within the body that can be felt as tingling or fluid-like movements throughout the body. This is the movement of potency and the phenomenon of primary respiration.

Awareness Exercise: Touching ourselves

1. Comfortable sitting position.

   - Come into an easy sitting position, with the full weight of your hands resting on your thighs.

   - Allow yourself to settle and relax. This exercise takes at least 5 to 10 minutes, so your comfort is important.

   - Notice your breathing. Notice body sensation. Say hello to your body.

2. Full weight of the hands in contact.

    - What do you notice under your hands?

    - Can you get a sense of the skin, the muscles and fascia, the blood and the bones?

3. 'Butterfly touch' contact.

    - Staying in contact with the thighs, make the lightest-possible contact with your hands.

    - Does the shift to a 'butterfly touch' contact change what you can feel?

    - Maybe you begin to get a sense of your whole leg, not just the area under your hands. Maybe differences between the legs or even the whole sides of your body begin to present.

4. Imagine your hands 30 to 50 cm away from the body.

    - Stay in physical contact but imagine your hands 30 to 50 cm away from your thighs.

    - This a perceptual trick, or shift, that will change what you perceive. What do you notice now?

    - Maybe you begin to get a sense of your whole body breathing and connecting up. Go slowly.

5. Dual circuit.

    - When we touch ourselves we create a dual circuit into our brain. There is the information coming from the hand and the information coming from the tissue being touched. See if you can appreciate these two circuits. Do they match up?

    - When we try to become aware of ourselves there is a similar dual circuit: the idea of what we should feel (more external, like the touching hand) and the moment-to-moment direct experience from the inside (more internal, like being touched). Frequently our idea of the body is quite different from what we can actually feel if we pay attention.

6. Bring the exercise to a close and try and write down what you felt.

Treatment Exercise: Where do we touch from?

1. Work in pairs.

    - This exercise is for working in pairs. Set up the space you are in so that you are either both sat down on chairs next to each other or one of you is on a treatment couch.

- Spend a while getting comfortable. Allow yourself to settle and relax.

- Notice your breathing. Notice body sensation.

2. Make contact at the shoulders.

- Gently bring one or two hands into contact with your partner's body. Try contacting their shoulders. Allow their system to get used to the contact.

3. Explore where you touch from.

- Bring your attention to your forehead and notice how it feels to listen to your hands and partner's body from this place. Stay with it for a few minutes.

- Shift your attention down to the centre of your chest. Do the same from here.

- After a few minutes let your attention move down to the centre of your pelvis. Again notice how this feels and how it changes the contact.

- Which place did you feel most comfortable listening from? Ask your partner which place had the deepest effect on them. Spend time experimenting with this. See if you can derive a contact that has internal connections to all three places.

1.2 WHAT IS BIODYNAMIC CRANIOSACRAL THERAPY?

Overview

Two big ideas go to the heart of cranial work: (1) the whole body expands and contracts in a rhythmic or tidal way; (2) there is an intelligence expressed through the whole body.

A skilled practitioner can interact with the rhythms and tides expressed by the body. The rhythms are very rich in information. If you were watching someone breathing and they were breathing quickly and rapidly in their upper chest you might learn to associate that with activity, excitement or anxiety. Similarly the tempo, strength and presence of the various tides in the body tells us huge amounts about that person. The founder of the work, W.G. Sutherland, initially described five key movements in the body: the mobility of the cranial bones; the fluctuation of cerebrospinal fluid; the motility of the central nervous system; the reciprocal tension membranes; and the involuntary mobility of the sacrum between the ilia. However, the tide is not limited to these five elements: it is expressed throughout the total human system; every cell knows the tide. Every cell breathes, inhaling and exhaling within cycles of what Sutherland called 'primary respiration'.

The smartest thing in the room is the intelligence expressed in our bodies. There are millions of years of evolution behind the shapes and forms and movements in the body. There are lots of coordinated self-regulating processes that respond to events and maintain an internal balance and flow. This intelligence defines the chemistry, nervous activity and alignment in the body. Biodynamic craniosacral therapy experiences this intelligence as an expression of a wider ordering principle in nature. Health is an active principle; it is a living breathing reality that can be palpated by knowing hands. Sutherland named the ordering principle as the breath of life. We will also use the term biodynamic health to represent this principle.

These central ideas will be explored in much more detail as the book unfolds. In any new paradigm, and biodynamic craniosacral therapy offers a radically different model of health, there is often a struggle to describe the insights in everyday language. When Sutherland was first struck with the thought that the bones in the head moved, this was against the accepted model of his time.[3] The next sections introduce a number of new terms; they will become familiar as you read on. There is a glossary at the end of the book to help.

A brief history of cranial work

The work grew from the pioneering insights of William Garner Sutherland. His identity was very much that of an osteopath and his writings are full of references to his teacher A.T. Still, the founder of osteopathy. He started writing about and teaching 'osteopathy in the cranial field' from the late 1920s. He died in 1954 at the age of 81.

Sutherland's early descriptions of the 'primary respiratory mechanism' defined five phenomena:

1. The fluctuation of the cerebrospinal fluid – the potency of the tide.

2. The function of the reciprocal tension membrane.

3. The motility of the neural tube.

4. The articular mobility of the cranial bones.

5. The involuntary movement of the sacrum between the ilia.

(Sutherland 1990, Chapter 2)

Towards the end of his life his writing underwent a shift in emphasis to include not just the mechanics and infinitesimal movements of the structures of the body, but also an increasing reverence for the breath of life. It was during the last few years of his life that he began to describe principles such as being a more passive observer and waiting for something to happen rather than just applying techniques, 'liquid light', primary respiration as being outside as well as inside the body and the power of stillness (Sutherland 1998, later chapters).[4]

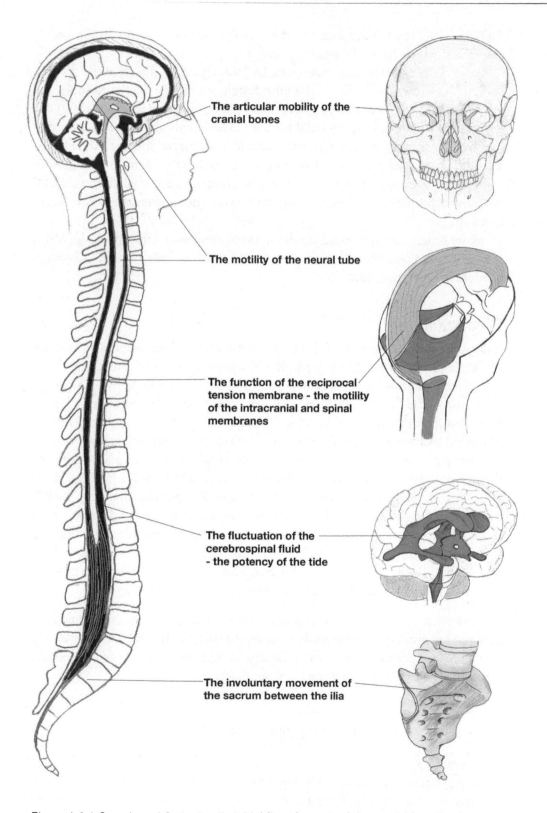

The articular mobility of the cranial bones

The motility of the neural tube

The function of the reciprocal tension membrane - the motility of the intracranial and spinal membranes

The fluctuation of the cerebrospinal fluid - the potency of the tide

The involuntary movement of the sacrum between the ilia

Figure 1.2.1 Overview of Sutherland's initial five elements of the cranial hypothesis

The cranial approach was passed on through a lineage of osteopaths, Rollin Becker and James Jealous being the most prominent.

In the 1970s an American osteopath, Dr John Upledger, observed the distinct, regular movement of a dural tube (the tough membrane that surrounds and protects the spinal cord) during surgery on a patient's neck (Upledger 2009). He studied the work of Sutherland, did his own experiments and caused a schism in the work by starting to train non-osteopaths in 'craniosacral therapy'. Upledger is a prolific writer and trainer and has done a huge amount to increase awareness of craniosacral therapy. Through his institute he claims to have trained over 20,000 people around the world. The training can be very short, often only a few weeks in length.

Many others have developed the discipline of craniosacral therapy. Hugh Milne is another craniosacral therapist and author of note; he calls his work visionary craniosacral therapy (Milne 1995).

Biodynamics

Jealous adapted the term biodynamic from his study of the embryologist Erich Blechschmidt. Jealous calls his work the 'biodynamic model of osteopathy in the cranial field'. He emphasizes the embryo as being ever present in the living organism (McPartland and Skinner 2005). He only teaches osteopaths. Osteopath is a legally protected term that can only be used by fully trained and registered osteopaths. The word biodynamic has connotations of holism and interrelationship.[5]

The biodynamic principles began to be applied to craniosacral therapy through the work of Franklyn Sills and the teachers at the Karuna Institute in the UK. There is now an International Affiliation of Biodynamic Trainings (IABT) consisting of eight schools. The biodynamic approach is one in which the main focus is the forces at work within the human system via mid tide, long tide and dynamic stillness (Ukleja 2009a). The work relates to insights from the later years of Sutherland's life. Franklyn Sills, Michael Shea and Michael Kern (Kern 2006) have all written defining books on biodynamic craniosacral therapy.

To review: there are cranial osteopaths and craniosacral therapists (sometimes described as having a biomechanical approach) (McPartland and Skinner 2005). There are biodynamic osteopaths in the cranial field and biodynamic craniosacral therapists. This book is about the latter approach.

Clinical Highlight: Cultivating patience and being present

In practice
The greatest qualities you can engender as a practitioner are the qualities of presence and patience. Sitting and waiting for your client's system to unfold

and communicate its health and history to you requires the ability to listen without any intention. This quality is what the body likes; it feels free to communicate openly.

- *Not being in a rush to know.* This requires you to let go of the need to analyse by searching or scanning using your mind and focus. Be a true Taoist and wait for the universe to unfold and inform you.

- *Not wanting to change things.* Do you really know what needs to change? The body is so complex that it's impossible to know exactly what is going on and what needs to change, what order it needs to change and in what way it needs to change to bring about greater health.

- *Not worrying about results.* The more you can let go of this anxiety the more you will be able to be present for what is actually happening in your client's system and only then will significant change take place.

It's important you give the body time to settle and reveal itself. Then give the body time to access the breath of life and for natural reorganization to take place. If you are too focused and intense you will stop this process from taking place. As your skills of differentiation develop you will feel the body more clearly and consequently notice when biodynamic forces are starting to assert themselves.

Useful intentions to bring to the body system:

- Establishing an optimal relational field.

- Looking for the health; 'Where is the health?' is a very useful question to ask yourself.

- Inviting the tide.

- Allowing things to unfold.

Breath of life

Sutherland discovered the existence of a movement in the body that he termed primary respiration. The animating force behind this movement he called the breath of life. He believed this was an energetic expression of an intelligence in the universe. The expression of primary respiration is a longitudinal fluid motion that has two phases of inhalation and exhalation, oriented around the midline of the body. Inhalation can be felt as an arising movement that expands laterally and exhalation as a complementary movement that recedes down towards the lower body and narrows side to side, very much like the ebb and flow of the tide. The qualities Sutherland attributed to the breath of life are:

- Basic constitutional energy of the body, having a potency and healing function.

- Conveys intelligence to every cell and tissue of the body and is the inner physician.

- Maintains order and integrity in the body.

The breath of life has several expressions that can be palpated by the skilled practitioner. One of the most common is the expression of primary respiration as a tidal movement, sometimes called the tide. Often you will be struck by its longitudinal expression which can feel very tidal. The flow is a potent surge of fluid potency that moves up the length of the midline to the head. A strong expression of this can feel as if it is pushing you out of your chair. The other expression is the lateral widening and narrowing that can feel like an expansion and contraction. Sometimes the head and body feel like a balloon that is inflating. Sometimes you have a full sense of the movement as a rising and widening and it feels like the balloon changes shape but not volume. It is interesting how you perceive it and how different aspects show themselves to you.

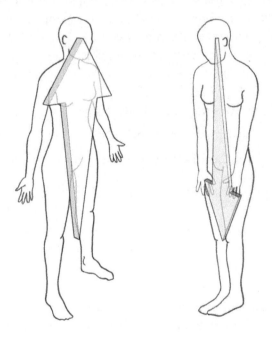

Figure 1.2.2 Whole body inhale and exhale
On inhale there is a rising, filling and widening side to side; on exhale there is a sinking, emptying and narrowing side to side

As you become more adept at feeling these expressions you can gain a sense of the nuances of the tide. These are the characteristic movements for that individual. So how the inhalation and exhalation phases are, the pauses at the change of the phases, the drive or amount of potency behind the movement, all define the body system and become the baseline for tracking change. Being in relationship to this force of life changes everything; there is a chain reaction that brings about a greater order of health. Watch the tide and see what happens. It's as if the body is made of sand and the movement of the ocean is reshaping and smoothing out the contours. The action of the tide itself highlights the body's forms and patterns and then brings about reorganization. In a treatment the tide may not reveal itself all the time. If you are following the inherent treatment process and relating to the body with an adaptable perceptual field, you will be in relationship to what the body wants to show you, that is, its priorities for treatment. Then, often the tide will reveal itself at key moments in the treatment and bring about deeper and more holistic changes.

1.3 KEY SKILLS 1: HOW TO COME INTO RELATIONAL TOUCH

Expanding your perceptual field

What separates us from each other as human beings? If aliens came to Earth we would probably all look the same to them. Just in the same way we look at a colony of ants and they all look the same. On the surface we have two arms, two legs, a head and torso. Obviously, there are differences in the detail, but these are minimal next to the gross construct of humans. So how do we differ? Are we all the same? Obviously no, our internal worlds are radically different. We all have similarly wired sensory nervous systems but we seem to process information in quite different ways. Perception is the view we have of the world around us. Perception is what makes us different. Two people can look at the same object and have quite different experiences of it; not just in terms of its dimensions and physical attributes but about its position in space and its relationship to other objects and to themselves. Try the perceptual field exercise below and see what happens for you.

Awareness Exercise: Exploring space and perceptual fields

- Find a room you are comfortable in. Make sure you are alone and the room is quiet. Start this exercise when you have established a state of balanced awareness (see p.31).

- Be interested in the space immediately around your body. Can you feel it? Even though this is beyond the margin of your body, you will find there is a strong palpable relationship to this space.

- Include this extra space in your balanced awareness. Stay with it for a while. Are there any changes that occur in your breathing?

- See if you can shift into relationship with a wider space around you. It's a 3D space, let's say the extended space that is the rest of the room you are in. Try being in your peripheral vision, not staring or focusing at any one object. Stay with that for a while.

- It's important not to strain. It's not an effort to do this. You aren't trying to spread your awareness into the whole room, just be in relationship to it. Notice what happens in your breath, in your mind and most importantly in your perception of yourself and the room. Nothing has changed in the room, the same objects are there. What has changed is your orientation.

- If someone came in now, would they be affected by your relational state? Notice body sensation and become aware of any changes of movement in your body.

- Notice stillness in the body.

- Notice how the space feels like it is enfolded around you, as if the space and your body and your mind are all part of one thing, in a natural way.

- If you feel you are becoming anxious, allow your perceptual field to gather closer to your body or come right back into the whole of your body sensations.

- Try relating to an even wider space, one that goes beyond the room and out into the space around the room and perhaps out to the sky and to the horizon. At first this will be a visualized thing, but you will notice that you quickly connect to something else.

- Sit with this for a while and simply observe.

- To finish the exercise you might need to come into a more immediate sense of your surroundings to avoid being disoriented.

As you can see there is a spectrum of experiences that results from the space and interconnectedness you view the object from. The perceptual field you orient to says more about your universe than any other aspect of you. A wide perceptual field reveals a very different universe than a narrow one. It naturally brings you into relationship with the implicit order of things, whereas a narrow field orients you more to the explicit, so that you see the object as separate and particular. A key skill in biodynamic craniosacral therapy is to be able to meet the client's system with a perceptual field they naturally orient to and to be able to hold open the door for them to enter a different perceptual field. This is like being on the same wavelength, and allows their system to be heard and met appropriately. Tissues, fluids and potency will then naturally mobilize and respond within this perceptual field. As reorganization occurs there is commonly an inner need of the client's system to shift to another perceptual field. It's important the practitioner has the ability to orient to and welcome this shift, so that the system is being heard and met with a different field of relationships.

A simple way of stating the relationship between perception and the body system is to acknowledge what is predominant in each perceptual field. For a narrow perceptual field, tissue is most expressed, so that you naturally find yourself in relationship to particular body structures and how these express primary respiratory motion as the cranial rhythmic impulse (CRI), the fastest of the three tides. Fluids and potency are also present, as these three elements are interwoven within the fabric of the body. As your perceptual field widens, it's natural to feel fluid as the most dominant expression within your perceptual field. The experience is of a body of fluid so that you are entering into relationship with the totality of body fluids and not just individual pools of fluid. This body of fluid is made up mostly of fluid within and around the cells. Primary respiratory expressions at this level of perceptual field would be mid tide. You can still feel the tissues of the body, but they are now more interested in relating to you as whole body patterns. As the perceptual field widens even more, our potency state becomes the most expressed element and primary respiration at this unfoldment is called long tide.

Awareness Exercise: State of balanced awareness

- Sitting still comfortably, allow yourself to settle and relax. Notice your breathing, notice body sensation.

- Become aware of movement in the body, and stillness.

- Notice how structures organize themselves around your central axis (spine and head).

- Feel your body in 3D, feel the front, back, top, bottom and sides of you.

- Your body occupies space. Staying with the sense of internal space, become aware of the space around you.

- Enter into the world of the senses by coming into your hearing. Notice smells. Slowly open your eyes and come into visual sensation. Experience these senses but stay in contact with your internal space/sensations.

- Try to find a state of balanced attention between external sensory experience and internal space/sensations. There is an interface where your attention is inclusive of both and feels at ease. This is a powerful place that will change from moment to moment; try to follow it so you stay with the state of balanced awareness.

- Notice what changes this creates in your body, mind and consciousness during and after the practice.

There seem to be three distinct unfoldments that represent, perhaps, the movement from potency through fluids to tissue or the movement we made when we were forming as embryos from energy to matter. That early organization of our body is still reverberating within us and still shows itself to the sensitive therapist as natural states of unfolding and enfolding through levels of perception and states of consciousness. Not only the body but the mind goes through profound changes as there is a deepening and widening of perception. The mind becomes quiet and free of thoughts as if it is connected back to a simpler state, perhaps back to a relationship to the early embryonic neural tube when the central nervous system was mostly fluid, or back to earlier forms before the body structures appeared. Anyone who has experienced long tide would say their sense of themselves as a body with a boundary and form often dissolves to be replaced by a sensation of lightness and expansiveness that might be more to do with the early shapes that life produces before the body even shows itself. These are mostly fluid-filled shapes. Perhaps these are a primordial meeting place of fluid, tissues and potency that we reconnect back to in the wider perceptual fields. So it's not so much that we go out and connect to the matrix of living things around us, but more as if we deepen into our original nature which is much more linked to the matrix of life.

Treatment Exercise: How much space do you need? Using 'Self, Other, Field' to help create space and a ritual of contact

1. Work in pairs.

   • This exercise is for working in pairs with one person lying on a treatment couch.

2. Self – state of balanced awareness.

   • As the practitioner, go through the state of balanced awareness exercise above.

3. Other – negotiate physical contact.

   • When a state of balanced awareness is established, gently bring your hands into contact with your partner's body.

   • Make sure the contact is pysically comfortable for both of you. The right contact space will vary from one person to the next and is very individual. Check in verbally as you negotiate the physical contact.

4. Field – negotiate perceptual space.

   • Play with your perceptual field to widen or narrow your awareness of the contact space. Some people might want a very expanded space; others might want a much closer space. This is a constant dance as sessions progress.

- Talk with your client about how the different perceptual fields feel for them. Negotiate with your client until you offer the right space for them. Only then will their primary system and respiration reveal themselves.

- In future sessions try bringing a consistent approach to making contact and setting up the relational field. A 'ritual of contact' will help you come into present time as you start each session.

Making contact from a state of balanced awareness

It is important to set the therapeutic and contact space up in a right way to facilitate the establishing of a relational field. Take your time doing this. Realize that from the moment your client walks into your room you are facilitating this process. In particular, when setting yourself up at the treatment couch you need to be comfortable so you can relax and listen. You will often need to stay in one particular hand hold for long periods of time during the session.

Typically you might make two or three hand holds during a treatment, so that's probably around 10–15 minutes in each position in a 35-minute hands-on session. Allow your hands to relax and offer a light touch. Make sure that the weight of your arms is being supported through your elbow contact into the couch. Your spine should be comfortably upright and the soles of your feet placed on the floor. Once these parameters are in place you can make contact anywhere on the body. Your posture is pivotal in creating an optimal contact. Being upright and balanced mechanically means you are at ease and available. Try to be oriented around your spine and pelvis as they are the main frame for weight bearing throughout the body. The important thing is to sit deep in your pelvis and sink into your sitting bones and soles of the feet. When you can do this well, the midline automatically becomes present and potent. Consciously allow your spine to stack along its length. You can spend some time doing this so that each section of the spine feels optimized in its position with the whole spine, and then each vertebra with its neighbours. The other crucial thing is to allow your head to balance as optimally as possible in relationship to the spine. The head is so heavy, just a slight side shift or rotation can have a huge effect on the spine and the rest of the body. Don't worry about trying to look aligned, it's best to feel aligned internally. Finally, always make sure your hands are supported by your body posture. This means pivoting on your elbows or your forearms. The art of offering a relational field requires you to be at ease all the time, so getting used to being in balanced posture through the length and breadth of your body is vital. Spend time using cushions and setting the height of your chair and table to make all of this easy. Once you have this in place get used to being still in your body. You can practise this by sitting or standing in meditations and of course through practise of the therapy.

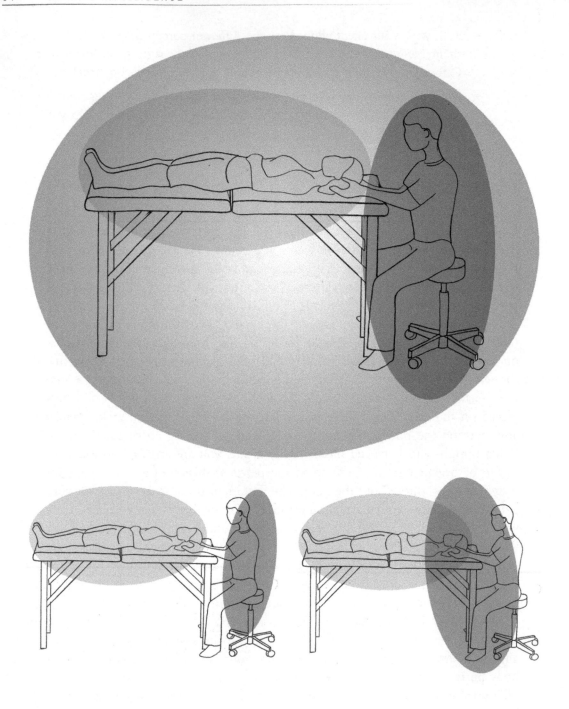

Figure 1.3.1 Making contact

Top: Ideal space, just meeting the biosphere of the client. This allows shared access to a much bigger space, sometimes called a 'third egg'. Bottom left: Too far away. Bottom right: Too close, resulting in a merging of the fields

Making contact and creating a relational field has a number of important components:

- Optimal posture.
- State of balanced awareness.
- Orientation to your midline.
- Orientation to your tissues, fluids and potency.
- Orientation to your primary respiration.
- Manifesting a still presence.

Being in relationship to all these aspects of your system acts as a huge resource for your client's system. How inspiring to have these qualities be in contact with you. As the practitioner you are operating from your biodynamic health. This is contagious and will open up a doorway to your client's body system to also access its deeper health and awareness. One of the main effects of this therapy is the creation of a greater sense of awareness. This in itself is healing and highly integrating of all aspects of us. The other huge influence is your ability as the practitioner to know your own system and its biodynamic expressions. Only then can you perceive it in others, only then can you be an intelligent, knowing listener. Otherwise you are blind to your client's body story and the underlying power of health and there will be a poor response. Only when these are in place does the body engage and reorganize itself from within.

The most important skill of the practitioner is to create a state of balanced awareness. This is an ability to simultaneously listen to your internal sensations and to be in relationship to your external sensory field. This is key to the safety and efficacy of the treatment. Spend time practising the state of balanced awareness exercise.

The inherent treatment plan reveals itself

When you have established a relational field sit back and listen. Become an interested, curious observer. Wait for the body system to reveal itself to you. That means not having a predetermined idea of how things are. Try to let go of any information you have received about your client's health and history.

Letting go of expectations is not any easy process and it can take time to truly sit in contact with no intention. It's important you cultivate this attitude as the body will then reveal its true health to you and its priorities. Touching with no intention is a huge force and is irresistible. Really try to have no expectations of what you might feel. What could come to you is a multitude of things, but to know what is being presented to you is what is important to the body. As you recognize the elements of the body anatomy presented to you there is a natural communication that takes place that leads to more revelations.

Initially the communication is about tissues and fluids local to your hand contact. These themselves may be the immediate priority or you might notice other movements taking place away from your hands in another part of the body, but again they are local. As the process of communication moves forward there is a gradual moving to whole body communication and expressions of primary respiration. When this happens you are communicating with the breath of life which starts to become active in the body and set more holistic priorities for change. Sills describes this as an 'holistic shift'.[6] Patterns of experience held in the body may start to reveal themselves. These will be generally something the body has held onto for some time.

Becker's three-stage process

Becker (1997) describes a three-step healing process that accurately defines what you feel when the body responds to relational touch.

1. *Seeking.* Step one involves many movements of tissues, fluids and potency and these movements naturally seek a state of balance where all the organizing forces of the pattern of experience come into relationship with each other.

2. *Setting.* Step two describes a pause or stillness that occurs when a state of balance is reached. Something happens.

3. *Reorganization.* Step three is when primary respiration resumes and there is a greater expression of health felt through a fuller expression of primary respiration and a balance and symmetry to tissue motion.

This is a wonderfully refreshing definition of what occurs under your hands or in relationship to your touch in every session. Becker was a true clinician and his definition is based on thousands of hands-on sessions. The other great thing is that he manages to keep the definition simple and based on what actually happens rather than a flowery idea of what occurs. Biodynamic craniosacral therapy is simple. The body's natural responses to this touch are clear and eloquent. You can easily become lost in the complexity of the body and miss the simple underlying responses. At the heart of this work is a relationship with the breath of life and your ability to be present with it. That's primarily what brings about deep change.

A state of balance is often preceded by common signs. The body intelligence is manifesting as if a new consciousness is trying to arise. This can be felt as an orientation to a particular part of the tissue field along with a perturbation in the local fluids. It's as if the potency/fluid/tissue relationship is trying to renew itself and only by all three coming back into relationship can there be a meaningful change. The important thing to understand here is that this process is a natural mechanism of the body. It's not something that needs inducing. What the body needs is a tactile knowing presence to be able to mobilize itself. It can't be any touch though, it needs to be a touch that can sense the underlying biodynamic health, know the anatomy and physiology that is being communicated and be holistic. The very reason the pattern has come about in the beginning is that it has lost its relationship to the whole and become separate. In a treatment session a healthy and potent body can go through many states of balance, some of them so fast you can't name them or so many of them going on at the same time you are not aware of them all. That's fine. All you need to know as a practitioner is that the body is shifting and changing and reorganizing itself and that if this is happening you are creating the right relational field. Bodies that are less potent will move through states of balance more slowly.

Differentiating tissues, fluids and potency

One of the core skills in craniosacral therapy is the ability to differentiate what you are feeling. Fluid and tissue move quite differently to each other. Each kind of tissue has its own unique way of expressing mobility and motility. There are four different kinds of tissue in the body: connective, muscle, epithelial and neural. Of course connective tissue covers a huge range of things like blood, bone, lymph, fascia, membranes, ligaments, tendons and joint cartilage.

All these structures have particular feels to them. When you are able to name what you are relating to and know what the body is showing you then a precision of listening enters your relational touch which acts deeply on the body. This allows the body to communicate with you more powerfully; suddenly you are hearing the words and the meaning behind them, not just an indistinct noise or vague meaning. The body likes this acknowledgement of its form and responds with a deepening into primary respiration. Often this accuracy in touch is followed by a surge of potency and defined changes take place.

It is very useful when treating to be able to distinguish between tissues, fluids and potency. Initially many people will naturally orient to feeling one of these three expressions of primary respiration in the body. Ultimately you will be able to feel the tissues, fluids and potency moving together as a unified tensile field. However, different routes into the whole will show you different things and support your ability to recognize and differentiate what you are feeling.

Tissues can be thought of as connective tissues, muscles and bones. They tend to exhibit pulls and twists and a classic sense of tension (like pulling on a jumper) more obviously. Nerves are also tissues; nervous tissue has its own particular feel, but often you can feel compression or stretching of peripheral nerves.

Fluids comprise all the water and fluid-based systems in the body. We are at least 65 per cent water, big, hairy, salty bags of fluid. All our cells are bathed in fluid. There are different compartments, to be sure, but the fluid body has a continuity of its own. It feels, well, watery. It is swirling, flowing, easily tidal, and it fills and empties. It is a very good route into the mid tide. In addition, fluids are also viscous; they are sometimes sticky and mucus-like. A body of fluid can hold twists and tension.

Potency is the cranial term for energy. It's a beautiful word, not degraded by common use; it speaks of a sense of potential and of inherent power. It can be experienced as light, fiery, windlike, a mist, tingling, to name a few common themes. Experience will give you your own language. It can commonly be an entry point into long tide and the first experience of field effects.

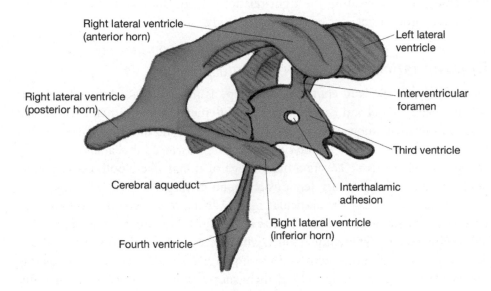

Figure 1.3.2 Oblique view of the ventricles of the brain

The ventricles are a unique meeting place of potency and fluid, cerebrospinal fluid is a very powerful mediator of potency

Treatment Exercise: Differentiating tissues, fluid and potency via the sacrum and occiput

1. Start at the sacrum.

   • Ritual of contact. Wait for the holistic shift. Orient to mid tide.

2. Tissues.

   • Without narrowing your awareness, see if you can feel the sacrum as a bone, then a bone held in a sock of ligaments and then feel its connections through the whole tissue body. Which words fit to your perceptions?

3. Fluids.

   • Shift your perception to fluids. Can you feel the fluid, blood-filled nature of the bone? Orient to the sacral canal and lumbar canal and then begin to get a sense of the cerebrospinal fluid (CSF). Can you get a sense of the whole fluid body expanding and contracting? How do fluids feel to you?

4. Potency.

   • Shift your awareness to include the potency. Liquid light, sparkling, shimmering, charged – see which words work for you. Can you feel the whole biosphere – the field around the body?

5. Move to the occiput.

   • Take time to settle and just see what speaks to you. Are you drawn to tissues, fluids or potency? Can you name what you feel?

   • Finish by trying to feel the body as a unified tensile field of tissues, fluid and potency, everything moving together.

Awareness Exercise: Feeling tissues and fluids

   • This exercise is a self-exploration, using experiential anatomy guidance.

   • Sitting calmly, place your hands on your thighs. Come into an awareness of sensations from the palms of your hands. Have an intention of feeling the tissue layers under your hands. First there is the skin. Can you feel the unique quality of the integumentary system? Do you get a sense of continuity?

   • Underneath the skin is a superficial layer of fascia. This is a different kind of tissue structure. Can you sense how different it is?

   • Underneath this are muscles with their individual fascial wrappings. Again, this is a different kind of tissue that you are feeling. What are the qualities of the muscles? Try using words to describe them.

   • Underneath the muscles is the long bone of the femur. Can you get a sense of this? This is a very different tissue. Can you feel the whole of the bone? At the centre is the bone marrow, a very active area of the body. Can you sense this? This is a very powerful place with lots of activity going on. Blood is moving throughout all of these structures, bathing all of the cells. Maybe you can sense its flow.

Biotensegrity and tissues

Tensegrity is the exhibited strength that results when push and pull have a win–win relationship with each other. Tension is continuous and compression discontinuous, so that continuous pull is balanced by equivalently discontinuous pushing forces. The term is well known in architecture. The American architect and inventor Buckminster Fuller (1961) explained that these fundamental phenomena were not opposites, but complements that could always be found together. Tensegrity is the name he gave for this synergy between co-existing pairs of fundamental physical laws; of push and pull, and compression and tension, or repulsion and attraction. Webster's dictionary has simplified the collective meaning as 'all things working together'. Biotensegrity is a combination of the words biomechanics and tensegrity; it is a useful term for applying the concepts to living things.[7]

The concept has huge applications in biology. Biological structures such as muscles and bones or rigid and elastic cell membranes are made strong by the unison of tensioned and compressed parts. The muscular skeletal system is a synergy of muscle and bone; the muscle provides continuous pull, the bones discontinuous push.

The rubber skin of a balloon can be seen as continuously pushing (against the air inside) while the individual molecules of air are discontinuously pushing against the inside of the balloon, keeping it inflated. All external forces striking the external surface are immediately and continuously distributed over the entire system, meaning the balloon is very strong despite its thin material. Similarly, thin plastic membranes such as plastic bags are often stronger when loaded rather than unloaded.

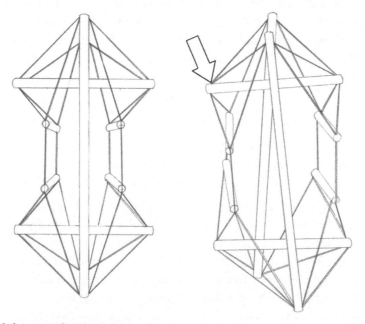

Figure 1.3.3 A tensegrity structure

On the left, neutral state. On the right, the whole structure distorts due to the conditional force represented by the arrow

Sutherland understood this concept well when he named the dural membranes of the skull and spine the reciprocal tension membrane system. It's a natural biotensegrity system, as are many other structures in the body. The spine is another structure that fits this model. When there is health there is a balance between the forces, but when there is a lack of health and strength the biotensegrity breaks down and the potency of the system decreases. When you feel the body you can tell if these forces are in balance. When the body resources itself in treatment the first thing to emerge is the feeling of biotensegrity. Biotensegrity is discussed more in Chapter 5.

Fluid form

Life in motion comprises shapes and patterns all having different qualities, expressing themselves in unique ways. Sometimes it can feel overwhelming, especially in a healthy system. There is so much life and life likes to express itself as motion. Where there is life there is motion. No motion means no life, which means death, so the more motion you feel in someone the more health there is.

Lots of the movements feel fluid-like, which is not surprising as we are mostly composed of water. Within the fluid matrix there is movement of the tissues of the body. That means cells and structures are all expressing the breath of life in their unique way, like the instruments of an orchestra. The entire piece of music represents the movement of the whole body system, yet within it are many individual sounds. However, all of this exists in a fluid tensile field and the fluid is water. Water is a molecule that is special because of hydrogen bonds. Oxygen is so much bigger than hydrogen that it pulls more of the electron cloud around it, creating a potential difference along the molecule and creating a V shape. This makes water electric and the hydrogen bonding creates a tensile field. This property produces water droplets. The surface of water has a strong tensile energy in it, creating a tension through the body of the water but also a surface tension. Water is a fundamental substance in the body, indeed we are water-based life forms much more than carbon-based, so the qualities of water are paramount within us. Not surprisingly our bodies show strong properties of tensegrity throughout all the tissues. Tissues are merely copying the property of water. All structures mirror this; not just membranes and fascia but also muscles and nerves and bone. Intrinsic to all these structures is the interstitial/extracellular space which is made up of water and collagen. The next most common substance in the body after water is collagen. Collagen is a triple helix molecule that is a hollow tube-like structure. The triple helix is held together by hydrogen bonds. The collagen tubes are hollow and interstitial fluids move through them. This fluid is like brine, water and salt, and the water molecules form an ongoing link to the collagen through hydrogen bonds. Therefore you have a fluid connective tissue tensile field as the substrate of the body. All cells exist in the interstitial fluid so the fluid is like a base substance for the whole body.

Let's add another property of water to this: its electric nature. Water is often called the universal solvent because so many substances can exist in it in their ionic states. Salt for instance easily dissolves in water and differentiates into its ionic form. Water can accommodate this. Not only does it allow molecules to exist in their electrical form, but it also allows chemical reactions to take place within it. So you now have an interesting set of qualities: naturally tensile, electric, continuous with collagen and the universal chemical solvent. When you put your hands on someone and set up a relational field many of the properties you are feeling are these. Sutherland described a fluid within a fluid; perhaps what we perceive is the electrochemical nature of water. When we attune to mid tide and sense a whole body of fluid motion, perhaps what we are coming into relationship with is the interstitial space. This is a discrete body of fluid that has a strong connection to the connective tissue framework.

Awareness Exercise: The fluid electric body

- Bring your awareness to your biosphere. Come into a sense of all that is contained within the sphere and your midline. Wait for the mid tide to show itself, and notice how the expression of the tide feels. What is the strong sense of fluid that is such a property of the mid tide? Where is the fluid? Can you feel the tingle that is often expressed in this tide? Can you also feel the sense of the fluid as being like a body of fluid? Literally it feels like the fluid has a tensile energy to it that feels as if it has a surface tension and an internal tension. Is there any sense of tissue in the tide? Often tissues within the mid tide are described as feeling like seaweed. Could this be the connection of interstitial fluid to the connective tissue framework of the body?

- At this level of connection to the body, not only changes in structure and alignment take place, but chemical balances can be affected too as a deeper ordering occurs within the molecular activity of the fluids.

- This is a level of the body where potency is more present. It infuses into the fluids of the interstitial space and acts upon the molecular balance and structural integrity. Therefore, just being in relationship to the mid tide can be a deeply beneficial state for the body order.

Stillness

A stillpoint is the temporary cessation of the expression of primary respiration in the body. Sutherland emphasized the importance of the stillpoint as a fulcrum for the action of the fluid tide. A fulcrum is an important concept in biodynamics – it is something that organizes or influences. Stillpoints can last from just a moment to many minutes; sometimes a whole session can be spent in stillpoint. Commonly it will last for a few minutes. During stillpoint the whole body becomes potentized with the breath of life, especially the fluids of the body. This is a natural resource for the body. Physiologically, fluid exchange is encouraged in stillpoint. Toxins may be discharged or eliminated.

The system will also attempt to process patterns of experience present in the body tissues and mind. The increased potency helps unresolved issues to complete their healing and resolve. Just think about that for a second. You have a natural mechanism in you that can bring about spontaneously more energy and more health without you having to do much. Lie on a couch and be touched by a craniosacral therapist, that's all it takes!

Dr Sutherland stated that there is a 'transmutation' of the potency of the breath of life within fluids which acts to convey this principle to the cellular and tissue world. The healing resource of the system is intensified and the drive and vitality of the system increases.

It's as if you have had a long, deep sleep, even though it has only lasted minutes. Often automatic adjustments can be felt in your body, as if a deeper intelligence is creating balance and a higher state of health. Many people experience creative ideas and automatically solutions to things in their lives simply appear in their minds. It must be similar to the state of discovery that many inventors describe.

Clinical Highlight: Cultivating stillness

In practice

When you are establishing a relational field, invite your system to become still. This means your mind, emotions and body start becoming still. The feeling of this is very pleasurable. Stillness of mind means your mind empties of thoughts, which is a relief as thoughts are in many ways tiring. With the emptiness comes expansiveness and timelessness. It's as if without thoughts we become timeless. This is a wonderful quality to manifest in your relational touch and will precipitate stillness in your client. This is a powerful thing as everyone needs stillness. It's a going back to our deepest nature before the mind and thoughts developed.

During sessions it might come to you that your client's system is busy and not settling. Simply sink into your internal stillness and see if this inspires your client's system to follow suit. You are suggesting stillness, and as stillness is such a strong state it's very difficult to resist.

In everyday life

Stillness is best derived from meditation practice. There are many approaches to meditation, but all of them have this as a common element. Practise stilling the body in a sitting or standing posture. As your body starts to be happy with not moving, you will notice the mind starts to follow. At first it might seem the mind becomes noisier, but that's because you are not distracted by your body movements any longer.

In time, with consistent daily practice your mind will be still too. Your thinking process will often stop. If thoughts do arise in this state of internal stillness they will not distract you, indeed they are often very creative thoughts that emerge in this space. You will notice that a permanent internal stillness becomes always available to you in whatever activity you are engaged with. You will also notice that the relational field you establish is much more effective and brings about powerful changes in your client's health in a short space of time.

Clinical Highlight: What happens when we feel nothing?

Ever had that moment when you put your hands on someone and you can't feel a thing? So you wait a bit more and still nothing is happening. Well you are not alone in this. Rest assured that thousands of practitioners before you have been in this situation. The main thing is not to panic. Setting off your sympathetic nervous system will not help anyone! The following are some of the most common reasons for what might be happening.

You have lost all your skills of touch
Actually very unlikely, though sometimes during the training when you are acquiring skills, abilities you had become proficient at suddenly aren't there for you any longer. This changes in time and is often an indication that there are unconscious transformations happening and a new you with new skills will emerge.

You aren't establishing an optimum relational field
Actually very likely. This takes some doing at first and can always prove tricky, especially at the beginning when you are starting to develop a sense of the subtle. This is a refined state to set up and takes a finesse that will come with time and practice. The best thing to do is check all the elements in the contact. A common difficulty is dissolving intention in your hands and in your system as a whole. This can be commonly felt as a pressurizing force by your client's system and they will naturally contract in response to that.

All of this may well happen at an unconscious level so that you aren't aware of what you are doing, and your client isn't aware they feel uncomfortable and are contracting. The important thing here is to get tutor help. An experienced set of hands will be able to tell that this is the case and help you meet the client's system in a more appropriate way.

Your client's system is shut down

Through a traumatic experience that has not been resolved your client's system may have shut down. Sometimes this can occur during a session but can also be a permanent state for some people. Lots of people in the world have suffered terrible traumatic experiences and this could well be the case for your client whether they have disclosed this to you or not. At a touch level their system will not exhibit any primary respiratory motion or motility. Often there will not be a sense of potency either, and tissues will feel fixed or frozen.

There are degrees of shut down. What is useful is to engage verbally with your client and explore what they are feeling in their body and mind. This may give you clues as to what is happening in the fluids and tissues, plus opening a dialogue often engages their primary system and suddenly there's some motion taking place.

Your client might be in stillpoint

This is quite different from a shut-down process. You will know this as there's a sense of spaciousness and potency in a stillpoint. Often your own system might be in stillpoint too. As you become more familiar with this state you will know it immediately. However, it's unlikely that your client has dropped into stillpoint from the first touch you make with them, but it could be that they are exhausted and their system is desperately seeking balance and new energy, both of which will take place in stillpoint.

Summary of Chapter 1

This chapter has introduced and explored some major themes in the biodynamic craniosacral paradigm: the phenomenon of touch and in particular the natural processes that take place when we touch with an inclusive and non-interfering contact. It looked at how listening and presence can bring about dynamic change to higher states of health and how stillness is a natural mechanism that comes about through craniosacral touch. It also explored skills to start to recognize underlying subtle biodynamic forces within the body anatomy and physiology.

The chapter has discussed a number of practitioner skills that will be established from practising the exercises described:

- Establishing a state of balanced awareness.

- Being able to achieve a settled state within your own system.

- Negotiating the contact space with your client.

- Being able to sit back and listen to how your client's system is.

- Establishing a clear relational field.

- Noticing expressions of primary respiration in your own body and others.

- Recognizing stillness in yourself and others.

- Inviting systemic stillness in your client's system.

- Offering a wide perceptual field.

Notes

1. Bowlby is the defining author on attachment theory. Holmes (1993) is a good introduction to Bowlby.
2. Schore (1999) charts changes in brain development linked to attachment processes. In addition, Sapolsky (2004, pp.104–105) describes dwarfism in stressed children in orphanages. There is an amazing, and well-documented, case of two nurses working in two different orphanages in post-war Germany. One nurse was warm, nurturing and comforting, the other critical and berating. The two growth rates in the orphanages were very different. The children in the orphanage with the comforting nurse grew more. When the critical nurse took over from the comforting nurse the growth rates in her former orphanage promptly increased; those in her new one decreased.
3. Sutherland was initially intrigued by the possibility of the skull bones moving when at osteopathic college at the end of the nineteenth century. He was looking at a disarticulated skull and a thought struck him that the temporal bone was 'beveled, like the gills of a fish, indicating articular mobility for a respiratory mechanism'. It took another 30-plus years of experimentation, initially largely on himself, before he published his ideas in *The Cranial Bowl* in 1939.
4. Jealous (2004) provides an excellent overview of the development of Sutherland's approach (CD series No. 4).
5. Biodynamic is also a term used by Rudolf Steiner.
6. Holistic shift is a phrase that emerged from the teaching of Franklyn Sills; see Ukleja (2009a).
7. Stephen Levin (2009) is an orthopaedic surgeon who runs one of our favourite websites (www.biotensegrity.com).

The Midline

2.1 THE EMBRYO, MIDLINE PHENOMENA AND ORIGINAL HEALTH

The embryo

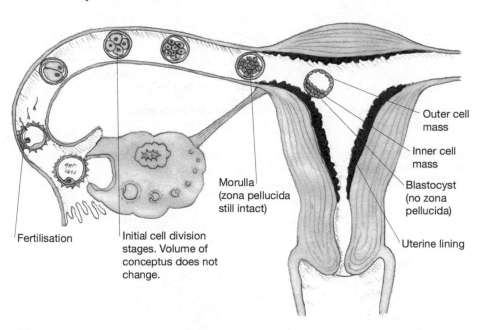

Figure 2.1.1 The passage of the conceptus towards the uterus

The forces of creation that form the embryo are the forces of healing. The directions and actions of the biodynamic forces that shaped the embryo are still present, and can still be perceived, in the adult. The embryo is a very powerful motif for biodynamic craniosacral therapy. There is an explosion of growth and movement in the embryo and within the first eight weeks all the major structures are essentially in place. After eight weeks the foetus grows and matures.

As cell division begins from the cell formed from the union of the ovum and the sperm, the new cells begin to have their own individual relationship with the environment. A cell in the middle will have different pressure on each side, may be further from the nutrient source and have a different relationship to the fluid, chemical surroundings.

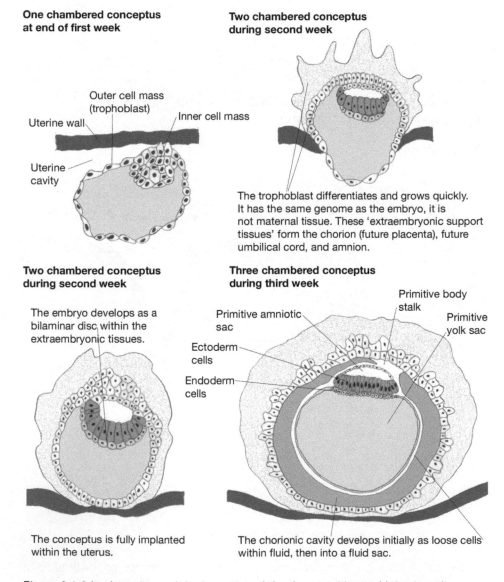

One chambered conceptus at end of first week

Outer cell mass (trophoblast)
Inner cell mass
Uterine wall
Uterine cavity

Two chambered conceptus during second week

The trophoblast differentiates and grows quickly. It has the same genome as the embryo, it is not maternal tissue. These 'extraembryonic support tissues' form the chorion (future placenta), future umbilical cord, and amnion.

Two chambered conceptus during second week

The embryo develops as a bilaminar disc within the extraembryonic tissues.

The conceptus is fully implanted within the uterus.

Three chambered conceptus during third week

Primitive body stalk
Primitive amniotic sac
Primitive yolk sac
Ectoderm cells
Endoderm cells

The chorionic cavity develops initially as loose cells within fluid, then into a fluid sac.

Figure 2.1.2 Implantation and the formation of the three cavities and bilaminar disc

These epigenetic (literally over or above genetics) experiences begin to change the development of individual cells and groups of cells. The position and movements of cells (their morphology) within this dynamic fluid field determine how they begin to differentiate. Groups of cells begin to have a shared history and begin to form different layers and dynamic structures. The insight of Blechschmidt[1] is that epigenetic field forces (metabolic fields) are significant formative, creative processes active in the embryo.

The biodynamic craniosacral therapy model recognizes an additional epigenetic force, an energetic field that is laid down at conception by the breath of life – the original matrix. The original matrix is both within and without cells; it is enfolded within the potency, fluids and tissues of the human form from conception.[2]

The in-depth study of embryogenesis (embryo formation) has led to many new insights within biodynamic cranial work. The growing shapes and the early intentions and gestures expressed by the embryo as it comes into form are still organizing the body as it is continually recreated in the present. Understanding and orienting to these underlying dynamic fluid and potency movements is a phenomenal way to support the process of healing.

The midline and early embryo

One cell becomes a group of cells following the imperative of cell division. A cavity forms within the group of cells and some of the cells clump together. This takes about a week and the structure is now called the blastocyst. The blastocyst contains two groups of cells, the inner cell mass and the outer cells, with very different fates. The outer layer, or trophoblast, will form the placenta. The inner cell mass will form the actual embryo. It is interesting that the embryo forms within a larger field of cells that originated from the cell formed at conception (see Figures 2.1.2 to 2.1.4).

The first cavity becomes the yolk sac. A second cavity then appears, the early amniotic cavity. Between the cavities a double layer of cells develops. This is the embryonic disc. This double layer of cells is where the embryo forms. The amniotic cavity is formed from the ectoderm germ layer. The layer of the yolk sac becomes the endoderm. As described below a third layer of mesoderm forms between the layers. The ectoderm becomes the nervous system and a layer of the skin; the endoderm becomes the gut tube and associated organs, epithelia and glands; the mesoderm forms all the connective tissue structures. These three layers are known as the germ layers. The tissues that derive from each of the germ layers maintain a coherent identity throughout life; they are very useful orientations in biodynamic cranial work. The ectoderm will be explored when we look at the nervous system in Chapter 9, and the endoderm will be covered under visceral intelligence in Chapter 8.

The primal midline starts life as a surge of cell reorganization in the ectodermal layer of the embryonic disc at the start of the third week after conception. A primitive streak appears from the caudal end of the disc, rising up over a day to produce a pit half way up the length of the disc (see Figures 2.1.5 and 2.1.6). This uprising movement is a movement that typifies the expression of the primal midline throughout life. Over the next few days there is an explosion of activity that results in a third germ layer being produced (mesoderm) through a process called gastrulation. Gastrulation involves the migration of ectodermal cells into the primitive streak and a conversion to mesoderm. The notochord process is formed out of this third middle layer of mesoderm. By day 17 after conception there is a hollow tube formed in the mesoderm that will become solid and be the reference for the neural tube and the gut tube. Therefore, the notochord is the first midline tube to be formed and the primitive streak is the first expression of midline motion. Over the next few days the action of differential growth means the primitive streak diminishes as the notochord becomes more prominent. It's as if the primitive streak represents an energetic surge or directional intention that creates a chain reaction of midline formations. The primitive streak is there for a day and gone the next, while the notochord becomes the first axis of the developing body.

It's understandable that this process could be viewed as a mystical expression which reveals the fundamental movement of life often referred to by the yogis as kundalini, the kabbalists as shekinah, the taoists as thrusting chi. The notochord is the central energetic channel of the body system that underpins all other channels and body physiology. The notochord, like the primitive streak, dissolves and becomes an energetic phenomenon at the core of the system. Remnants of the notochord are precursors of the nucleus pulposus of the spinal disc joints and the ligaments connecting the dens of the second cervical vertebra to the occiput. The vertebral bodies form around the notochord as do the body of the sphenoid and the ethmoid. This is taken therefore as the line of the primal midline. Thus a relational field that has an orientation to the primal midline will bring about an absolute centring, and is often regarded within the biodynamic field as coming into an original intention.

Being able to appreciate the early organizing nature of midline phenomena is a key skill within biodynamic craniosacral therapy. The midline is a fulcrum for all development and healing. It can be experienced as a still centre where health is returning into relationship with the midline.

It is useful to differentiate two main expressions of the midline:[3]

- The fluid or posterior midline: it starts as the neural grove; it is located within the spinal cord through to the lamina terminalis at the front of the third ventricle. Inhale and exhale through the fluid midline can frequently be felt as a mid tide (and long tide) phenomenon.

- The primal or anterior midline: it passes through the coccyx, sacrum, vertebral bodies and cranial base ending at the sphenoid body/ethmoid.

A continual (therefore non-tidal) uprising surge, it follows the path of the notochord.[4]

Any experience of midline phenomena is always significant. To distinguish between the different midlines will take time. At this stage we are concerned only with a general appreciation and exploring of the fluid midline and primal midline.

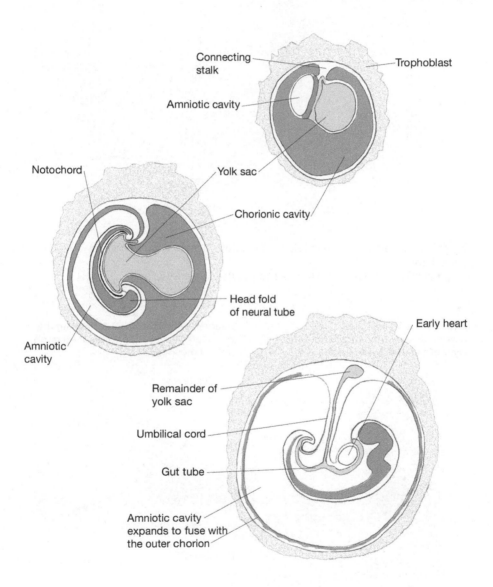

Figure 2.1.3 Embryological development of the three cavities

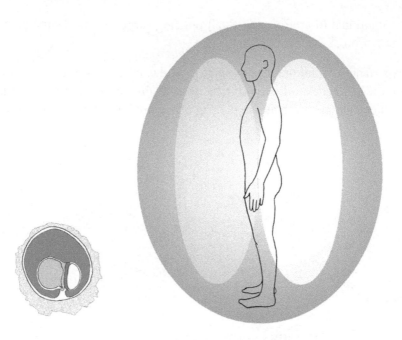

Figure 2.1.4 Schematic diagram relating the three cavities and trophoblast in an embryo to the adult body
The 'extraembryonic support tissues' can be equated to the biosphere

Amniotic cavity removed looking down on the ectoderm layer of the disc (end of week 2)

Enlarged section at level A showing the migration of cells to form the third germ layer of mesoderm.

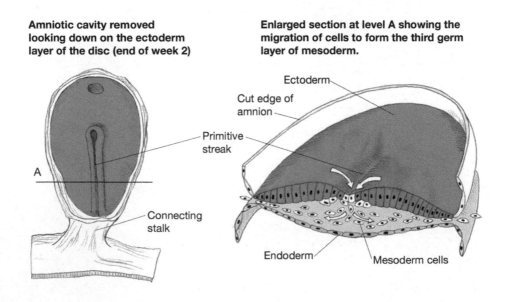

Figure 2.1.5 Embryological formation of the primitive streak and the third germ layer of mesoderm

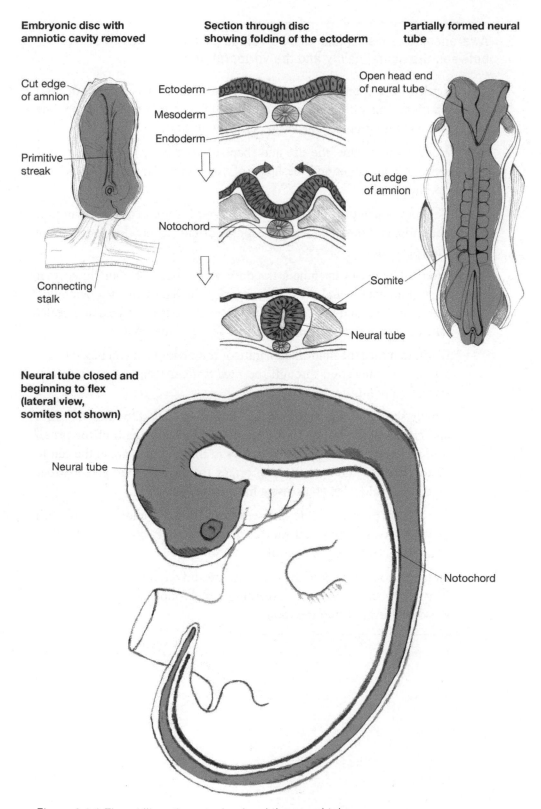

Embryonic disc with amniotic cavity removed

Cut edge of amnion

Primitive streak

Connecting stalk

Section through disc showing folding of the ectoderm

Ectoderm

Mesoderm

Endoderm

Notochord

Partially formed neural tube

Open head end of neural tube

Cut edge of amnion

Somite

Neural tube

Neural tube closed and beginning to flex (lateral view, somites not shown)

Neural tube

Notochord

Figure 2.1.6 The midline, the notochord and the neural tube

Awareness Exercise: Fluid midline versus primal midline – moving between the neural cavity and the vertebral bodies

- Settle into a comfortable sitting position. Feel your contact with your chair via your sitting bones and the earth via your feet. Take some time to come into present-time awareness of your body.

- Notice your outline, the size and shape of your body. Try to get a clear sense of your edges and the limits of your body. This is the space you occupy.

- Begin to notice your breathing, follow your breath, in and out, through your nose and throat and into the lungs. Briefly acknowledge the whole thoracic cavity.

- After a few cycles imagine a trapdoor at the back of your throat that opens into your neural cavity – the space bounded by the neurocranium, vertebral canal and the sacral canal. Deepen your awareness and really take time to notice the space and get a sense of the cavity.

- Begin to notice the fluid-filled nature of the cavity. Can you begin to get a sense of connection through the *fluid midline*? Can you sense a tidal rising and falling?

- Slowly shift your awareness forward into the vertebral bodies, the discs and cranial base through to the ethmoid. This is the path of the *primal midline*. Remember the vertebral bodies in the abdomen are in the centre of the body. Settle more deeply, orient to the long tide and a wider perceptual field. Can you sense a light rising quality?

- How is the primal midline different from the fluid midline? Play with moving forwards and backwards. Take your time, go slowly. Midline awareness can be very powerful.

- Finish by coming back to the neural cavity and out through the trapdoor in your throat. Notice your breathing for a couple of cycles and then slowly come back into the room.

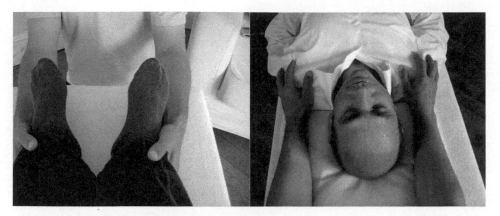

Figure 2.1.7 Contact at the feet and shoulders

Treatment Exercise: Primal midline with client sitting

1. Start with client sitting upright.

   • Stand (or sit) behind your seated client.

   • Follow your usual rituals of contact. Spend some time deepening into your fulcrums and pay particular attention to any impressions of your own midline as you start.

2. Make contact at the shoulders.

   • Start with your hands resting lightly on the client's shoulders. Orient to their whole body and then their spine. Settle with any initial impressions.

3. Orient to the primal midline.

   • Allow the possibility of feeling a continual rising upwards, like a shaft of air or heat. It rises up from the sacrum through the vertebral bodies and through the cranial base. It can almost feel like stepping into a lift.

   • Notice any areas where the rising seems impaired or hard to contact. Sometimes you can feel gaps or discontinuities in the primal midline. These are very useful diagnostic clues. Keep a sense of the whole midline and the whole biosphere. Enjoy.

   • Slowly disengage.

Original health

A fundamental concept within biodynamic craniosacral therapy is that we are self-regulating organisms. Enfolded within the flesh of the body is a blueprint, or recipe,[5] for life – called the original matrix or original health in biodynamics. It is an inherent knowing or a wisdom of the body.

The breath of life, the animating force, interacts with this recipe to create an individual form. The original matrix is laid down at conception. The information and a potential for health, as such, is always present. This is much more than genetics, though genes are certainly part of the mechanism of expressing the intelligence of the body. William Blake, an English poet, is useful here:

> To see a World in a Grain of Sand
>
> And a Heaven in a Wild Flower
>
> Hold Infinity in the palm of your hand
>
> And Eternity in an hour.
>
> (Blake 1803)

This somehow speaks of original health being enfolded within every part of the whole. Franklyn Sills (2001) uses the holographic paradigm developed by David Bohm to further explain the concept of original health.

Clinically we can say that the existence of the original matrix means that optimum health is always an underlying possibility. Given space, time and resources, healing occurs through an ongoing interaction between the breath of life and the original matrix. Becker calls this a balanced rhythmic interchange.[6] Furthermore the health available from within is far greater than anything we can apply from the outside.[7] The work is about facilitating the conditions where this interchange can occur – ultimately we cannot impose some external model of what needs to happen.

Treatment Exercise: Fluid midline from feet and shoulders

1. Start at the feet.
   - Follow your usual rituals of contact. Spend some time deepening into your fulcrums and pay particular attention to any impressions of your own fluid body and midline as you start. Wait for the holistic shift. Orient to mid tide.

2. Orient to fluids.
   - Use the image of your hands being immersed in water. It is as though the tissues you are touching are seaweed being moved by the tide of the

ocean. See if you feel the whole body as a bag of fluid expanding and contracting.

3. Orient to the fluid midline.

- Within the fluid whole see if any impressions of midline phenomena appear. After a while see if you can deepen your awareness and orient to the dural sac containing CSF – a very special midline bag of fluid.

- Can you notice a longitudinal surge and then receding of fluid through the posterior/fluid midline?

- After a few cycles move to the opposite end of the body and try again from the shoulders.

2.2 KEY SKILLS 2: STATES OF BALANCE

States of balance

A state of balance is a very important therapeutic principle. It can be considered as a settling of the motion of the whole system in relationship to a particular pattern of experience. It is as though the whole system has deepened enough to allow all the resources to be focused on one place. All the opposing forces around the organizing centre (or fulcrum) of the pattern of experience – the pushes and pulls, the eccentric motions, the twists and swirls – slow down and balance out. Something happens (Becker 1997).[8] There is a shift in the field as the nature of the fulcrum changes.

The attempt to find a systemic neutral, where the whole field settles in relationship to a fulcrum, is the biodynamic approach and leads to a deeper, more significant shift. If working biomechanically the focus is not on the whole; there is a local reorganization called a point of balanced tension, often felt solely within the tissues.

Sills describes a state of balance as a mysterious gateway (Sills 2001). There are often clear surges of potency and a crescendo of stillness at the moment the conditional forces organizing a pattern of experience are dissipated. In a state of balance the complete focus of the resources and the tide that can manifest, given the current relationship, is on a primary fulcrum. It is a momentous event. If you can be present at the precise moment a state of balance happens it is possible to drop further into stillness, into long tide or into dynamic stillness.

Treatment Exercise: State of balance via a spinal segment

1. Start from the occiput.

- Ritual of contact. Wait for holistic shift. Orient to mid tide.

2. Orient to the fluid midline.

- Allow the detail of the fluid midline to come through. Track the tide. Notice any discontinuities in the midline – similar to the session holding the occiput and sacrum in side position.

3. Two-handed contact at sacrum and on the spine.

- Reorient and see if the discontinuity or inertial area/s feel the same. Place your non-sacrum hand under one area that stands out. If it is higher than the lower/mid thoracic spine you will need to remove your sacrum hand. See if you can orient to a particular disc between two vertebrae that feels inert – that is, not in relationship to the midline. The discs are the natural fulcrum for the vertebrae and all the dermatomes, myotomes and sclerotomes that grew from that embryological segment.

- Stay in relationship to the whole midline and the whole field. On an inhale there is a natural creation of space in the structures of the body. See if you can track an inhale and support a natural disengagement of the inertial fulcrum and a coming back into relationship with the midline. It may be useful to slow down any eccentric motions of the vertebrae to help a state of balance, a systemic settling around the inertial site. Do not narrow down – let the tide do the work.

- Finish in side position or at the sacrum or occiput. How does the midline feel now?

How to support a state of balance

Sometimes the system seems to flirt with change. A pattern presents but does not seem to resolve. Things keep circling around a particular point. Sometimes we lose awareness and, instead of the system dropping through a state of balance, things go mushy and we come out of relationship. A good rule of thumb is 'do not stay with something that does not deepen'. If you have been there longer than 10 or 15 minutes without some form of clarity emerging in the relational field, it is probably time to renegotiate the contact. Go through the process of making contact again and re-establish your state of balanced awareness; you have either spaced out or become too narrow. It is amazing how often just changing your hand-hold and going to the other end of the body recharges the space and allows more possibilities.

There are a number of historical and classic approaches to support a state of balance, sometimes called augmentation or conversation skills. It is possible to augment the natural movements of potency to facilitate a state of balance. It is important not to be overactive in your intentions here; useful skills that we use are:

- Supporting space and disengagement.

- Orienting to stillness and slowing things down.

- Resonance with the intentions of the breath of life.

- Orienting to the midline and natural fulcrums.

- Spacious intentions of acceptance, recognition and acknowledgement. Try not to get hooked into needing things to change.

- Differentiating tissues, fluids and potency.

- Orienting to the whole and a wide perceptual field.

Orienting to tides

Sills has done some incredible work articulating clues as to how to differentiate the different tidal unfoldments of the breath of life. This section is a brief summary that draws heavily on his insights (Sills 2001).[9] Mid tide is the most frequent tide that we feel, so we shall outline skills to orient to mid tide first. We will then explore skills for long tide and then finally acknowledge perceptions that seem to accompany cranial rhythmic impulse (CRI) awareness.

In mid tide it is easiest to feel the embodied resources of the system. There are two strands of thought in biodynamics about starting orientations. Shea, for example, prefers starting at long tide;[10] Sills' preference is for the more grounding, fluidic space of mid tide. We have observed that it can be very easy for practitioners to space out and dissociate when using long tide as the starting orientation. Both approaches are valid. We notice how powerful it is to meet the client's system with a perceptual field that acknowledges the present time unfoldment of their system, in which case it could be any one of the three tides.

In mid tide the hands feel as though they are immersed in fluid. The tissues are moved like seaweed in water, a long, slow undulation. The perceptual field widens to hold the whole of the body and the biosphere. The mind is relatively quiet and is in relationship to the whole person. Fluid tide, the posterior fluid midline and fluid drive are often easily felt at mid tide. You can be aware of the tide breathing at a rate of 2.5 cycles per minute, approximately 25 seconds to rise and fall. It is relatively stable. We do not encourage you to count the rate; the other perceptual clues are much more important. If you are truly with mid tide then, nearly always, 'something happens' within two or three or four cycles of it manifesting; a state of balance will occur, a priority emerges via the inherent treatment plan that may require a more specific contact or there will be a stillpoint and a deepening into stillness or the system will drop into long tide. Mid tide is a state of wholeness you can feel in relationship to another; there is a tone, texture and tempo to the other person that you can relate to and be present with. You are in relationship at a being-to-being level. It is a very powerful place, a place of enormous therapeutic efficacy.

In long tide the hands feel as though they are immersed in potency; your hands become translucent. The perceptual field widens to the whole space in the room, the space outside the room and out to the horizon. The mind is very expansive and still. The awareness and quality in the field goes very quiet and slow. You become very aware of the whole space around you and the possibility of a 'rhythmic balanced interchange' with the breath of life as an environmental force. The long tide comes from somewhere and returns to somewhere; we hitch a ride as it moves through the space. Long tide is frequently about potency; there can be a shimmering or wind-like quality in the space. (It should be noted that you can feel tissues, fluids and potency at each tidal level we do not want to imply that long tide is only about potency, mid tide about fluids and CRI about tissues.) Long tide is always a gift. The therapeutic power of long tide occurs when it emerges as a decision from within the client as priority of the breath of life. The practitioner orienting to long tide is useful, and a very skilful thing to be able to do consistently, and it can allow the client's systems to express long tide, but this is quite different from long tide emerging spontaneously. Long tide is a very stable tide that is described as taking 100 seconds to complete a cycle.

In CRI the hands feel as though they are floating on corks on water. The perceptual field is relatively narrow and focused on local dynamics of bones and soft tissues. The practitioner's mind is interested in individual structures and frequently has a plan. Sutherland and Becker would have spent large parts of their careers working at CRI and getting great clinical results. Their books are full of techniques emphasizing biomechanics. We see the CRI as a true unfoldment of the breath of life and not an epiphenomenon. It is, however, a very variable tide, strongly influenced by the conditions present. Sometimes it is essential to meet the client at the only tide they can present, whilst holding the door open for deeper tides to come through. When resources are low, often the only unfoldment they can present is CRI. CRI is described as 8 to 14 cycles a minute, approximately 6 seconds to complete a cycle of inhale and exhale. That is still a very slow awareness for most people.

Treatment Exercise: Primal midline and long tide

1. Start establishing a relational field before getting on the table.

   - Our ability to be in relationship to primary respiration can be seen as our ultimate resource. This exercise is about offering up the possibility of relating to the long tide via the primal midline.

   - Start with both you and the client in sitting position. Take time to settle and to create a relational field. Use some verbal skills to draw out where the client is starting from. Help the client find and orient to something that tells them they are OK.

2. Contact the feet with the client on the table.

- Move to the table. Start from the feet. Explicitly renegotiate the relational field. Wait for the holistic shift. When you are ready move to either the occiput or sacrum.

- Initially orient to mid tide. Allow any impressions of midline phenomena to present themselves. It may be useful to keep checking in with your own spine and midline.

3. Widen your perceptual field.

- Slowly widen your perceptual field. A useful image might be how far you can stretch the elastic of your awareness out from the client's midline. Try doing this in stages, from the dural sac and fluid midline, to the whole body, to the space around the body, to the edges of the room, out to the horizon. Find your comfortable perceptual space – your comfort zone. Do not move out of this too quickly. Be very aware of spacing out. If you have lost relationship to the client's midline or your own midline, you have gone too far. Re-establish your state of balanced awareness and slowly try again.

4. Orient to the primal midline and long tide.

- In the wider perceptual field see if you can feel the primal midline – there may be a light, continual rising, it may feel like a still centre, you may feel cycles of the long tide. Let your hands be immersed in potency. Let whatever comes to you just be there.

5. Negotiate ending.

- Slowly come back to mid tide awareness. Maybe finish at the feet. Make sure to verbally check in with your client. Slowly disengage.

Clinical Highlight: Sacrum and occiput holds

Sacrum

- The sacrum fits very neatly into the palm of the hand. It can help to have your chair by the knees so you are facing the head.

- To help someone lift their pelvis evenly, ask them to bend their knees and place both feet flat on the table, then to lift their pelvis, then slide your hand in to make contact. Get them to drop back down and then straighten their legs again. Sometimes it is good to keep the knees up as this softens the back – the client can let the knees fall together to make it easier for them.

- Nearly everybody needs a pillow or cushions under the knees. This flattens and softens any lumbar lordosis and supports the knees. If you can slide your non-sacrum hand easily under the low back in supine, it is an indication there is holding in the whole body and/or low back/psoas tension.

- Try and make sure your elbow is as close to the midline as possible (it helps if the table is not too wide) – this often means moving the pillow under the knees towards the feet.

- Use a soft hand. Try to think of your hand as a bag of fluid with no bones; this somehow helps prevent the feeling of being crushed.

- Imagine your hand below the table to help create space within the negotiation of contact.

Occiput

- The cradle hold is one of the classic cranial holds. Generally it's a very comfortable, supportive hold.

- Try to have your forearms, and optimally your elbows, resting on the table. It is generally OK for feet to hang off the end of the table to enable this.

- Nearly everybody needs a cushion or pillow under the head to prevent hyperextension of the neck. A good sign of overextension is that the Adam's apple looks prominent.

- You can have the little finger sides of your hands touching. Your first and second fingers can often reach down, if required, to contact the atlas and axis. Similarly, the fourth finger can rest on the mastoid and the thumb can reach up to the squama of temporals.

- Soft, fluid hands as above – commonly compression can be felt by the client via the heels of the hand medially or pushing inferiorly.

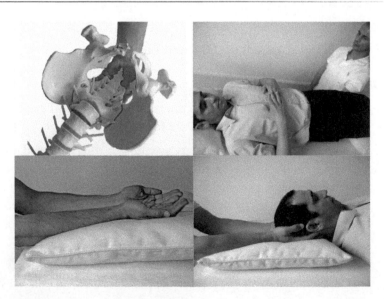

Figure 2.2.1 Sacrum and occipital cradle holds
Top: Contact at the sacrum. Bottom: The cradle hold at the occiput

2.3 THE SPINE

Overview

The spine is a very clear and obvious anatomical expression of the midline. It is a fearsomely complicated arrangement of bones, discs, ligaments and muscles. It is intimately related to the functioning of the nervous system. Its connections into the dura mean it is an integral part of the reciprocal tension membrane system. It is limited at the top end by the neurocranium via the occiput and at the bottom end by the sacrum and coccyx as part of the pelvic bowl; with these structures and the ribs it forms the axial skeleton.

There are many theories on how the spine functions and how best to treat the spine. A brief list of some primary treatment models gives some idea:[11]

- Only treat the upper cervicals and the whole spine will follow; this can be refined to just treating the atlas – 'hole-in-one adjusting'.[12]

- Treat the sacrotuberos ligament between the sacrum and inominate bones. The sacrum is seen as key to the health of the spine.[13]

- Treat sacroiliac joint dysfunction (some chiropractors and osteopaths can list 10, 20 or more listings for the position of the sacrum and pelvis).

- Treat the junctions of the spine – the occipital atlantal junction (OAJ), cervical thoracic junction (CTJ), thoracic lumbar junction (TLJ) and lumbar sacral junction (LSJ).

- Treat the arches of the spine defined by function and changes in shape in the vertebrae C5, T9 and L5 are seen as important 'interarch pivots' in this model (Stone 1999, p.129).

- 'As above so below' dysfunction at one end of the spine is mirrored in the other end.

- Various muscles are implicated – 'the multifidus solution', core stability and psoas and trapezius imbalances.

This is by no means an exhaustive list; all of the above approaches can be useful at certain times. The many models reflect how remarkable the spine is and how it is a compromise serving many functions. Maybe, also, no one really knows what is going on.

The biodynamic focus on the spine as a midline is a beautifully simple and elegant way of working. It allows a profound deepening into the spinal motion dynamics as part of the whole body. Each segment of the spine is potentially significant, and the spine is not seen in isolation from its embryological roots.

When orienting to the spine it is useful to consider the spine as a whole organ. The goal is to always try and get a sense of the whole spine, to really invite the spine into the relational field. There can be moments when the whole of the spine suddenly appears to you – cherish them; something useful will have happened or will be about to happen.

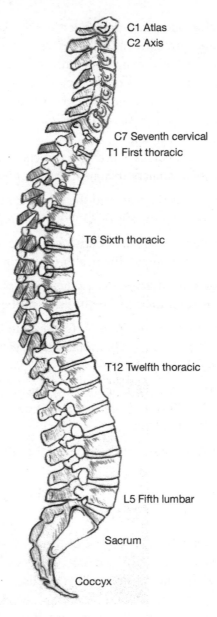

C1 Atlas
C2 Axis

C7 Seventh cervical
T1 First thoracic

T6 Sixth thoracic

T12 Twelfth thoracic

L5 Fifth lumbar

Sacrum

Coccyx

Figure 2.3.1 Lateral view of the spine

Each vertebra has the ability to move in relation to the vertebrae around it. Sometimes they get fixated in certain positions. You will frequently find that fixation of one vertebra is the primary inertial fulcrum for the whole spine and the whole body. Different vertebrae in different parts of the spine have different ranges and possibilities for movement (for example, you can rotate your neck much more than your lower back). Throughout the whole spine it is common for vertebrae to be fixed in rotation round the vertical axis. Other possibilities are for the vertebrae to bend sideways (lateral flexion), move forward or backwards and tilt up or down (for example, the spinous process is tilted superior) or combinations of all these movements. In health, vertebrae inhale and exhale in a similar way to the sacrum and occiput. On inhale, as well as feeling the inner motility of the vertebrae in relationship to the midline, you can feel the spinous process move inferiorly as the body of the vertebrae tilts superiorly.

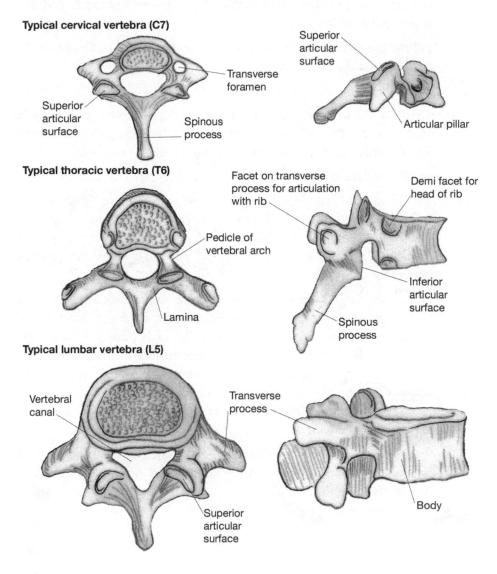

Figure 2.3.2 Superior and left lateral views of typical vertebrae

Treatment Exercise: Fluid midline from the occiput and sacrum – side position

1. Start in side lying position.

   - Start in side lying position, one hand on the sacrum and one hand on the occiput. To support your elbows it can help to make sure your client is as close as possible to the opposite side of the table. For narrow tables bolsters can be useful for resting your elbows. It can take a while to find the right position of the chair so that your wrists are not too angled. See some options below.

   - Follow usual ritual of contact and wait for holistic shift. Orient to the mid tide and the fluid midline.

2. Can the sacrum and occiput move together?

   - Orient to the possibility of the sacrum and occiput moving together in inhale and exhale – this is a clear sign of health. Frequently one or both will feel quite inert and move in a disjointed, fragmented way.

3. Orient to the fluid midline.

   - The fluid midline passes through the neural cavity bounded by the cranium, vertebral canal and the sacral canal. At the sacrum and occiput are relatively large amounts of CSF – the superior and inferior 'waterbeds'. Wait for the possibility of a surge of fluid and potency between your hands.

   - Notice any areas where the fluid midline seems disjointed or hard to contact. It can feel as though the surge of fluid gets stuck along the spine; sometimes it feels as though the fluids bounce back from a restriction – this can happen anywhere, but the lumbar thoracic junction and the cervical thoracic junction are common places. As you practise this you will be able to identify individual segments of the spine (it is useful to think of the disc as a centre of a segment rather than individual vertebrae) that are inert.

   - Deepen into your own midline and the awareness of the waterbeds between your hands to support a settling in the system and a sense of wholeness through the midline.

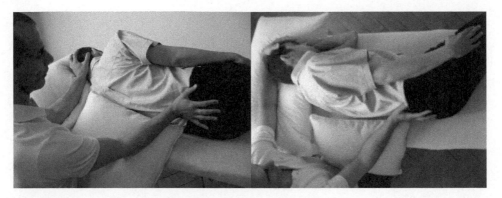

Figure 2.3.3 Treating in side position
Note the different possible hand positions and the cushion to support the arm

Awareness Exercise: Surface anatomy of the axial skeleton

Some descriptions of the essential lumps and bumps on the back and the front of the body, and how to find them, are given below. Figure 2.3.4 shows the landmarks described for the back of the body (see p.69). Practise finding them on a partner.

Back of the body: cervical spine landmarks

- C2 (axis): Moving inferiorly from the inion on the occiput, C2 is the first spinous process that you can feel. C1 (atlas) does not have a spinous process and there is a hollow between the inion and C2 spinous.

- C3–5: It is often hard to differentiate each of these bones. The spinous processes can be bifid.

- C6: Disappears under your finger on hyperextension/tilting the head back. This is useful to differentiate C6 from C7 as the C7 spinous does not disappear on tilting the head back.

- C7: Running your hand inferiorly down the neck (in supine it is usually clearer) the first big bump you feel is usually C7. The majority of the time it is the most prominent spinous process at the base of the neck. This is a very useful landmark.

- C1 (atlas): C1 has wide transverse processes. Palpating from behind with the client sitting and the head slightly tilted back, they can be felt midway between the angle of the mandible and the mastoid. In this space you can feel the transverse processes as hard lumps, especially when the head turns.

Back of the body: thoracic spine landmarks

- T1: Sometimes T1 spinous is more prominent than C7. You can differentiate T1 from C7 as T1 does not rotate as much as C7 when the head turns. Also, the spinous process of T1 should move if you press on the upper sternum due to the connection to the first rib.

- T6/T7: T6 or T7 are roughly at the inferior angle of scapula.

- T12: T12 is the first blade-like spinous process (the spinous processes of the five lumbar vertebrae are also blade-like). You can also trace upwards and inwards on the floating 12th rib to find T12 or count upwards from L4.

Back of the body: lumbar spine and pelvic landmarks

- L4: L4 spinous is at the level of iliac crests. This is an extremely useful landmark. You can find the iliac crests by placing the sides of your forefinger/hand in the fleshy part of the waist at the level of the umbilicus. Move inferiorly and the first hard lumps you feel on each side are the iliac crests. Counting up and down from L4 helps find the other lumbar vertebrae.

- Sacral spines: The sacral spines can usually be felt easily on the midline.

- Coccyx: Take your time and negotiate with your partner to feel the outline of the coccyx in the cleft of the buttocks.

- PSIS (posterior superior iliac spine): In prone, this is easily found by moving superiorly and medially from the mid part of the fleshy part of the buttocks. Use the thumbs to try to feel up and under the PSIS on each side. You are at the level of S2. Another extremely useful landmark.

Front of the body

- Throat landmarks: The hyoid bone is roughly at the level of C3. You can feel it move when someone swallows and it should easily move from side to side. The thyroid cartilage surrounding the larynx (Adam's apple) is at the C4–5 level.

- T9, T12 and L3: The xiphoid process at the inferior end of the sternum is roughly at the level of T9. The umbilicus is usually at the level of L3. Midway between the xiphoid and the umbilicus is a good guide for the level of T12.

- ASIS (anterior superior iliac spine): In supine, from the anterior midline of the thigh, move superiorly. The first lump you feel will be the ASIS of the pelvis.

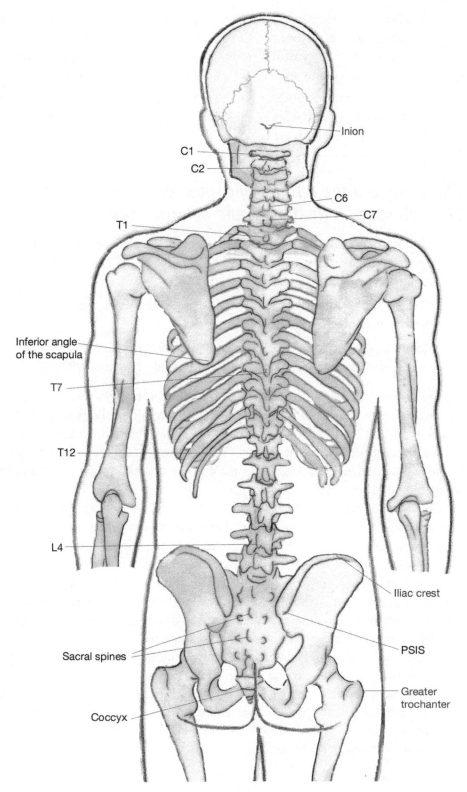

Figure 2.3.4 Surface anatomy of the back

- Greater trochanter of the femur: Palpate inferiorly from the iliac crests, down the most lateral part of the hip. The first hard lump you feel is the greater trochanter of the femur. You can check by asking the client to rotate the leg and you will feel the greater trochanter move.

- Pubic symphysis: Palpate inferiorly from the umbilicus; it will initially be soft and then you will eventually feel the bones of the pubic arch. Often it is easier to get the client to find it for you.

The discs are the natural fulcrums for the innervation of myotomes, dermatomes and sclerotomes

> The nucleus pulposus becomes the point of orientation for the development and growth of all the life force fields related to that segment, all the tissues, and all the fluids. (Jealous 2004)

> There is more embryology under our hands when we're treating than there is anatomy. (Jealous 2004)

> Before a bone can have a relationship with another bone on either side of it, it must first have a relationship within itself. (Jealous 1994, p.3)

All the structures that grow from the somites in the embryo retain a segment identity. Somites are masses of mesoderm distributed along the two sides of the neural tube that will eventually become dermis (dermatome), skeletal muscle (myotome) and vertebrae (sclerotome). The reference point for the segment in healing is the nucleus pulposus, the remnant of the notochord found in the centre of the intervertebral discs.

The centre of the disc is the natural fulcrum for the two surrounding vertebrae. The vertebrae are formed from two different somites combining as cells migrate to surround the notochord. Orienting to the discs naturally takes your awareness into the anterior midline and allows a deepening into the contact.

In addition, when contacting peripheral structures you can orient to the disc as the natural fulcrum for the muscles, skin, bones and connective tissues that formed from the somite surrounding the notochord at that level. This is the 'segment identity' of the myotomes, dermatomes and sclerotomes.

When treating place your finger tips on the spinous processes of two adjacent vertebrae and orient to the centre of the disc between the vertebral bodies. With your other hand contact the peripheral muscles, skin, bone and connective tissue that grew from that segment. This awareness has a slower quality than nerve flow; it is about embryological intentions. The orientation of the limbs budding out from the somites can be very useful.

Jealous (2004) calls the nucleus pulposus a nodal point on the midline. He states that these points also become the fulcrum for the orientation of the segmentation of the autonomic nervous system.

Each vertebra is potentially significant when treating the spine

> The cranial concept does not overlook spinal lesions. In fact, techniques that apply to the entire body and its mechanical problems are demonstrated at courses of instruction in cranial technique. (Sutherland 1998, p.219)[14]

Think of the keystone of an arch. The whole structure is dependent on the keystone being correctly aligned. Every vertebra within the spine has the potential to be the 'keystone' for a particular pattern of experience at a given moment in time.

Each vertebra has the ability to move in relation to the vertebrae around it. Sometimes they get fixated in certain positions. Different vertebrae in different parts of the spine have different ranges and possibilities for movement (for example, you can rotate your neck much more than your lower back). Throughout the whole spine it is common for vertebrae to be fixed in rotation round the vertical axis.

Other possibilities are for the vertebrae to bend sideways (lateral flexion), move forwards or backwards and tilt up or down (for example, the spinous process is tilted superior) or combinations of all these movements. Due to the mechanics of the joints in the spine, the vertebrae do not move in one plane alone. There are coupled motions. If there is some rotation there will always be some sideways bending. To complicate things further the direction of sidebending changes for a given rotation from the top to the bottom of the spine. In the neck, if the spinous process is rotated to the right, the vertebra sidebends to the left (think of a spiral staircase bending at the centre). In the lumbar spine if the spinous process is rotated to the right the vertebra sidebends to the right. There is a point of transition somewhere through the thoracic spine.

Coupled motions can be confusing (and have been the subject of much debate within the history of manipulative therapies). It is strongly recommended to work with the rotation of the vertebra, felt via the position of the spinous process relative to the vertebra above and below, as the primary orientation.

In health, vertebrae inhale and exhale in a similar way to the sacrum and occiput. On inhale, as well as feeling the inner motility of the vertebra in relationship to the midline, you can feel the spinous process move inferiorly as the body of the vertebra tilts superiorly. Again this is slightly confusing as during inhale, if you are only aware of the spinous process, you will feel the spinous move inferiorly whilst tracking the tide surging in a superior direction towards the head.

It is useful to differentiate between the different areas of the spine. Having stated that all vertebrae are potentially significant in the previous section, certain vertebrae are treated more frequently than others. ('All vertebrae are equal, some are more equal than others', to borrow from George Orwell.) Try not to forget that each vertebra could be the key to unlocking the whole pattern of the spine. Below are some thoughts on different areas of the spine.

Cervical spine

C7 is a useful vertebral segment to orient to for most clients. The cervical thoracic junction, including C6 and T1, provides a huge amount of afferentation to the central nervous system (CNS). This area seems to be involved in the majority of cases of musculoskeletal pain and organ dysfunction. This area is often quite buzzy and throbbing. It often feels as though there is a real grab and tightness in this area.

C3 to C5 are also very important. They are frequently related to breathing issues as the phrenic nerve emerges in this area ('C3, 4, 5 keep the diaphragm alive'). These three vertebrae can be harder to palpate and can feel a little hidden as they are relatively anterior due to the lordotic curve of the neck.

Working with the occiput, especially intraosseous patterns, nearly always clears issues in the occipital triad of occiput, atlas and axis. It is easy to overtreat the atlas; it is its nature to move and it is relatively free to rotate. It is not much use inviting a bone that acts as a washer to move.

Thoracic spine

The thoracic spine is often relatively hard to treat. It can be awkward getting the hand under the shoulder blades especially. The ribs also confuse things a little. The thoracic spine is very linked into the organs, breathing and the sympathetics. It is very easy to pick up on a sympathetic hum when working in this area due to the closeness of the chain ganglia to the rib heads. Holding the T4 area can be a wonderful route into making a relationship to the heart. Stubborn shoulder issues often require attention to the ribs and the thoracic vertebrae.

Lumbar spine

The lower lumbars often seem to give out a long low moan. Perhaps it is all that weight they carry. They can often feel hidden and difficult to contact. It is very common for all the lumbar vertebrae to hold strong inertial patterns. The body of L3 projects the furthest forward into the abdomen; it is sometimes closer to the abdominal wall than it is to the rear of the body. The root of the mesentery hangs off L3. The body of the pancreas passes in front of L1. Making friends with the psoas and being aware of its route down onto the lesser trochanter of the femur is often very useful for the lumbars.

Facilitation of vertebral segments

Each vertebra is associated with peripheral somatic nerves on either side and a more complex peripheral visceral nerve relationship through the sympathetic chains. The musculoskeletal system is directly innervated by the somatic nerves and the organs are sympathetically activated through the visceral nervous system. For example, all the intercostal muscles in the T5 segment are innervated through the intercostal nerves, one on either side. However, T5 visceral innervation is about the heart along with fibres from T2, 3 and 4. It is a common occurrence in practice that irritation will develop in these segmental relationships, so that the peripheral nerves become over-excited and the whole segment starts to be affected. This can stem from the muscles or organs or from their surrounds of fascia or membranes. If this is not resolved in the short term, the overstimulation can spread from the peripheral segment to the spinal cord fibre tracts and start to affect the length of the spinal cord. Other nerve fibres become affected by this, so there is a shift from local disturbance to spinal cord disturbance. At its worst the brain becomes affected and there is a general facilitation of many centres of the brain that become more active and less able to settle. So now the whole system is affected and along with this has come a lowering of the activation potential for nerves which means that nerves fire with much less stimulation than in a healthy state. The system is now hypersensitive and intolerant of sensory overload. This stress response is now heightened.

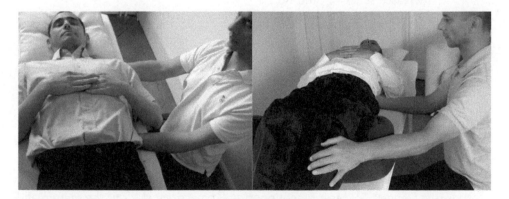

Figure 2.3.5 Two-handed contact at the spine and between the spine and a limb

From a craniosacral perspective as the nervous system is progressively irritated there is a reduction in healthy expressions of potency and whole system relationships start to decline. Intervening through establishing a relational field has a powerful therapeutic effect that stems the spread of nerve excitation. Through acknowledging the relationships along the nerve pathway and its associated segment (i.e. the nerve itself, the spinal segment, the muscles, bones, connective tissue and organs involved) there is the possibility of the health of the whole segment re-emerging and bringing about a resolution of the pattern. This often occurs in chronological order, so the original effect will be the last to resolve.

Clinical Highlight: Two-handed contact on the spine

We recommend that the two-handed contact from the side is as familiar to you as holding the cranium or the sacrum or working from the feet. Using the finger tips allows you to touch three, sometimes four, spinous processes quite easily. This direct contact with the vertebrae really aids clarity and precision in the treatment process.

In shiatsu training we were always taught to have a 'mother' hand and a 'working' hand. The mother hand had a calming, grounding influence and could be used to monitor changes. The two-handed spinal contact can use this idea and allows you to feel how one end of the spine responds to shifts in shapes and patterns at the other end. It really facilitates awareness of the whole midline.

Some useful indicators of change:

- The vertebrae under both hands inhale and exhale together.

- The midline lights up. Potency surges.

- There is a sense of flow between the hands along the midline. An increased sense of fluid tide.

- The spinous process derotates and comes back in line to the other spinous processes.

Being able to contact three or four vertebrae at a time allows you to directly contact manageable 'chunks' of the spine as you wait for the primary fulcrum to present. Holds we use a lot are a combination of C6, C7 and T1 (cervical thoracic junction) or C3, C4 and C5 with the upper hand and L3, L4 and L5 or T11, T12, L1 and L2 (thoracic lumbar junction) or T8, T9 and T10 with the lower hand.

Intraosseous work at the occiput is the key to this triad of occiput, atlas and axis (see Chapter 7). Most practitioners will have great skills at the sacrum and working with the lumbar sacral junction. It is important to feel confident with the sacrum and occiput alongside your direct skills on the spine.

There are some other huge advantages of working with the two-handed contact:

- Being under the junctions (CTJ and TLJ) really allows you to tune into the spinal cord and more easily orient to facilitation throughout the whole cord (see the debate on the flexor withdrawal response in Section 9.6).

- You will frequently pick up on the sympathetic chains; there is a characteristic buzz to the sympathetics that is unmistakable once felt. Similarly it is easy to pick up on the adrenals and the solar plexus.

- The anatomy above the thoracic lumbar junction is phenomenal – you are in contact with every major physiological system in the body; organ issues, the diaphragm and soft tissue pulls often pop up when making this contact.

- Dynamics organized around the ignition centres of the heart and umbilicus can be clearly felt (see Section 7.3).

Clinical Highlight: Treat the spine more often

Why treat the spine more often? Because it is incredibly effective in clinical practice is the simple answer. Our firm belief from running a teaching clinic for CSTs in London, of observing and talking to other CSTs, of supervising students and practitioners and being involved in teaching at four different biodynamic schools is that many practitioners hugely undertreat the spine.

There are many exciting strands emerging in the field of biodynamic craniosacral therapy: embryology, pre- and perinatal work, trauma, neuroscience and a deepening into stillness often tied in with notions of spirit. However, often we feel that BCST practitioners can forget to do the simple things and can be overly cautious in orienting to the structure. As osteopaths, Sutherland and Becker would have had fantastic skills in relating to the spine.

In clinical practice it is a rare session where we do not orient to the spine at some stage. Primary fulcrums in the spine present during session work at least as much as the cranial base and pelvis combined, probably more often. This may be because we are disposed to look for them but we also work with plenty of birth stories, embryological intentions and expansive states of stillness. It is not either/or but and/both. Being confident with the structure and particularly the spine is a very powerful doorway into the work.

We have presented a neurological and a biomechanical case for treating the spine. We are deeply aware that biodynamic work is so much more than defacilitating the nervous system. However, our experience is that clearing the facilitation and the flexor withdrawal response (see Section 9.6) in tandem with settling fight or flight and/or freeze responses (see Chapter 3) works wonders in practice. Orienting to the spine as a function of the midline is the other big treatment focus. Can you find the stillness within the midline and allow the vertebral segments to come back into relationship to that stillness?

Summary of Chapter 2

We explored the spine as a unit of function and natural fulcrum for the whole body's health as well as a conductor for the primary energies of the body mind system. The chapter looked at how natural adjustments take place around this axis. The aspects of the midline covered in this chapter include the embryological origins of the primal midline; the holistic nature of the spine; the two poles of the midline, the sacrum and occiput, spinal motion dynamics; and the fluid midline.

From practising and digesting the material you will learn how to:

- recognize how the health of the spine affects the health of the whole body

- become familiar with recognizing expressions from the primal midline

- listen to the spine as a whole unit of function

- relate to the health of the spinal curves and the continuity through the spinal column, helping you to identify spinal joint patterns

- recognize the horizontal relationships of the spine, that is, facilitated segments and irritability in visceral and somatic nervous arcs, and how to meet them therapeutically

- learn skills of assessing your client's health.

Notes

1. Blechschmidt (2005) discusses metabolic fields at length. It should be noted that for Blechschmidt the forces are within the embryo and are an imperative that emerges from the morphological changes in the growing embryo. He did not describe external environmental forces, such as long tide, as described by the biodynamic craniosacral model (Maitland 2008).

2. Maitland (2008) critiques the original matrix as a platonic ideal. It may be that the original matrix is an emergent property from the internal complexity of cells talking to cells. Complexity theory shows how extraordinary intelligence and coordinated behaviour arises from many, relatively simple, parts interacting. No external central coordinator is required. Swarms of birds swooping and moving as one unit exhibit emergent behaviour. See, for example, Johnson (2001) and Newell (2003).

3. Other midlines are described in the biodynamic model: the quantum midline, a horizontal midline via the umbilicus, a midline through the gut and even a blood midline through the aorta. The quantum midline is a descending surge associated with the breath of life coming in at conception; it can be experienced as a shaft of light anterior to the spinal column.

4. The end of the notochord is a powerful place and the area is formed from neural crest cells (ectoderm) as well as mesoderm. 'The vertebrate cranial base is a complex structure composed of bone, cartilage and other connective tissues underlying the brain; it is intimately connected with development of the face and cranial vault... Neural crest cells contribute to all of the cartilages that form the ethmoid, presphenoid, and basisphenoid bones with the exception of the hypochiasmatic cartilages.

The basioccipital bone and non-squamous parts of the temporal bones are mesoderm derived. Therefore the prechordal head is mostly composed of neural crest-derived tissues, as predicted by the New Head Hypothesis' (McBratney-Owen *et al.* 2008, p.121).

5. Dawkins (2009, Chapter 8) makes a convincing case for any plans of the body to be described as recipes rather than blueprints. A recipe implies much less external control and design and an irreversible process unlike a blueprint.

    Dawkins is talking about DNA as a recipe, but the processes he describes also apply to the biodynamic model of the original matrix (see note 2 above). He describes how emergence and local interactions are sufficient to account for the generation of the form of the embryo and the final shapes of folded proteins such as enzymes.

    For Sheldrake (2009) the consistent formation of complex 3D shapes from chains of amino acids is not yet adequately explained.

6. Sutherland uses the phrase in *Contributions of Thought* (1998, p.218). Becker expands on the theme in *The Stillness of Life* (2000).

7. 'Osteopathy is a science with possibilities as great as the magnitude of the heavens. It is a science dealing with the natural forces of the body. We work as osteopaths with the traditional principle in mind that the tendency in the patient's body is always toward the normal. There is much to discover in the science of osteopathy by working with the forces within that manifest the healing processes. These forces within the patient are greater than any blind force that can safely be brought to bear from without' (from the cover of Sutherland 1990).

8. As he developed as a practitioner Becker describes how he just wrote 'SH' in his clinic notes to describe the session.

9. In the work cited, see Chapter 23 'Skills and the Tides', and Appendix 1, 'Perceptual Levels and Skills', for an in-depth exploration.

10. 'The Mid Tide is not sought out because of the exceptional amount of trauma imprinted in it except in certain circumstances noted throughout the book. In the post-9/11 world, the Mid Tide is so compressed that it requires "resuscitation," according to one osteopath. Thus it is critical for the practitioner to dramatically slow down and stop the movement of her mind and body and synchronize with Primary Respiration. Throughout this book the term Primary Respiration is used as a principal aspect of the Long Tide' (Shea 2007, p.xxii).

11. Stone (1999) has a good discussion on some of the different models of spinal biomechanics within osteopathy. There are also many models of how to approach the spine in chiropractic. Redwood and Cleveland (2003) is a good place to start.

12. Upper cervical techniques have a long history in chiropractic. Two newer examples (one from chiropractic) are www.atlasprofilax.ch and www.atlasorthogonality.com. It is easy to over-adjust the atlas; it is its nature to move and it is relatively free to rotate.

13. For example, see www.alexanderbase.fsnet.co.uk and Logan Basic Methods.

14. This quote is from a talk given in 1948, in the latter part of Sutherland's life.

3

Resources and Overwhelm

3.1 RESOURCES

Resources are essential to health and healing

Resources can be defined as anything that supports health. All healing occurs in relationship to the amount of resources that we can bring to bear in a given situation. ('No resources equals no get better', Perrow 2005.) In clinical work the first priority is often to establish someone's ability to find their resources, and in addition, whether they can manifest present-time, embodied awareness of those resources.

It is very different treating someone who is in a stable and happy family/relationship environment, has a strong network of friends, is fulfilled in their work, is able to express their creativity, likes where they live, has a relationship to the natural environment and has a strong sense of their body, from someone who is isolated, feels unsafe, is disconnected from their body, has no contact with the natural world and has very little stability. Interestingly you do not get many of the former presenting with chronic pains in your clinic.

Resources are very personal. They are a mix of external events or objects and internal beliefs or frameworks. They tend to generate body sensations of ease, calm, warmth, space and stillness. There is an inner sense of being alright, strength, hope, vitality and safety when we are in relationship with our resources. As resources are so personal, these words will not work for everyone – for example, a sense of cool rather than warmth or dynamic energy rather than calm may be important. Resources are not fixed and cannot be imposed from the outside. The right fit of resources will emerge through the therapeutic relationship and will evolve as session work progresses.

Developing resources needs to be handled creatively and with a light touch. Too much insistence, and a formulaic approach, on the part of the therapist on finding a resource can get in the way. If the clinical highlight suggestions below do not work, then the negotiation around physical space and coming into relationship and contact can be very useful to revisit (see Chapter 1). Helping someone take control of how the room is organized (they know where the exit is, it is not too bright, the blinds are drawn) and take control of where, when and how contact is made can be incredibly productive negotiations that can be played out over a number of sessions.

Given all the above, often it is important to just sit with your hands on wherever you are and let your quality of touch and presence be the resource.

Pain and suffering act like a magnet that grabs our awareness. The journey to embody our experience is a big step in developing resources. The body gives a whole new theatre in which our experience and emotions can be played out. We can move towards and away from sensations, slow things down and control what is centre stage in our bodies in a way that is not possible with mental functioning alone. Learning that we have emotions and sensations and that we do not need to become them is very important. Pain is unlikely to be the only sensation possible. Stepping back and finding a wider context and other sensations is often a transformational shift.

Clinical Highlight: Resources

In clinic work it is always slightly worrying to meet someone who says there is nothing that makes them feel good. Unfortunately it is not uncommon. To help someone struggling to find something that tells them they are OK, you can use the following simple framework.

Present-time, embodied sensations as resources

- 'What are you aware of in your body right now?' Often you will get a string of aches and pains. You can ask someone to see if there are any other sensations present – something not painful even if it is the tip of the nose or the elbow. Humour and ordinary language can be useful here. ('Can you feel your bum in the chair? It's all painful, even your little toe?')

- 'Can you find any sensations in your body right now that speak of warmth, ease, comfort or a sense of being OK?'

- 'Can you feel your feet right now – if not can you try and feel your feet and a connection to the earth or table?'

Memory of resources

- 'Can you remember a time when you felt really good?'

- 'When was the last time you were not in pain?'

- 'When was the last time you can remember feeling well?'

- 'Can you pick a peak time in your life when things were going better than normal?'

- Objects and places can be useful – a favourite toy, a book, a picture, a familiar walk, a room.

- Pets can be fantastic – sometimes the unconditional love experienced in relationship to a favourite pet is a bedrock experience.

Fantasy of resources

- 'Can you imagine what it would be like to feel really well? Try and picture yourself in a completely safe situation where you have total control. See if you could imagine what you could hear or smell or how your skin would feel, as many body sensations as possible. How would your body feel on the inside in that safe place?'

- You can support people to be very creative here – remember it's a fantasy or ideal. We have had clients create completely empty white rooms, castles, islands, sitting in an armchair cosied up in front of a fire, sitting in top of a huge tree, running on grass.

Awareness Exercise: Finding places of health in your body

- Spend time on your own doing this exercise. Let your awareness spread through your whole body as if it's a fluid. Are there any places that feel good? Try to find these places. They might be an area of the body, a particular structure or just one spot. When you've found one of these places simply be with the sensations of it for a while. How does it make you feel and what effect does it have on your body and mind?

- Practising in pairs, get your practice partner to contact you while you lie on a treatment couch. It doesn't matter where. Let them establish contact and then find your healthy place and go through the process above. Stay with this for 5–10 minutes and ask your partner what their experience was of you being in relationship with your place of health.

3.2 A FIRST LOOK AT TRAUMA

Introduction to the trauma model

Trauma can be defined as anything that overwhelms our resources (Levine 1997). When we are overwhelmed we rely on very primitive responses that are hard-wired into our physiology. A simple version is that we go into fight or flight mode or we freeze. Understanding our responses to overwhelm is clinical gold dust.

I heard a shout; starting and looking half around I saw the lion just in the act of springing upon me... Growling horribly close to my ear he shook me as a terrier does a rat. The shock produced a stupor similar to that which seems to be felt by a mouse after the first shake of the cat. It caused a sort of dreaminess in which there was no sense of panic or feeling of terror, though I was quite conscious of all that was happening... This peculiar state is probably produced in all animals killed by the carnivora; and if so is a merciful provision by our benevolent creator for lessening the pain of death. (The explorer David Livingstone giving a classic description of dissociation, in Kandel, Schwartz and Jessell 2000, p.489)

Much of the research on trauma emerged from the identification of post-traumatic stress disorder (PTSD) as a distinct condition. Van der Kolk identifies core symptoms of PTSD as intrusions (thoughts, dreams, flashbacks), hyperarousal and numbing (Van der Kolk, McFarlane and Weisaeth 1996). Levine (1997) compares living with overwhelm to driving a car with one foot full on the accelerator (hyperarousal – sympathetic overwhelm) and the other foot full on the brake (hypoarousal – parasympathetic overwhelm) or rapid switching between the two states.

Van der Kolk *et al.* (1996) suggest that, with time, some people's PTSD may become subclinical and yet continue to influence their ability to function. There is a whole continuum of responses possible from ongoing panic attacks or severe withdrawal and depression to a mild sense of disconnection or an inability to feel parts of the body. We feel treating dissociation in particular is always a clinical priority. Not much healing can occur if someone is not embodied.

One of the most basic questions human animals operate around is 'Am I safe?' If the answer is no, our physiology prioritizes its resources to fight or flight or freeze. If the underlying physiology continues to respond as if there is no safety, and this can happen for days, weeks, months, years or, tragically, whole lifetimes, this has huge consequences for health and healing. To facilitate the healing process it is essential to help promote flexibility in the range of possible physiological responses, to help the system orient to safety in the present and down-regulate the fight or flight or freeze reflexes.

There is a hierarchy of responses if we are threatened

We have quick, instinctive responses in the presence of any threat to our integrity. The polyvagal theory of Stephen Porges develops the basic trauma model and lists a hierarchy of responses, each involving progressively older evolutionary responses of the autonomic nervous system (ANS): communication, mobilization and freezing (Porges 2003).

Initially, with any perceived threat there is a communication or orienting response, an engagement with our environment to gain more information. In the orienting response, the person locates and assesses the source of the threat. There may then be a communication; for example, using negotiation or social skills to address the threat. In this stage a mouse may sense a hint of cat and sharpen its hearing and smell, open and move its eyes and turn its head to gain more information. There is a temporary stilling of the heart, breathing and posture. In humans this orienting response is highly developed and frequently includes communication. This is based on our previous experiences of attachment to figures of safety; we can soothe and reassure ourselves in contact with others. This response comes from a newer part of the parasympathetic nervous system. Porges calls it the social engagement system. It is mediated by cranial nerves V, VII, IX, X and XI and involves the nucleus ambiguus. Neck issues and eye strain may be rooted in a prolonged orienting response. The orienting response may also explain why we can also talk a lot when we get nervous.

The next level of response are the fight or flight mechanisms; they come into play if the orienting response still signals danger. The mouse sees the cat and, in this case, the mouse runs as fighting is not an option. Humans can get confused at this stage as we have been both predator and prey in our history. The sympathetic nervous system goes into overdrive and causes the release of large amounts of adrenaline and later cortisol. We breathe more quickly to get more oxygen, the heart beats faster and more strongly to pump as much oxygen-rich blood as possible to the large muscles, the pupils dilate to take in more light, the blood supply to the periphery (hands, feet and skin) is reduced and the digestive functions are reduced.

The final response is the dissociative or freeze response. If the mouse is caught it goes limp, floppy and plays dead. Its body is flooded with endorphins, the body's natural painkillers. If it is going to die the release of endorphins mean it will feel no pain. There is another evolutionary advantage: the predator may be put off, as it may have instincts against eating carrion. The cat may lose interest in playing with the mouse and the mouse can then move to safety. This fundamental survival response is inherited from reptiles and is mediated by an old part of the parasympathetic nervous system: the dorsal motor nucleus of the vagus, slowing down the heart and breathing. Reptiles are good at feigning death as they can maintain long periods with highly reduced blood circulation. (One of our clients told a story about a cat bringing in a frog. She thought the frog was dead but put off clearing it up for a few hours – suddenly she saw it come back to life and jump off, apparently unharmed.)

Fight or flight is the most commonly known phase. It is the phase where we get anxious or aggressive and is frequently misunderstood to be the whole of the response to overwhelming events. The freeze response is a significant but often-overlooked factor. The insight of defining authors in the field such as Van der Kolk

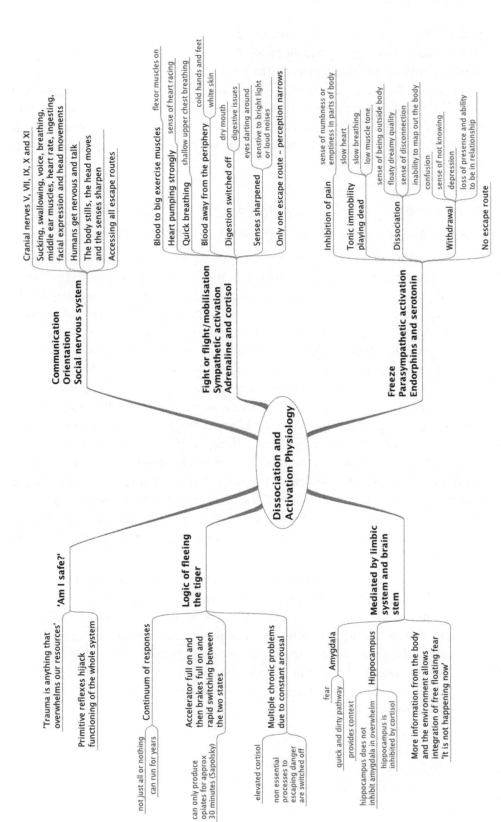

Figure 3.2.1 Dissociation and activation physiology mindmap

et al. (1996), Levine (1997), Rothschild (2000) and others working with trauma is that trauma has huge implications for the body; it is not just a psychological, hysterical, hypochondriac construct. The body makes these decisions really quickly, more quickly than conscious thought. Our thinking and understanding lag behind what is going on in our bodies. This is frequently confusing for humans; we lose touch with the stories our body is trying to tell us. It is not until an overwhelmed aspect of the system begins to collapse that we realize that our physiology has been working like crazy.

In overwhelm implicit memories are coupled with body states and emotional charge and a loss of context

Levine and Rothschild stress that knowledge of the relevant physiology is essential to understanding the symptoms of trauma. It is initially a preconscious experience, involving primitive parts of the brain – the brainstem and limbic system (especially the amygdala and hippocampus) – and the ANS. In PTSD there can be free-floating, highly charged emotional responses where the initial context is hidden.

It appears that there is a loss of communication between the amygdala, which provides the emotional charge and implicit memory, and the hippocampus, which provides the context and explicit memory (explicit memory can be thought of as easily accessed memory as opposed to the more hidden implicit memory). In overwhelm the hippocampus does not inhibit the amygdala. The strong emotional charge associated with the amygdala may initiate fight, flight or freeze.[1]

The storage of implicit memories often involves emotional states, the right brain, the amygdala and the rest of the body. This encoding of memory in the internal environment and structure of the body is very relevant to bodyworkers. A particular posture, muscle tension, smell or sound, in fact any somatic trigger, may lead to the activation of a memory and emotional response – flashbacks or 'state-dependent recall'.

> Though usually discussed in reference to internal states, state-dependent recall is exceedingly relevant to postural states… The somatic nervous system carries out the trauma defensive reactions of fight, flight and freeze through simple and complex combinations of muscle contractions that result in specific positions, movements and behaviour. In co-operation with proprioception, the somatic nervous system is also party to encoding traumatic experiences in the brain. (Rothschild 2000, pp.55–56)

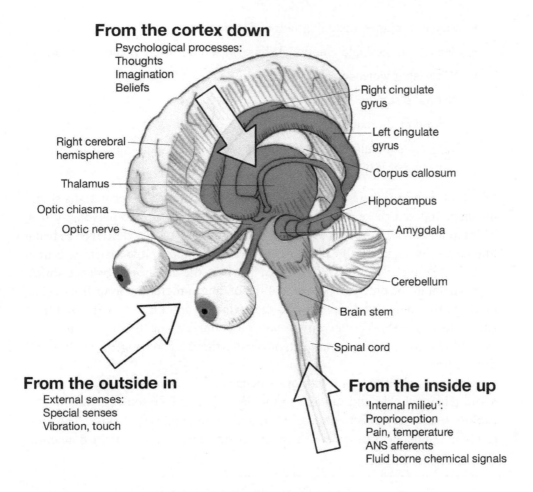

From the cortex down
Psychological processes:
Thoughts
Imagination
Beliefs

Right cingulate
gyrus

Left cingulate
gyrus

Right cerebral
hemisphere

Corpus callosum

Thalamus

Hippocampus

Optic chiasma

Amygdala

Optic nerve

Cerebellum

Brain stem

Spinal cord

From the outside in
External senses:
Special senses
Vibration, touch

From the inside up
'Internal milieu':
Proprioception
Pain, temperature
ANS afferents
Fluid borne chemical signals

Figure 3.2.2 Information flow into the deep brain centres

The brainstem, limbic system, thalamus and hypothalamus assess incoming information for danger and can trigger overwhelm responses that hijack the functioning of the whole body

Trauma can be caused by big single events or be a cumulative process

Our resources can be overwhelmed by one big event or an accumulation of smaller events. Dissociation seems to be particularly connected to the experience of feeling helpless. Levine (1997) lists the following common traumatic antecedents:

- Foetal trauma (intra-uterine).

- Birth trauma.

- Loss of a parent or a close family member.

- Illness, high fevers, poisoning.

- Physical injuries, including falls and accidents.

- Sexual, physical and emotional abuse, including severe neglect or beatings.

- Witnessing violence.

- Natural disasters.

- Certain medical and dental procedures.

- Surgery, particularly tonsillectomies with ether and operations for ear problems or lazy eye.

Sills (2004, p.383) states that low-level chronic nociception (pain signals) and inflammation can cause overwhelm responses in the autonomic nervous system. This model develops the idea of a facilitated segment (typically described as being limited to the spinal cord) to include the brainstem and limbic system (a central sensitized or maladaptive state in the CNS where the autonomic balance shifts). Overwhelm in the older deeper parts of the brain can therefore occur from below up (from the spine and periphery into the brainstem and limbic system) and from above down (cerebral cortex down into the brainstem and limbic system). This means low-level continual joint pain or organ irritation can trigger activation and dissociation.

The initial skills to work with overwhelm we have covered so far are creating a safe relational field and supporting the development of resources. We will also explore other, very effective verbal tools and more craniosacral skills. The tools can help trauma held in someone's system dissipate in a slow, contained manner.

Clinical Highlight: Signs of sympathetic activation – fight or flight or hyperarousal

The difference between stress and trauma is a matter of degree. Below are listed some of the signs of ANS activation that are associated with overwhelming experiences. We tend to respond to stressors in line with our historical responses. Early overwhelming experiences (for example, birth and early development) therefore set the pattern for how we respond to all subsequent stressors.

- Faster respiration (to get oxygen in).

- Quicker heart beat and pulse (to supply blood to the large muscles).

- Increased blood pressure.

- Dilated pupils (to take in more light and information).

- Pale skin colour (blood is diverted away from the periphery).

- Increased sweating (there is an expectation of heat being generated in the mobilization response, so sweating can be seen as a pre-emptive response to cool the body down).

- Cold, clammy skin (especially hands, due to less blood in the periphery and increased sweating).

- Decrease in digestive processes (including a dry mouth and contracted sphincters).

- Tingling muscular tension.

- Startle response.

- Increased flexor tension.

- Emotionally this may be experienced as anxiety/panic, terror, aggression and everything happening too quickly.

Clinical Highlight: Signs of parasympathetic activation – freeze or dissociation or hypoarousal

- Tonic immobility.
- Numbing.
- Dissociation.
- Analgesia – this may be in the whole body, one side or one limb or a part of one limb.
- Inability to move a limb, dreams of not being able to move (one client called this 'sleep paralysis').
- Inability to perceive the outline of the body (for example, hands or feet feeling too big or too small or too close or too far away).
- Inability to feel the skin as a sharply defined edge.
- Sense of floating (this may be the whole body off the treatment couch, legs higher than the body or vice versa, or a sense of tilting from one side to the other).
- Sense of disconnection (commonly from below the neck or diaphragm or pelvis or feet).
- Low muscle tone (hypermobility).
- Emotionally this may be experienced as depression, withdrawal, feelings of unreality or not knowing, and lethargy. Dissociation can be a very frightening experience but can also be experienced as a dreamy, floaty, pleasant event – it is a place where you feel no pain.

Patterns of experience are imprinted on the body

Sometimes we meet events in life that we cannot deal with because they are too overwhelming. These experiences are then held in the bodymind as imprints and memories and create physiological effects. We use the term *patterns of experience* to describe how the body centres and responds to the conditional forces of life events. Inertial fulcrums and shapes are equivalent terms. Biodynamic forces represent the inherent adaptability of the body, its continual striving for health. How much you are affected by an event depends on your resources and your relationship to biodynamic health. We all do the best we can, given our history and current circumstances. Many of our responses are deep reflexes embedded in our personality that are based on previously successful strategies. Bringing awareness and choice to our habitual responses and our deepest imprints is a huge part of biodynamic craniosacral therapy. This is necessarily an embodied awareness as most of our defining experiences are encoded non-verbally and non-consciously in our bodies.

Patterns of experience can be created by:

- physical trauma – injuries

- birth process – foetal distress, interventions

- nutrition – deficiencies, toxicity

- emotional trauma – abuse, neglect, lack of support

- belief systems – strong beliefs/attitudes can fix the body

- environment – air, water, light

- hereditary factors – genetic influences.

They are formed when the potency of the breath of life is unable to dissipate the effects of an overwhelming experience. Often these patterns emerge and resolve themselves by coming into a new relationship with the breath of life. However, sometimes the system needs help with this and a powerful way to help is for your client to come into a deeper connection with their own health. Patterns of experience are places of resistance and fixation in the body. They are formed by the inability to recover from an overwhelming experience. The following is a typical sequence of events:

- Threatening event.

- Contraction.

- Experienced as overwhelming.

- Frozen state/fixation.

- Fragmentation and compartmentalization.

- Unable to express the primary respiration.

- Lowering of potency and craniosacral motion expressed with altered shape.

Force vectors can be generated by impacts

One kind of trauma is an impact injury through a forceful event such as falling or being hit by an object. These kinds of events have a momentum and trajectory to them that is absorbed by the body's tissues and generate what is called a force vector. If it is a strong force then the force vector can travel deep into the body before its energy is diffused. This force has an energy and a direction. When you are treating someone with this kind of injury in their history, you might notice that, as the body starts to process the trauma, the tissues along the force vector pathway start to activate and sometimes in the reorganization there is a migration of the force back along the pathway out of the body.

Sometimes the pathway in the body is not linear, perhaps because the impact force was not linear or perhaps because the force vector hit a bone in the body and bounced off it along another direction. Then you can get complex ricochet pathways that reveal themselves. Sometimes the force vector passes right through the body and comes to a stop in the field surrounding the body.

At first the force from these events feels like a charged force held in the body unable to discharge itself. This is an active state. In time, though, it starts to wind down and go into a frozen state, so that the tissues and fluids in the associated areas become immobile. As the body accommodates to the external force there is a kernal of biodynamic potency, a still core, to the new shape that emerges. This still core centres the conditional forces and organizes the body's response. After a state of balance, where the conditional forces are dissipated, the biodynamic potency that was at the heart of the pattern is free to do much more interesting things and you can often feel a surge in potency along the midline.

Shut-down is a closing down when overwhelmed

If the force is completely overwhelming then the body can shut down as a whole. The body has gone into a contracted state that it is unable to shift out of.

Shut-down can take place through a whole range of events that the body recognizes as too much to deal with. Therapeutically one of the most powerful things you can offer is listening to and acknowledging the body's state. At first you can feel as a trainee practitioner that you need to do something to bring about motion. Be patient and recognize that the body is simply not going to shift out of this state in a short time. It will take time for the body's resources to emerge. You will need to spend time with your client helping them to re-associate through verbal contact. Using language to help your client come into a felt sense of their body or part of their body can be an essential tool for re-animating the body intelligence.

Your client's system will need to feel safe in order to do this. It will need to know there is no present danger. Helping people out of shut-down isn't a technique, so be patient and know that small changes are big things. The beginning of fluid motion can be a huge step for that person's system to make and will almost always bring along with it trauma expressions. Don't expect their system to leap into primary respiration; that takes time and the creating of a safe therapeutic space and relationship.

3.3 DISSOCIATION

Some themes on how to treat dissociation, in a biodynamic craniosacral therapy context, are explored below. It is important to note that the model offered is that dissociation is not an all or nothing experience. Also it is much more than a pure psychological withdrawal. Dissociation has many nuances and graduations and has huge consequences for the experience of being embodied.

Orienting to the outline of the body helps perceive dissociation

An extremely useful skill to learn as a practitioner is to check whether you can perceive the whole outline of the body in front of you. This is not a given. The first place to start practising this is on yourself. In your own meditations and treatments work through the Weight, Outline, Skin, Inside (WOSI) sequence (see below). Can you really inhabit the whole of your body space?

Rothschild (2000) is very keen on feeling the boundary of the skin. It helps differentiate who we are. Our skin is a transition place between me and not me. A layer of the nerve-rich skin grew from ectoderm; we can engage with the skin as an outpost of the nervous system. It is very powerful to come into relationship with your skin and take up occupancy in the whole space of your body.

Once you have some consistent sense of your own outline, you can use it as a reference to feel the whole of the body of the person in front of you. Frequently there will be bits that are very hard to feel: missing or tiny legs, very diffuse bodies, absent abdomens and pelvic bowls, one side or one limb being absent.

How is your brain mapping out your body?

Below are some sample questions that can help you draw out a client's ability to feel their body. Initially it can be useful to go through them as a sequence, using the mnemonic WOSI: Weight, Outline, Skin, Inside. With more experience you can be much more flexible. Often the simple question 'How does x compare to y?' can open up a realization of an incomplete mapping of the body.

Weight

'How does the weight of your body feel on the table?'

'Do your shoulder blades, hips, knees and ankles feel even on the table?'

Outline

'Can you feel the outline of your body, the silhouette it makes?'

'Does the outline feel the same from the inside with your eyes closed as it would if you were looking at your body or touching it?'

'How close or far away are your hands and feet? They are not too big or too small or too close or too far away?'

Skin

'Can you feel your skin as a clear boundary between the inside and the outside?'

'Does your skin feel sharply defined and easy to contact or is it a bit blurry or amorphous?'

Inside

'How does the inside of your body feel?'

'Does the inside of your body feel full, flowing, alive or are there bits that feel empty, fixed, numb or hard to contact?'

Other useful orientations for dissociation

Bones

Bones are very grounding. The minerals in bones can be related to the solidness of the earth. In a light spacey diffuse system trying to make a relationship to the bones and the skeleton can be very useful.

Floating is not necessarily good

The pleasant, dream-like quality in dissociation is often confusing. Clients frequently enjoy being dissociated. As a young child, a client of one of the authors learnt to dissociate when her parents were arguing. When the author first started treating her, and did not understand this model, we both thought the sessions were productive because she consistently reported a warm, floating quality, a space where her body did not constrain her. However, her symptoms never changed. It took over a year to work out what was going on. Her healing started when she made friends with her 'boring' body.

Many people can misinterpret the dreamy floaty quality of dissociation as an expansive, spiritual, healing experience. We have treated many long-term meditators, yoga teachers and spiritual searchers. The relationship to the body offered through biodynamic craniosacral therapy has been surprising and beneficial for many of them. It is essential to not be too quick to let go of the body. Before we can transcend our body we have to have a body. For most of us there is a lifetime of work involved in exploring our flesh.

Deepening into our bodies is the necessary step that allows us to widen our perceptual horizons and drop into deeper tides and stillness. It is true that the sense of the body can become much more diffuse and fade into the background. However, the form is never lost, as in dissociation, and is always available for our return.

Clinical Highlight: Dissociation

Some simple questions in case history taking can help draw out how overwhelmed someone's system is:

- 'Do you get cold hands or feet?'
- 'Are you sensitive to bright lights or loud noises?'
- 'Do you bump into things or are you clumsy?'
- 'Do you ever have a sense of being detached or feeling dreamy or have you been described as having your head in the clouds?'
- 'Are you more anxious than you would like?' (Can follow up with: 'Have you ever had panic attacks?')

Clinical example on dissociation

One of the authors was referred a client by an osteopath who had treated a 40-year-old woman for chronic low back pain and pain in her right hip. She had treated the client for approximately ten sessions with little improvement. The pain varied between the right hip and lower back, but rarely occurred together. On referring, the osteopath said of the client, 'Her pelvis has not got a brain': the pattern of biomechanical dysfunction was always shifting.

In the case history she said yes to cold hands and feet, yes to sensitive to bright lights, yes to feeling a bit spacey and yes to being clumsy. She experienced periods of anxiety and ground her teeth. On asking her to focus on simple body sensations she felt withdrawn and not connected to her body. She could not really feel anything below her hips.

We started working primarily with body awareness and craniosacral therapy. In the second session there was a clearer sense of connection and feeling in her legs but an absence of feeling around her right hip. Over five sessions her pain levels decreased as her ability to map her internal environment increased.

The adjusting she had received previously had not worked as there was a clear dissociative element to her condition. If the nervous system cannot map the somatic structures because of analgesia then the motor output to maintain the correct tone will be confused. This often leads, as in this case, to bizarre migratory symptoms that are hard to relate to biomechanics.

Treatment Exercise: Working with dissociation

1. Start at feet.

   - Establish resources, wait for holistic shift, orient to mid tide. Negotiate moving your hands during the session as required.

2. Orient to the outline of the body.

   - Deepen into your own outline and use it as a guide for what is possible to feel.

   - Notice the bits that are hidden or missing or hard to contact. Most commonly one of the legs will be missing but there are many possibilities: including shoulders, no abdomen, one side hazy or fixed or floating or sinking, head only or very small legs, everything very diffuse.

   - Compare top to bottom, left to right, middle to periphery.

3. Check in verbally – 'How is your brain mapping out your body?'

   - Short version: 'How does your left leg (arm/side, etc.) feel compared to your right leg?'

   - Longer version: WOSI (see p.86).

   - Use a light, responsive approach here. The goal is develop awareness of present-time sensations for both you and the client. Try to draw out simple words. Slow down too many stories; encourage differentation of sensations.

   - 'So that's interesting, your brain is mapping out your left leg differently. Can you just notice that for a bit, try not to want it to change.'

4. Orientation skills.

   - Expand your descriptive awareness so that it is safe enough for the whole to become present – the third egg model of the biosphere can be useful (see Figure 1.3.1).

   - Orient to the bones and the skeleton.

   - 'Being to being, midline to midline' (a phrase used by Franklyn Sills).

5. Negotiate ending.

Appreciate the hidden parts as organizing centres

The noisy, painful bit of the body, the part that is screaming for attention, is frequently not the primary fulcrum. The organizing centre of a pattern of experience is often hidden and hard to contact. Commonly, in clinical practice, there can be a choice between paying attention to a tight, hard, dynamic part and a quiet, inaccessible part. We strongly recommend considering the bit you cannot feel as the inertial fulcrum. The obvious part is often like the end of the flag flapping in the wind. What is organizing the dynamic of the flag is the still part, attached to the pole.

Any work you can do to support the hidden parts coming back into relationship to the whole and the midline will be beneficial. For example, it is very common to feel one leg as fixed and held and not moving well. The other leg may feel quiet and not troublesome. Try deepening into the quietness and check that it is not an absence. Primary respiration will often start expressing simply by acknowledging an absent quality in the quiet part.

Treatment Exercise: Working with what is hidden

1. Start.

    • Establish resources; spend some time doing this before putting your hands on. Use the outline from the resources section above.

    • Wait for holistic shift, orient to mid tide. Move your hands during the session as you feel.

2. Orient to the outline of the body.

    • Deepen into your own outline and use it as a guide for what is possible to feel.

3. Check in verbally – 'How is your brain mapping out your body?'

    • 'How does x compare to y?' or use WOSI.

4. Awareness of signals coming up – 'How do you know you are not wearing shoes right now?'

    • 'Can you try something for me – slowly move your foot (or muscles in hip, abdomen, pelvic floor, arm, wrist). Can you feel the skin stretching, the bones moving, the muscles contracting?'

    • 'Let your ankle go still. Even though it is not moving there are lots of signals still coming up from the foot. How do you know that you are not wearing shoes right now – not the idea but the direct sensations that tell you that?'

- Keep tracking your awareness of the outline, any changes in distortions in the field, the client's experience of their body, changes in primary respiration. It may take a few cycles within a session; it may take a number of sessions. Go slowly, be creative.

5. Orient to the hidden, empty parts.

   - If your client sails through the above, is present, aware of their whole body and you can feel the outline clearly then try the following:
     - Orient to the relatively hidden, empty, quiet, hard to feel parts as inert fulcrums.
     - Can you support the most hidden part to come back into relationship to the whole?
     - Maybe make direct contact. It is often useful to go to the boundary of the hidden area.
     - Support Becker's three-stage process.

6. Negotiate ending.

3.4 ACTIVATION

Activation is used here as a general term to describe sympathetic activity. There is much that is useful on activation in the models around stress (for example, Sapolsky 2004; Watkins 2008) as well as the research that comes under the heading of trauma or post-traumatic stress disorder. The stress model and neuroendocrine–immune responses are covered in Section 9.5.

Autonomic nervous system coordinates overwhelm responses

The autonomic nervous system controls the organs, glands and smooth muscles of the body. Included in the control is a huge sensory feedback to the CNS from the ANS. The ANS is usually classified as an involuntary system; control is automatic and outside our conscious experience. One of the great gifts of bodywork is to open up the world of the autonomic nervous system to conscious perception; we can learn to feel the sensory input from the ANS. The skilled awareness developed through giving and receiving craniosacral therapy is an incredibly powerful tool. We can access the tunes played by the inner orchestra of the body. The autonomic nervous system is a central player in the orchestra. The music is the felt sense, the emergence of emotions and intelligence from the physiology.

The neurology of the autonomic nervous system is extensive. It is classically divided into the sympathetic nervous system, concerned with mobilization and excitation, and the parasympathetic nervous system, concerned with rest, recuperation and regeneration. There is a dynamic balance between the divisions of the ANS to maintain homeostasis.

Sympathetic ganglia and the vagus nerve

A feature of the ANS is that there are two nerves to carry the signal from the CNS to the target organ. In the somatic nervous system there is only one nerve. A ganglion is the name of the structure where the two peripheral ANS nerves synapse. These ganglia are particularly significant in the sympathetic nervous system. They form interconnected chain ganglia anterior and lateral to either side of the spine, and various plexi in front of the aorta, in the neck, thorax and pelvis. It is common to feel the highly charged sympathetic ganglion in overactive, stressed systems in clinic work. Along with the adrenal glands, an active brainstem and a buzzing ganglion impar (coccygeal ganglion), these structures contribute to a characteristic sympathetic hum.

The sympathetic nerves are also called the thoracic lumbar division, as the nerve roots of the sympathetic nervous system leave the central nervous system between the spinal vertebrae T1 to L2.

The parasympathetic nerves emerge from the cranial base and the sacral segments S2, 3, 4. Consequently they are also called the cranial-sacral division. (The parasympathetic nerves also form ganglia but in a different way – the ganglia are much more dispersed and closer to the target organs and therefore much less significant as a clinical awareness. The parasympathetic ganglia in the organ walls contribute to the characteristics of how we perceive individual organs.)

The big player in the parasympathetic nervous system is the vagus nerve, cranial nerve X. It is a huge nerve emerging bilaterally from the jugular foramen, hitching a ride alongside the major arteries and spreading to connect to all the major organs. It is classically influenced by supporting space at the jugular foramen. The sacral parasympathetic nerves are also significant clinically. They supply the lower large intestines and the organs of reproduction and elimination.

Treatment Exercise: Portals into the sympathetics

1. General points.
   - The following steps are about exploring the quality and feel of the sympathetic nervous system from different portals. They are used mainly in a diagnostic sense; they are useful to confirm that the system is busy or that it has changed. With experience a characteristic sympathetic buzz will become very familiar.

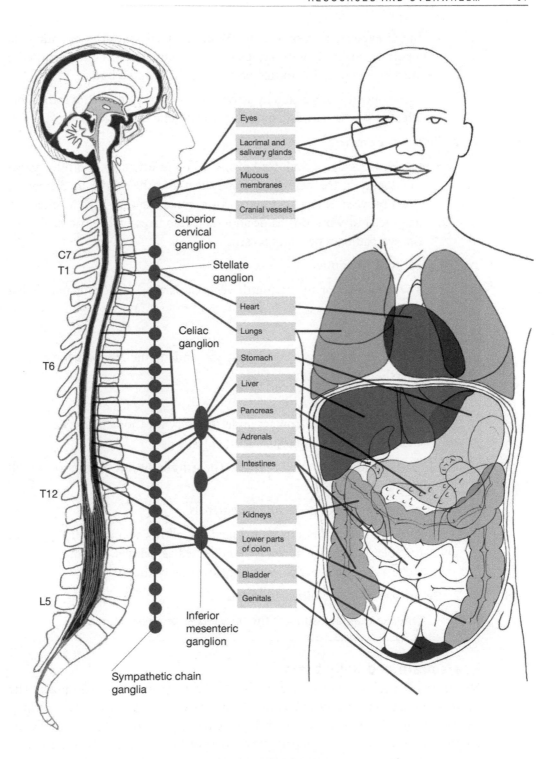

Figure 3.4.1 Schematic of the sympathetic nervous system

The chain ganglia are bilateral; one side only is shown. They are located lateral to the vertebral bodies and anterior to the rib heads. Also not shown is the coccygeal ganglion where the two chains link inferiorly, just in front of the coccyx. The ganglia, chains, adrenals and brainstem are powerful portals into the sympathetic nervous system

- In our experience in only about 50 per cent of cases does orienting via a portal actually slow the sympathetic response down. The sympathetics are active in response to fulcrums held by the whole body.

- Remember that inhibition by activating the parasympathetics is the most effective way of downgrading the sympathetic action.

2. Start at the cradle.

- Establish resources, wait for holistic shift and orient to mid tide. Assess the quality in the whole nervous system and the whole fluid body. Is this a busy system or a diffuse, hard-to-contact system? If the latter you may need to work on dissociation and resources before the quality of the sympathetics becomes present.

3. Orient to the brainstem.

- The area anterior to the fourth ventricle is the location of nuclei that govern the ANS.

4. Contact the coccyx.

- Orient to the ganglion impar at the end of the sympathetic chains, directly in front of the coccyx.

5. Holding the junctions.

- Make a two-handed contact under the cervical thoracic junction (CTJ) and the thoracic lumbar junction (TLJ).

- Orient to the sympathetic chains. The ganglia sit just in front of the rib heads.

6. Orient to the various plexi and the adrenals.

- The two-handed 'holding the junctions' allows you to easily orient to the solar plexus, the adrenals and the cardiac ganglia. You may want to make a direct contact above and below one of the plexi.

7. Be curious about the different portals.

- Offer settling and support the three-stage process as required.

Heart brain and belly brain

New science is showing that we can talk of a heart brain and a belly brain. The nervous connections around and within the heart (thoracic ganglia and its intrinsic nervous system) have their own independent circuits (Armour 2008). Similarly the enteric nervous system and sympathetic plexi, coordinating gut activity, have their own independent processing outside the CNS.

These new mind–body connections are very exciting for bodyworkers. The heart brain is particularly well researched. It has been shown to have primitive memory. Heart rate variability research shows that the prefrontal cortex is switched off when the heart rate begins to race under stress because of sensory vagal input (Watkins 2008). There is no doubt neurologically that the body talks to the brain and frequently leads the conversation. The language of the conversation is frequently what we call emotions – the informational chemicals of the neuroendocrine–immune system (or molecules of emotion, Pert 1999).

In health parasympathetic activity inhibits sympathetic activity

The dynamic balance between the two arms of the ANS is largely maintained by inhibition of the sympathetics by the parasympathetics. The vagus nerve, especially, acts to inhibit the sympathetic nervous system. The sympathetics are set to run in overdrive all the time; health depends on an active vagal brake.

There is lots of research showing that ANS imbalance (causing anxiety, poor attention and immune disorders as shown by proinflammatory cytokines plus other conditions) is due to low vagal tone. The vagal brake not working causes the sympathetics to be dis-inhibited and the system to become much less flexible in its responses (Porges 2003; Thayer and Lane 2000).

Clinically this means that any inputs that allow the parasympathetic nervous system to function more effectively will inhibit the sympathetic nervous system. One of the most powerful ways of doing this is to offer stillness and space and allow the system to orient to resources and the environment in present time. The extra information from the whole body and the whole field will allow contextualization of cycling and speedy stories and slow down the stress response.

In overwhelm the sympathetics and flexor muscles are switched on and the extensor muscles are inhibited. The extensor muscles are associated with the parasympathetics. The extensors allow us to come into a softer, upright, open and receptive posture. Supporting this posture, and the reflexes to maintain it, can be a useful tool in clinic work. In a treatment session asking the client about their contact with the table helps engage the back of the body and the extensors.

The organs, especially the heart and gut, utilizing the heart brain and belly brain, are also very powerful tools in stimulating the parasympathetics and inhibiting the sympathetics.

Information flows from the body and the environment can inhibit overwhelm

The quick response to the question 'Am I safe?' is mediated by centres deep in the brain. Simply, we can talk of the limbic system and the brainstem controlling dissociation and activation. These deep brain centres receive information from three sources: from the cortex down; from the external senses in; and from the body coming up. Figure 3.2.2 attempts to show this flow of information.

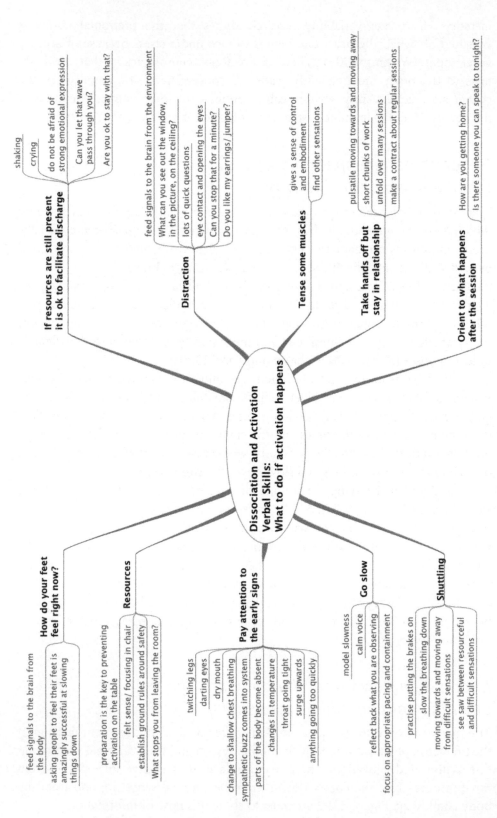

Figure 3.4.2 Mindmap giving overview of verbal skills that can help if activation occurs

Finding your state of balanced awareness and giving more space are often essential alongside the verbal skills given above

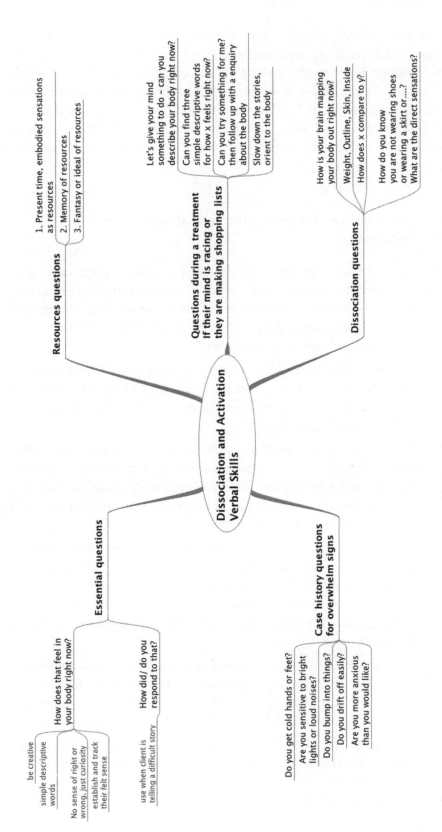

Figure 3.4.3 Useful general questions for dissociation and activation

If we are overwhelmed, wherever the information comes from, the amygdala will trigger communication, mobilization or freezing. Orienting to the flow of information from the body (the internal milieu) and from the environment (the external senses) are much more powerful ways of inhibiting the sympathetics than using the cortex-down route. It is very hard to think your way out of anxiety; it is much easier to orient and feel your way out. Biodynamic cranial work can use these pathways from the body and the environment to help the system come into present time.

Awareness Exercise: Tuning into the sympathetic and the parasympathetic

- *Sympathetic nerves* emerge from the thoracic spine and upper lumber spine (thoracolumbar division) and form an interconnecting chain of ganglia on either side of the spine in front of the rib heads. The chain extends all the way down to, and joins up at, the ganglion impar, in front of the coccyx. It also extends up into the neck.

- The nerves also form additional ganglia – the most famous being the solar plexus – that innervate the gut and organs. Using your awareness, try tuning into the sympathetic chains and then the visceral nerve network including the plexi.

- Feel the quality and motion within the ganglia and the interactions with the organs. The brainstem and adrenal glands are other important hotspots of the sympathetic network. Frequently there can be buzzy, dynamic, quick, hot qualities to tuning into these structures – which words and impressions work for you?

- Now tune into the *parasympathetic nervous system* (also called the craniosacral division); start from the cranial nerve nuclei in the brainstem. See if you can imagine and follow the vagus nerve down through the cranial base and the neck into the thoracic chamber and down through the diaphragm into the abdomen though a series of plexi into ganglia at the organs.

- Notice too the pelvic nerves exiting from the sacrum into the pelvic space and viscera. Try orienting to nervous activity geared towards rest and recuperation at the base of the skull and in the pelvic bowl at the same time. How does this feel? Is it different to the sympathetic system?

- Try being attuned to both the sympathetic/thoracolumbar division and parasympathetic/craniosacral division systems together and notice how the two interact.

Clinical Highlight: Using Allan Wade's concept of resistance
in a bodywork context – 'How did you respond to that?'

> From the beginning you had some life force that refused to buckle
> under and submit to his authority. (Allan Wade, psychotherapist)[2]

The above statement holds deep resonance for our work as bodyworkers. Many forms of bodywork and alternative medicine emphasize the concept of a life force – 'vital force' in homeopathy, 'innate intelligence' in chiropractic, 'breath of life' in craniosacral therapy or just simply energy (qi) in shiatsu. As a craniosacral therapist the aim of the work is to engage with the embodied movements and expressions of this life force. It is a living, breathing, palpable, experiential reality. Most simply, the work is supporting people to become aware of and become more skilled in allowing this life force to express itself.

Reading Allan Wade's paper was hugely exciting for us. It brought together a number of themes from our training and practice that allowed a real deepening of our understanding and skills in working with people. Along with 'How does that feel in your body?' 'How did you respond?' has become a stock question. It gives a very spacious model with which to support clients to explore difficult experiences. Focusing on the response allows an acknowledgement of whatever story you have just heard or are hearing but subtly shifts the space to a proactive, empowering debate. It can allow you to feel much more comfortable in talking with people who disclose abusive, violent or overwhelming experiences. Without this it can be easy to get lost in the pain of someone's story whilst making the commitment to keep engaging verbally with their process. The primary method of working with people in cranial work is through touch. Listening skills and verbal skills, such as the questions above, are part of the training and are wonderfully valuable. However, we are drawn to the simplicity and power of working through touch, because it sidesteps lots of issues with explaining, interpreting and the drive to understand.

The experience of emotion always involves a bodily response. In many ways the background tensions, the nagging pains, the vague sensations of discomfort are emotions. The felt sense of Gendlin (1981), Damasio's (1999) construction of the consciousness and emotion, Pert's (1999) molecules of emotion all support this view. Authors such as Levine (Levine and Frederick 1997), Rothschild (2000) and Sills (2001), and even Shapiro (2001) to some extent, all place the body's responses (particularly the autonomic nervous system) at the forefront of working with shock and trauma. We feel Wade adds to this body of work by allowing us to see the inherent but often hidden acts of resistance that form people's response. He also places a strong emphasis on the body: 'I find it useful to ask persons to describe their facial expressions, tone of voice, posture, and so forth, in responding to mistreatment. Such questions frequently yield a description of disguised or indirect expression of protest.' In the cranial framework these responses shape and form people's bodies. The forces activated as resistance can easily be held in the body and continue to generate tissue and body patterns throughout someone's life. The understanding of these forces as necessary attempts at resistance to being overwhelmed can be a very powerful shift to resolution.

When discussing the autonomic system response to being overwhelmed it is easy to slip into jargon and pathologizing. Wade makes a timely reminder to avoid this and focus on the creativeness of people's response. Dissociation is a term to be careful with; instead you can talk of a place of withdrawal and/or the ability to find your own internal untouchable world – 'the only possibility for the realization of resistance may be the privacy afforded by the mind'. For one client her felt sense of being trapped in a white room of no feeling became the place of her ultimate truth where the walls were protecting her rather than imprisoning her. It became a safe place where she could choose to go to. This understanding was so much more useful to her than labelling it as a dissociated state. (To repeat: dissociation can be a resourcing and a very necessary state. However, it is very important to be able to spot it is happening – not much healing can happen if people are not present.)

Below are two clinical examples involving the concept of resistance.

1. The client suddenly looked up and said, 'Do you think I am toxic?' Her father was physically abusive to her; one of the things he used to do was to hit her around the back of her head and dismiss her. Contacting the tension in the back of her skull triggered a memory of some of the messages she used to get from her father. In some way she still felt that her contact with people 'pollutes' them. Solely reassuring her that she was not toxic somehow felt inadequate, so discussion moved on to how she used to respond to her father hitting her. She said she became extremely sensitive to his moods. She used to be able to prepare herself because she knew what he would do before he knew himself. She then immediately flowed into explaining how she was always sensitive to how other people were. In her first job she had been a teaching assistant. She knew what the children wanted and was able to respect and meet their needs quickly. She was told by the teacher that she was the best assistant they had ever had. It was wonderful to feel her body soften as she said this and to invite her to hold the knowledge of her sensitivity next to her belief that she was toxic.

2. Another client was continually frustrated with her sense of being rebellious and destructive. As an example of her destructiveness she told a story of how as a child she was a good athlete and how her emotionally abusive father, who was also sporty, liked to show her off. When she was 11 she was due to run in a race and her father brought his friends along expecting

her to win. Before the race she sabotaged her ability to run by eating lots of pickled onions. She threw up during the race. By using Wade's framework it was possible to view this act of rebellion as an extremely clever way of humiliating her father. Even though outwardly she had very little power in relationship to her father she was still able to find a way to publicly defy him. Her ability to see her rebellion as a powerful act of resistance to abusive authority was incredibly helpful.

Summary of Chapter 3

This chapter define the key concepts of health and resources along with the mechanisms of shock and trauma. The chapter discussed how the body responds to threat and overwhelm. The body has a natural ability to activate and dissociate in order to protect itself; this happens through the autonomic nervous system response. Understanding the biological and psychoemotional mechanisms is an important feature of working safely with trauma and trauma resolution. The biodynamic approach offers a contained and neutral space to allow the body to access its own health and resources to change from within at its own pace and timing. Verbal skills of bringing the client into felt sense are explored.

Notes

1. Excess cortisol, a major long-term stress hormone, is implicated in inhibiting the explicit memory of the hippocampus; for example, see Sapolsky (2004). High levels of cortisol are strongly associated with the fight or flight part of the stress response.

    The relationship of cortisol to PTSD is complex. 'Neither low basal concentrations nor enhanced suppression of cortisol are consistent markers of a PTSD diagnosis' (Lindley, Carlson and Benoit 2004, p.940). Many researchers however seem to indicate low-level cortisol in PTSD; for example, Mason *et al.* (1988).

    Dissociative disorders are categorized differently from people suffering from PTSD. In subjects with dissociative disorders Simeon *et al.* (2007, p.966) found 'significantly elevated urinary cortisol' compared with the control group and no difference between PTSD and the control group.

    The above demonstrates that the differentiation of the neurobiology of stress, traumatic stress and dissociation is complex. When we are overwhelmed it is safe to say that there is disruption to the normal function of the neuroendocrine–immune response, specifically the HPA axis and the autonomic nervous system.

2. This and all other Wade quotes in this clinical highlight are from Wade (1997).

4

Stillness and Potency

4.1 LONG TIDE

Why can't many people express long tide? Is it because their systems are not capable of it? Perhaps there's too much congestion and trauma in their systems to be able to access it. Or perhaps the practitioner is not able to offer the right space and orientation to facilitate a long tide expression. Maybe it's all of these things.

All a practitioner can do is to be open to long tide. This means that your system needs to be in relationship to it. Thus, it is possible that within the relational field you create you may enable your client's system to shift into a long tide state. Becoming familiar with long tide will change your practice, change your state of awareness and bring you into a more immediate relationship with the breath of life.

Cellular potency

> Single cells…must have some sort of fractal supply network. This is radical as it implies that there exists a whole echelon of biological organization that we have not yet detected, and even proponents feel obliged to talk about a 'virtual' network, whatever that might be. Even so, many biologists are receptive to the possibility, for the cytoplasm is now seen to be far more organized than the amorphous jelly that is passed off in text books. The nature of this organization is elusive, but it is clear that the cytoplasm 'streams' through the cell, and that many biochemical reactions are more carefully defined in space than had been assumed. (Lane 2005, p.163)

> One cannot help but suspect that the great stream of energy that passes across the earth plays a larger role in biology than our current philosophy knows: that perhaps the flood of power not only permitted life to evolve, but called it into being. (Lane 2005, p.103, quoting Franklin Harold from *The Vital Force*)

What happens to the body in long tide? There is that mysterious shift from a fluid field that has a containment of the body and the space immediately around the body, to a very light and air-like space that is much more expanded and has only a vague sense of the body. The experience is exhilarating for both client and practitioner. As the practitioner, the nature of your body has changed. You have become lighter and more rarefied and much more present.

The whole state is one without effort. It often steals upon you during a treatment. As a practitioner you know there is a wonderful freeing up in this state. The body system is charged up and you feel rejuvenated from it. The force of presence is so strong in this state that the body is automatically aligned. Presence and potency seem to co-exist here and every cell tingles in your body. It's as if the body has gone into a much more original state beyond the body systems.

Could it be that potency is now forming a connection as it did at the beginning of our lives in utero to the individual cells? The body is still there but it's now a connection to the very building block of life, the cell itself. Now the infusion of potency is directed to every cell in the body and no wonder there are automatic shifts in structure in this state. Each cell now creates a new alignment to the breath of life so that there is a renewing of original health along with an optimizing of the cellular organization and function. The cell membrane is important for the expression of biodynamic motions, particularly motility, and it's essential that this primary motion is re-established through a connection to long tide and the potency field.

Follow long tide and notice how the body responds. As a practitioner you notice how your hands have moved out of fluids and start to feel air-like. This is the 'hands in potency' experience that Sills describes (Sills 2001, p.423). The bioenergetic field is light and expansive and the tissue and fluid fields feel as if they are less structured and contained. The body goes back to a simpler relationship with the breath of life as each cell re-potentizes. Do some cells have a stronger connection to the potency field? Perhaps. Neurons are the oldest cell in the body and the longest lived and there is commonly a strong potentization of these cells so that the central nervous system feels particularly charged up from the shift into long tide. However, the all-abiding experience is of all cells coming into a direct relationship with the breath of life and moving to a higher state of health and order. Try this next exercise to explore this phenomenon.

Awareness Exercise: Cellular intelligence

- Close your eyes. Settle into an embodied state and use an image of a cell to help you orient to the cells in your body. There is a feel to this that will emerge as you hold the intention that is not easy to describe but nevertheless is a distinct experience in your body. Open up to the natural motility of the cell.

- Open up to the potency field in and around your body so that you can notice the interaction of potency and cells. What happens to the cell in its direct relationship to potency?

- Now bring your attention to the cell membrane. How does that change the experience? Now bring your awareness to the nucleus of the cell. Is there a change when you do this?

- Finally, invite your cells to shift into a stillpoint and notice the response within the cell.

Awareness Exercise: Hierarchy of levels

- Close your eyes. Be with a sense of your whole system. This is the integrated you. Now shift your perception to a sense of individual systems within the whole such as the nervous system, or the GI tract. Stay with this state of perception for a while.

- Now shift your perception to the world of individual organs and structures. Notice the kidney, or individual bones. What is the quality of this?

- Now shift to the tissue field. Notice the different kinds of tissues in the body and how they blend together. Be interested which tissues show themselves to you. Again stay with this for a short while.

- Shift again to a sense of the cellular level of the body. Try visualizing the cell as a way to connect with this level of organization. See if you can come into a sense of the cell through the interstitial space, that is, through the extracellular fluid. This should open up a relationship with the intracellular fluid and of the cell membrane. Stay with this for a few minutes.

- Shift again to the molecular world within you. This is the world of chemical activity. The cell is a factory of intense chemical activity. See if you can relate to this. What comes to you?

- Shift again to the smallest unit within you, the atom and the subatomic world. Do you have a sense of the energy held within the smallest unit of the body and the universe? Has the potency changed? Wow! Now wonder why we ever get tired.

The uncarved block of wood

p'u (Chinese: 'simple,' 'in primordial condition'), in Chinese Taoism, metaphorical expression often translated as 'uncarved block' and signifying the primordial condition of the mind before it has been affected by experiences. In the state of p'u there are no distinctions between right and wrong, black and white, beautiful and ugly. Taoists desire to return to this state of childhood by abandoning conventional knowledge and by suppressing desires that bind them to the world. Because truth becomes relative, ideas have no value and all contradictions are resolved. The goal is thus to restore the human mind to the state of an 'uncarved block.' Individuals who achieve this state of mental unity thereby align their existence with the unity of the Absolute Tao, the mysterious, undefinable, transcendent reality that, according to Taoists, produces all things. (Encyclopedia Britannica 2009)

Imagine for a moment that you are an accomplished woodworker. You look at an uncarved block of wood with a certain affection, knowing that here is uncreated potential. As an uncarved block it can be anything – the possibilities are infinite. No one can name it because it has not yet become something except what it is in its natural, untouched state, much like the Tao.

The Taoists believe that if we could return to a state like the uncarved block of wood, p'u, we find the Tao. Human beings are often in a hurry to acquire the finished product, the carving. But once the item is produced, the limitless Tao is lost. A carving of that object is only that one thing. It has a name. It has come into existence. Eventually it will become worn, broken, or lost, going through its cycle of existence–non-existence.

But the original uncarved block is nameless, beyond definition, quietly open. The sage tries to be like an uncarved block, open to potential without being limited to one definition. What Taoists are trying to encourage is for people to find their way back to their natural being before it is influenced and shaped by culture. There is a simple, pure nature in all of us, and this nature is one with the Tao. Through society we learn to be limited. We experience restraints and norms and have many events that shape us. We form arbitrary and relative definitions of ourselves, alienated from our inborn nature.

Awareness Exercise: Long tide

- Come into body awareness. Get a sense of the depth of your body so you come into connection with your intero and extero receptors.

- Become interested in your skin and the boundary of your body. Does your system stop here? See if you can feel beyond your skin into the space around you.

- Feel subtle movements of air and temperature fluctuations but also see if there is a sense of a potency field which surrounds and invests the body. As you open up to this field you will naturally feel light and be more expansive.

- Try opening out to the potency field in the whole of the space that is contained by the room you are in. There's something subtle and satisfying about this aspect of ourselves.

- Now try relating to your midline. You will notice how energetic the midline feels, much more so than fluid or tissue.

- See if you can sense how far the potency field extends. Don't let the boundary of the room prevent you from being open to a wider field. As you do this there is a sense of a connection to the universal, where you as an individual unit within creation become less felt and there is more of a sense of involvement and connection with a greater scheme.

- Now check in with your midline and invite the tide. Be patient and wait for the tide to show itself. It might take a while to identify it as it moves very slowly but it moves very powerfully. Stay with the long tide and notice how your body and mind respond. You are in contact with the breath of life as itself. How does this make you feel?

4.2 DYNAMIC STILLNESS

Stillness keeps going. There is an endless depth to the experience of slowing down, becoming present and resting in stillness. Like the apocryphal person who asked 'Is this cool?' (or 'Is this jazz?'), if you have to ask about it you are not quite there yet. The depths of stillness have to be experienced. They are frequently obscured, but always available. Think of the times you have gazed at the stars, listened to the ocean, smelt the clean air on top of a mountain and felt the hum of life in a forest. Stillness is ever present, it is the essence of the teaching within biodynamic craniosacral therapy.

Working within the biodynamic paradigm, as teachers, practitioners and clients, has, for us, consistently and uniquely opened the door to profoundly still places. Dynamic stillness is a phrase – jargon if you like – that is used in cranial work to try to describe deeper states of stillness. The word dynamic is useful to indicate that stillness is not a void of nothing, but an experience teeming with life, information and potential.

The model of dynamic stillness, which is perceived to underlie all phenomena, is useful as a challenge to not be content with the depth of healing and engagement that can occur at such wonderful states as mid tide and long tide. Stillness is endless.

When, as practitioners, we become still, the client's system will resonate with the stillness we offer and that we can embody. The stillness that centres us is no different from the stillness in other people. In such a contact we could say that stillness meets itself, again. As we stay in relationship we then discover that the stillness we share connects to a stillness in all living things and a stillness that pervades everything.

Transcendental, numinous experiences are essentially very personal, embedded as we are in particular spiritual, religious and cultural frameworks, but they also speak to all that is universal. To not engage with awe and wonder at the phenomena we can perceive is to strip ourselves of something fundamental about being conscious humans. The biodynamic paradigm offers that stillness, dynamic stillness, is at the core of everything. It is the centre, the reference that allows form to generate.

> It is the stillness of the Tide, not the stormy waves that bounce upon the shore that has the potency, the power. (Sutherland 1990, p.16)

The metaphor of depth is an interesting way of trying to articulate going into the heart of stillness. There are many others; we can talk of going higher, wider, being more connected, more open, being more refined. By using the image of dropping through layers of the ocean, depth allows one way of linking dynamic stillness to the tides experienced in cranial work. The CRI is the unsteady, variable rocking of the waves on the surface, mid tide is like the surge and fall of the tide underneath the waves, long tide is the slow, deep currents of the ocean streams, dynamic stillness is the dark, still, mysterious ocean floor.

We strongly recommend reading Rollin Becker and Franklyn Sills.[1] Some quotes that give a flavour of stillness are given below.

> You have asked the question, What occurs at a stillpoint? That's a good question and I'll try to elaborate, but this isn't the answer – because there is no answer for what occurs at stillpoint (Becker 1997, p.69)

> The stillness is that which centres every molecule of being of that living body. The body physiology is the outward expression of that stillness. They are in total unity, in balanced interchange. (Becker 2000, p.68)

> As soon as I am aware of stillness as the motive power that is in command of this case, then my hands begin to palpate and feel the shift of the elements of the body physiology and their response to this motive power coming from the stillness. (Becker 2000, p.69)

> The deeper you can access stillness inside yourself, the deeper you can access the person's system…and recognize the deep intelligence at work which holds everything together. (Sills 2004)

It is an endless journey to be in stillness. In modern life it is frequently only a fleeting experience, but even glimpses of stillness can be breathtaking as we meet such simplicity and potential. When we touch dynamic stillness we cannot help but be changed.

4.3 BIODYNAMIC POTENCIES
The underlying force of life

Potency is the underlying force of life in the craniosacral therapy paradigm. It is the motive force behind biodynamic movements. It's the stuff of life, its vital energy that embodies through the fluids of the body. This is the brilliance of Sutherland's discoveries that the vital force connects with the body through the medium of fluid. It manifests through all fluids in the body. All fluids in the body are water-based substances, so the property of water is a key element in understanding the nature of potency. Water's structure and function gives many clues to biodynamic effects and expressions.

In the early days of cranial osteopathy, the orientation was to the tissue field and making adjustments. This gives rise to a perceptual field that is oriented to specific structural relationships and is therefore CRI in essence. At this level the cerebrospinal fluid is the carrier of potency and that's why the approach was concerned with the movements of CSF and longitudinal fluctuation along the craniospinal axis, along with adjustments of cranial joints. As the work has become more biodynamic and practitioners have approached the body with a wider perceptual field, the experience of the body has changed from tissue to fluid, and in turn from fluid to potency. There is an understanding that tissues, fluids and potency are part of a matrix of relationships that include the body and the body energetics through the interface of fluid or water.

As you widen your perceptual field to include the biosphere, the body shows you its fluid nature. At this level potency infuses into the interstitial fluids around the cells of the body. There is a strong relationship between the interstitial fluids and the connective tissue framework, so that changes that occur at this level create body-wide changes.

As you widen out to more expanded fields of perception the body shows you its potency expressions more clearly, so you start to have a stronger sense of the field around the body more than the physical body itself. At this level the potency is infusing into the body through the intracellular fluids, so each cell is going into a direct relationship to potency. This produces a wonderful organizing of the body at a cellular level and a deeper intelligence emerges that originates in the early embryonic phases when cells were coming into being and organizing themselves into the first structures. This cellular potency is like a stem cell energy and brings about a freshness to cell organization that allows the body possibilities of making huge shifts in relationship at all levels of the body and the mind.

Alongside all of this there is a deepening into the midline phenomenon. As the orientation to fluids from tissues takes place, the midline shows itself as a much more fluid-like phenomenon, as if the whole spinal column has become fluid. Along with this comes a stronger drive within the inhalation phase and a slowing down of primary respiration. This is the fluid midline. As the body shifts to the potency state the midline becomes more primal. Primary respiration is changing throughout this so that mid tide and long tide reveal themselves in the fluid and potency spaces.

It is a remarkable phenomenon that the midline can change its state during a craniosacral treatment and go from matter to energy in the space of 30 minutes. At one point in the treatment it can feel like the midline is the spinal column, then it can feel like a fluid tube and then it can feel like an energetic midline as if all structure has dissolved and the body is now a subtle energy body with a glowing centreline. If you can offer the right relational field then your triune nature of tissues, fluids and potency will readily reveal itself.

The potency field of the body

This is expressed in the space around and permeating the body. It is also known as the biosphere. The potency field came first before the midlines and before the body structures. During the embryonic development of the body, fluid spaces came into being through the energetic stimulation of the potency field. The intelligence within this field brought about a gathering of potency to create an energetic midline through the primitive streak and then the notochord. So when you orient to the midline remember that it is intrinsically linked to the potency field which not only permeates through the body's fluid and tissue fields but out into the space around the body. And at the risk of repeating things, the field came first. It was there before the midlines. Just look at the early embryonic sequences and you will see fluid potency spaces emerging as the first structures as precursors to the embryonic midlines and the formation of the body. So opening up to and acknowledging this is connecting with a more original health. From conception the dividing early cells are expressing primary respiration as motility, a natural breathing from within the cell structure. This is the earliest and oldest expression of biodynamic health in the body. So when you are feeling this motility expression within structures know there is an original potency here. Often when the body system is traumatized and there is no tide, there will be some motility. Only later when the embryo has developed a neural midline and the enfoldment process has occurred is there a longitudinal fluctuant movement along the midline.

The body expresses potency in different ways. As a practitioner you can feel a multitude of these. The most common is a sense of potency as an emanation from the body tissues and fluids. It's like a light shining from within. It's the vitality expression that we so often talk about around health. It's the glow of life that can be seen in the skin and the eyes and the aura. What is that? It's a vibrational quality of potency which increases as the body system becomes more deeply resourced. You can feel potency as something fluid electric that builds up in your hands. You can feel it as a lateral fluctuation somewhere in the body with all kinds of different-shaped movements from circular to swirling to figures of eight. You can feel potency as the tide. You can feel it gather around a state of balance; as the body moves towards reorganization, potency often starts streaming through the body.

The potency field is a resource for you and for your client. As you start to familiarize with the potency expressions in your system there is an embodiment that emerges and naturally orients you to this aspect of yourself. So you start to feel deeply resourced and more complete within your system. When you set up the relational field you will therefore attract this into the contact space with your client and engender a connection to the client's own potency state. You will notice how your client's system moves with greater potency. Potency enables natural mechanisms of change and balance to come about.

Awareness Exercise: Connecting to your potency field

- Come into whole body awareness. Let your system settle. Shift your awareness to your skin and become interested in the space just out from it. Gradually let your awareness be open to relating to more and more of the space out from here.

- Take your time. Let the space invite you into it. You will wait at boundaries sometimes before other layers of the space open up to you. Track your body sensations as you explore and notice how your mind is affected. What is the feeling quality of the potency field?

- Can you feel how it interacts with your body, in particular your skin, the body cavities and the spine?

4.4 SPIRIT AND CRANIAL WORK
Know your own model

The more a therapist feels supported by the creative forces of life, the more she/he can reflect this in the clinical holding environment. I believe that it is imperative for the therapist to have a spiritual context in which to hold the deep suffering that surfaces in clinical work. The particular spiritual orientation of the therapist, *as long as it is not imposed on the client*, is not as important as the intention to hold a spiritual level of truth. I do it through my meditative practice, application of Buddhist principles, Taoist practices, and also the contemplative understanding found in the writings of Christian mystics… However, *a simple humility and awe in the presence of the creative forces at work in human-beingness is all that is really necessary.* (Sills 2009a, p.133; italics added)

Religions frequently tell the best stories. The myths and archetypes that are part of the major religions form a defining part of the identity of most humans. If you are drawn to work in healthcare then at some stage you will meet clients who will have radically different spiritual and religious beliefs from your own. How nimble you can be in meeting your client's beliefs, and to not start imposing your own, becomes very important, especially given the inherent power imbalance of the therapeutic relationship. However, healing that cannot encompass some notion of spirit and the transcendental, whether from a place of belief or non-belief, will always be limited. To be an effective practitioner we recommend an explicit awareness of your own spiritual framework and an awareness of different models.

As authors, teachers and practitioners attempt to articulate and explore the depths of the biodynamic approach, a number of strands of spiritual thought are influencing the work. The authors feel spectacularly unqualified to teach on spiritual matters. We are cautious about some of the language that is emerging in the field. For us, cranial work is so much more than an act of prayer and the creation of a sacred space.

Our sensibilities have been affected by running a busy, low-cost, teaching clinic for a number of years in an inner city area of North London. Many practitioners offer low-cost treatments or volunteer in schemes run by mental health organizations, brain injury charities and old people's homes, to name a few. Working with people who would not normally access paid-for healthcare is quite an eye opener. The cranial field is still a very small profession, trying to carve out an identity. In private practice, the majority of clients will be middle class and able to afford often significant fees in order to receive cranial work. The chaos that can exist in low-cost clinics, where you are trying to see as many people as possible, strips away many of the luxuries around creating a sacred space. Biodynamic craniosacral work is an eminently practical and clinically effective approach.

Around the world, health depends at least as much on politics, economics and social justice as it does on pursuing individual meanings and personal connections to spirituality. It is important not to forget the social context of health. Wilkinson and Pickett argue very convincingly that people in societies that have equality, fairness, trust and strong communities are healthier.[2] Spirituality is of course important, sometimes the most important thing, but we observe that it can easily become the ultimate explanation for what happens in the cranial field and this makes us a little suspicious. Below we highlight various beliefs relevant to notions of spirit in cranial work. These are more prompts to increase awareness than attempts to define a position. Engaging with other people's spiritual beliefs is a skilful process. Trying to dissuade people of deeply embedded ideals is rarely time well spent. There is often a real safety and untouchable quality to such beliefs. William James urges us to focus on the 'fruits, not the roots' of religious experience, the intensely personal nature of religious experiences and the consequences for the individual rather than the dogma and rules of the various institutions.

> Religion shall, arbitrarily, mean for us the feelings, acts, and experiences of individual men in their solitude, so far as they apprehend themselves to stand in relation to whatever they consider divine.
>
> (James 1902/2008)

'A higher power'

Alcoholics Anonymous has a relatively neutral phrase: 'a higher power'; it allows participants to engage with a transcendental force but does not railroad people into a particular religious view. Christianity, Islam and the Jewish faith describe an all-powerful God. Within these religions the 'passions of the flesh' are frequently to be mistrusted and overcome through ritual behaviour.

Religion often supports reflective practice and discipline in its disciples. Being held in a community, adhering to codes of behaviour and regular acts of contemplation can lead to wiser and more responsible community-oriented behaviour.[3]

A higher power can also be framed as an order in nature. Things work more elegantly when we are in harmony with this principle. In chiropractic this is called innate intelligence, in cranial work we use the breath of life, whereas homeopaths refer to the vital force. Sutherland in his later writing talks of the natural agencies. The Taoist descriptions of the Tao offer many simple ways of coming into relationship with this ordering principle. The model of following the path of least resistance and the power of non-doing described by Zen and Taoist texts[4] fit very closely with the authors' experience of biodynamic craniosacral therapy. We spent years in our early bodywork careers sticking our elbows in people's shoulders to release tight muscles. However, it is probably the most exciting thing we know to feel a shift emerge from the inside, or outside, of the client and for the tightest tissues to melt with no effort.

Sills and Shea write extensively on issues of spirituality and biodynamics. They have done an amazing job of synthesizing many different traditions from both an intellectual and experiential basis. Sills' new framing of Source, Being and Self is a wonderful model (Sills 2009a). Source is the transcendent cause, Being is a universal quality inherent to all humans and Self is the individual stories and forms. As a therapist, the ability to relate in a being-to-being manner, recognizing the universal being needs of acceptance, recognition and acknowledgement, is key to supporting change.

The soul

Many people are used to the debate about whether God exists or not and have found their own answers. In 2009 organizations representing atheists and Christians offered versions of the probability of God on the sides of London buses. Often concepts of the soul are much trickier. An immaterial essence that continues after the death of the body is one way of defining the soul. There are many. Soul is sometimes used interchangeably with mind. The soul is a central tenet of Christian belief, though that does not extend to notions of reincarnation offered in some eastern traditions.

In the biodynamic field many of the writers have been strongly influenced by Tibetan Buddhism which describes various stages of 'ensoulment' and the ability of adepts to track the soul as it leaves the body. The model of pre- and perinatal dynamics is gaining increasing influence in biodynamic craniosacral therapy. Teachers of pre- and perinatal work talk extensively about factors affecting the incarnation of the soul.[5]

In clinic work it is not uncommon to hear the statements 'I did not want to be born', 'I do not want to be here' or even, 'My soul did not want to incarnate'. People can perceive themselves as only reluctantly incarnated in physical form. This can be a very painful belief. We have especially noticed it in people who have done pre- and perinatal work. It can be a hard belief to engage with in a therapy that encourages embodied awareness as a route to health. Other than becoming an expert on models of the soul, Shea[6] offers one route of support. Dissociation is often a feature of struggles around incarnation. Shea describes how we can be flexible in the act of presence and how dissociation can be a skill to be appreciated. He describes how 'we can maintain a flexible attention and attunement', shifting between the midline, the body and the horizon. Ultimately we can learn to let our awareness breathe at the tempo of the primary respiration, moving between a sense of being inside and outside of the body. This may allow people who struggle with the idea of their soul, being in a body, in the world, more choice and skills in being with that story.

'It's all energy'

Information, in the form of energy, streams in simultaneously through all of our sensory systems and then it explodes into this enormous collage of what this present moment looks like, what this present moment smells like and tastes like, what it feels like and what it sounds like. I am an energy-being connected to the energy all around me through the consciousness of my right hemisphere. We are energy-beings connected to one another through the consciousness of our right hemispheres as one human family. (Bolte Taylor 2009)[7]

Physics describes four fundamental forces in the universe: the gravitational force, the electromagnetic force and the subatomic forces called weak and strong. All the weight we experience is the result of the gravitational force. Electricity, magnetism and chemistry are all the results of the electromagnetic force. The explosive release of nuclear energy is the result of the strong force. Some forms of radioactivity are the result of the weak force. Energy is also a technical term to describe the amount of work done or potential stored in a given state.

Events at subatomic levels quickly become counter-intuitive viewed from our macro-world view of nature. We simply do not have the perceptual reference points to make sense of quantum science. Quantum mechanics precisely describes the interaction of subatomic particles; it has not been shown to apply to larger particles (Al-Khalili 2003). It is very strange. Having been deeply impressed by *The Tao of Physics*,[8] we would still offer that a good rule of thumb is to investigate thoroughly before accepting any explanation of human behaviour that uses the word quantum.

Many alternative medicine forms have much more flexible definitions of energetic forces. There is good and bad energy, auras, we are beings of light, energy that can be transmitted by distant healing and there are psychic phenomena accessible to and interpreted by the gifted. All these models draw on some sense of an energetic connection that is often linked to a notion of spirit.

Chi or prana has a much longer history as a cultural norm in Asia. In the west there can be a tendency to be seduced by the exotic, energetic powers of eastern mystics, enlightened beings and yogis.

How to make sense of all this, particularly in a clinic situation? Field is a useful concept we can borrow from physics – it describes a zone of influence. There are packets of energy moving through the atmosphere that interact with other packets of energy. Matter appears solid because the field of energy generated by particular arrangements of particles affects the movement of other particles, even though we know that the atoms are more space than particles. Energy can be equated to information moving through a field, whether that is electrochemical information in fluids, tension in structures or potency in an energetic field. We live in a gravitational field. We are used to things falling to earth depending on their position in the gravitation field. We do not theorize mystical magnets or wavy lines of energy, we just accept the field exists. The idea of a field of electromagnetic energy is readily understandable to most of us as well. If we stand in the sun's rays we become hot; if we tune our radio to the correct frequency we will hear music; magnets will repel or attract depending on their arrangement in the field. A number of writers describe electromagnetic fields of living things and organs (for example, Mae Wan Ho 1999; Oschman 2000; Winfree 1987).

Clearly the authors think there is something interesting about the relational field. Without resorting to energy, we can understand that there are real-time changes in the physiology of both client and practitioner as they respond to each other's presence. By being in a room together they have entered into a relational field. However, in biodynamic cranial work we go further than that. This is one of the big conceptual and experiential hoops that it is very helpful to step through in biodynamics. You can do great work without believing in environmental forces; however, it is generally much easier to expand your awareness to include as wide a zone of influence as possible. Primary respiration is something in nature, as well as something experienced as a tidal form within the body. Franklyn Sills, whilst showing pictures from the Hubble telescope, is fond of saying that the forces that created the universe created us. Long tide is a movement in the natural world that we can learn to perceive, an energetic movement. It is maybe one of the four types described above, or maybe it is a particular set of information moving through the electromagnetic field. The four types of energy describe types of communication between particles, but not what is actually communicated. Maybe the long tide is a constant reminder to breathe.

Science and research

> There is nothing that living things do that cannot be understood from
> the point of view that they are made of atoms acting according to the
> laws of physics. (Feynman 1998, p.20)

The prevailing scientific view of spirit is that it does not exist. There is no God and no soul. Stephen Pinker gives a good overview of some of the defining events that are the basis of current scientific thought; Newton breached 'the wall between the terrestrial and the celestial'. Charles Lyell showed the earth was sculpted over 'immense spans of time'. William Harvey showed that the 'human body is a machine that runs by hydraulics and other principles'. In 1828 Frederick Wöhler 'showed that the stuff of life is not a magical, pulsating gel but ordinary compounds following the laws of chemistry'. Darwin gave us evolution and the pioneers of DNA showed how natural selection can emerge from replicating genes.[9]

Objective reasoning enshrined in science is only one way of knowing the world; art is another, subjective knowing is another – and they may all give different truths. Subjective, experiential knowing is the rigour of biodynamic craniosacral therapy. In the field of human relationships and health, things are not as knowable as some scientists would have us believe. Consciousness is still a great mystery despite the huge advances of neuroscience. Consciousness is explored more fully below. Here we will briefly look at some ideas about research, the cornerstone of the scientific approach, that are relevant to cranial work.

There is a very limited amount of research into cranial work. There are one or two interesting studies within osteopathy and from the Upledger Institute.[10] A culture of research does not really exist. The authors took part in an study organized by Sylvia Neira (Neira, Elliott and Isbell 2006). It was a lot of work for the organizer and in the end statistically inconclusive. As of 2010 the UK Craniosacral Therapy Association is beginning to obtain the resources to organize some research, including an MSc project. These are small but useful first steps. Cranial work relies on expert opinion, anecdotal evidence and the cumulative wisdom of our own practice.

There are many valid critiques of alternative medicine. *Bad Science* is a great book, one of the fairest, as Goldacre trains his guns at the pharmaceutical industry, the media as well as alternative medicine (Goldacre 2008).[11] Goldacre essentially argues for clear thinking and evidence. The lack of an evidence-based approach is a concern in craniosacral therapy. Goldacre describes the importance of all research and particularly meta-analysis as carried out by the Cochrane Review. Goldacre describes the general puzzlement about the widely researched placebo effect (otherwise named as the 'meaning effect').

Taleb (2007) argues for empirical scepticism over statistics.[12] The patterns of how we heal, particularly in low-level chronic illness, do not easily emerge from the research data so far. All the variables in events involving humans make them very difficult to predict and to research. Human relationships are not rational. In the real world, it is meaningless to say that people do not change in relationship to other people. Cranial work is essentially very simple; we come into a present-time relationship, we put our hands on, something changes, we take our hands off. Touching other people will cause a change in their physiology. Our direct experience, our empirical research that we trust, is that biodynamic craniosacral therapy supports long-lasting changes more quickly and more effectively than any other discipline we know. Viewed from pure science, we would celebrate that cranial work is particularly good at creating the 'meaning effect'.

The perceptual problems described in the next section mean there needs to be an ongoing rigor in trusting your own experience of human relationships, particularly where the therapist needs to become an expert in the act of perceiving other bodies. The act of touch and embodiment is elevated to an art form. Below is a quote from Yuasa that argues for experience over theory. For Yuasa mind–body unity is something to be achieved and a state to be acquired rather than something innate or essential.

> …in the east one starts from the experiential assumption that the mind–body modality changes through training of the mind and body by means of cultivation (shugyo) or training (keiko). Only after assuming this experiential ground does one ask what the mind–body relation is.

That is, the mind–body issue is not simply a theoretical speculation but it is originally a practical lived experience (taiken). (Yuasa 1987, p.18)

4.5 PERCEPTION AND CONSCIOUSNESS
Phenomena and perception

A raven soaring in the distance is not, for me, a mere visual image; as I follow it with my eyes, I inevitably feel the stretch and flex of its wings with my own muscles, and its sudden swoop toward the nearby trees is a visceral as well as visual experience for me. (Abram 1996, p.61)

My divergent senses meet up with each other in the surrounding world, converging and commingling in the things I perceive. We may think of the sensing body as a kind of open circuit that completes itself only in things, and in the world. The differentiation of my senses, as well as their spontaneous convergence in the world at large, ensures that I am a being destined for relationship: it is primarily through my engagement with what is *not* me that I effect the integration of my senses, and thereby experience my own unity and coherence. (Abram 1996, p.124)[13]

There are phenomena and there is perception of those phenomena. The accurateness of our perceptions of phenomena have been argued over for centuries. Perception is the interpretation of incoming sensory information; it is also goal oriented and dependent on our ability to act. We extract meaning from the world according to our history, habits and evolutionary imperatives. A sense of a consistent player in the continued act of perception emerges: our sense of self. How and where we locate the sense of self can be useful to play with. This section describes some shifts in the act of perception that seem to allow more choice and flexibility in our responses.

Many of us locate our sense of self, the perceiving I, behind the eyes and in the brain. The fantasy of cryogenically freezing our brains so we can return after the death of the body speaks to this sense of self in the brain. A mind that is separate from the body is an expression of this view, as is Descartes' statement: 'I think therefore I am.' A huge step in becoming a bodyworker is to appreciate that consciousness is not just about the brain but is also about the body. We can locate ourselves not just in the brain but actually in our whole bodies. The sensory information that is used as the basis of awareness for consciousness comes from all the cells in the body. To reframe Descartes: 'I have a body therefore I am.'

However, biodynamics takes us a step further. The information we use to create our sense of self is not just coming from the body but is also from the environment around us. Who we are is shaped by being in the physical world with certain rules and constraints. Individuality emerges from particular bodies and particular environments.[14] However, all humans have certain assumptions about our bodies and about the stability of the external world that are essential to a coherent sense of self. There needs to be some stability in the phenomena that we perceive; this stability is provided by the consistency of the physical world (there is weight, the sun comes up, I can move, there are other living things) and by the consistency of the body. One of the reasons dissociation is so fundamental is it strips us of our relationship to the body and the environment, we become fragmented and isolated. David Abram, quoted above, provides a wonderful introduction to the world of embodied perception. We are an open circuit and complete ourselves only by being in the world.

We can often get the act of perception wrong. The nervous system is a bag of tricks that privileges speed over accuracy. There is an evolutionary imperative to be quicker and smarter than our predators. In interpreting the events we perceive 'we favour the sensational and the extremely visible', we 'impose narrativity and causality' and we simplify (Taleb 2007, pp.89 and 70). Magicians can exploit our habits. Derren Brown describes one such habit that is quite scary for craniosacral therapists. He calls it 'ideomotor movement'; 'if you focus on the idea of making a movement, you will likely end up making a similar tiny movement without realizing it' (Brown 2006, p.45).[15] He describes how this is the basis of spiritualist phenomena such as ouija boards and table tipping that 'spread like wildfire in America and the UK in the late 1800s'. The challenge for craniosacral therapists is to learn our habits, practise, practise, practise and separate our projections from what is actually there.

Consciousness

> There is no separate 'mind stuff' and 'physical stuff' in the universe: the two are one and the same. (The formal term for this is neutral monism.) Perhaps mind and matter are like the two sides of a Möbius strip that appear different but are in fact the same. (Ramachandran 2004, p.32)

How do we go from a group of cells to something that has consciousness? The idea of consciousness just emerging from cells talking to cells is very challenging, so challenging that many people think it must be something extra, hence we get an immaterial and separate mind. Consciousness can be defined as knowing that we know. It is much more than responsiveness, emotions, intelligence and memory.[16] In this section two features of consciousness that are helpful to understand in clinical practice are explored: (1) How much and what types of information are important to being conscious? (2) Where does the information come from that provides the basis for consciousness? We have already named the body and the environment as primary sources of information in the section on perception. Here we will go into more detail on the importance of the flow of information through the body.

Taylor (2001) argues that at a critical level of information processing in the nervous system we became conscious. He likens the shift from non-conscious to conscious to the difference between stumbling around on solid ground with skates on, to skating on ice. The elegance, speed and creativity of the skater are a world away from the previous state. Animals have many of the building blocks in place for consciousness but not the required complexity to make the leap of self-awareness exhibited by humans.

Becoming upright (Diamond 2005)[17] and socialization (Attenborough 2002) are two candidates for the drivers for increasing complexity in the development of the human brain. Humans have a very particular posture. We managed to switch off our flexor muscles and use our extensor muscles to stand up and be human. Essentially this is a parasympathetic mode; optimum posture is about being soft, open and receptive at the front of the body. A huge portion of activity in the nervous system is about movement and staying upright. Movement feeds the brain and is essential to the overall level of activity in the brain. Primates' brains also became bigger as the social networks they maintained grew. So, in addition, we can say that social interaction stimulates the brain. Supporting the structures and nerve flow involved in movement and communication, and helping orientation to the surroundings from a receptive posture, helps the whole person be more aware and improves the flexibility of the brain in responses to the demands of its environment.

Consciousness is modular. Interaction between the modules creates the subjective feeling of awareness. The incoming sensory information is processed in discrete packages (for example, short- and long-term memory, movement, emotion and many more) and then assembled into a whole. Brain sciences are increasingly showing how the loss of functioning of certain modules and connecting pathways between the modules begins to strip away normal behaviour. We can identify our wife as a hat to quote a famous example.

Damasio makes a very convincing case for consciousness as something that emerges from the body. The modules involved in processing information on body states (proprioceptive information from the tissues and fluid chemical information) are key. The gap between an historical and learnt sense of the body and the ongoing orientation to the present moment is one of the defining relations in the emergence of consciousness. Our sense of self is constantly being remade. 'You are the music whilst the music lasts.' The body provides the stable reference point. 'Emotion, feeling, and consciousness depend for their execution on representations of the organism. Their shared essence is the body.' The phylogenetically old midline structures in the brainstem and limbic system involved in 'some aspect of body regulation or representation' are essential to a sense of self (Damasio 1999).[18] So clinically we can see that supporting the free flow of information through the body to the brainstem and limbic system is useful to our whole ability to be aware.

Perceiving the whole body

> My body is an object in the physical world. But unlike other objects I
> have a special relationship with my body. In particular my brain is part
> of my body… My first mistake is to think that there is such a clear-cut
> distinction between my body and the rest of the physical world. (Frith
> 2007, p.61)

Researchers have recently been able to produce a consistent illusion of being
outside of our bodies. Extending insights from research into phantom limbs they
were able to fool volunteers into believing they were in a phantom body. They fed
the brain two types of information to generate the illusion. First, visual information
from a camera attached to the head of a lifelike dummy was relayed to screens
in goggles over the participant's eyes. The only incoming visual information to
the participant's brain was equivalent to the first-person view of the dummy.
Second, they provided rhythmic, tactile stimulation coherent with the view from
the camera. They directed the camera to look at the dummy's abdomen and they
stroked the abdomen of the dummy and the abdomen of the participant at the
same time. The first-person view of the dummy's abdomen being stroked plus the
synchronous feeling of their own abdomen being stroked were enough to give the
illusion of the participant being located in the dummy's body.

If that was not enough they were able to extend the illusion to being inside
another person's body. The camera was placed on the head of the other person.
The participant shook hands with the other person. The camera on the other
person was directed to look at the shaking hand contact and the other person gave
a rhythmic squeeze to the participant's hand. Incredibly, the participant, seeing
only what the other person could see and feeling rhythmic contact coherent with
the visual input, experienced themselves as inhabiting the body opposite them.
The brain created a 'body swap illusion' of inhabiting the whole body behind
the hand they were shaking, even though they could actually see their own hand
being shaken.[19]

This is a very rich experiment. There are at least three parts that can be drawn
out that are relevant to cranial work. First, the experiment strongly confirms that we
create and continually recreate a sense of self from incoming sensory information.
Second, we need to constantly assess the sensory information. Third, there is a
module in the nervous system for perceiving whole bodies. The participant did
not only locate themselves in the arm of the person they were shaking hands with
but they recreated a whole body to occupy.

This latter perceptual habit is very useful for craniosacral therapists. We
inherently orient to whole bodies. Fragments do not make sense. When we put
our hands on someone else's body and have the skills to stay in a state of balanced
awareness, we can begin to pick up sensory information from the whole body in
front of us. By using our knowledge of what a whole body feels like, from our

self-exploration, from other bodies we have palpated, and from our innate ability to orient to whole bodies, we can begin to interpret what is happening in the space in front of us, occupied by another person. We have direct access to the shapes and patterns held in the space in front of us, it becomes part of our perceptual circuit. In the same way that we have learnt to know that a chair is in the centre of a room when we enter the room, when we put our hands on someone we can know the pulls and twists, the ebbs and flows and tones of the inside of their body space.

Some of the circuits that may be involved in this ability to perceive, experience and mimic what is happening to bodies in our perceptual field are the mirror neuron circuits (the 'ideomotor circuits' described by Brown may be similar). When we watch a beautiful dancer, or a raven soaring in the Abram quote above, we reproduce the sensations in our own brain and our own body. This reinforces the essential nature of self-awareness; our bodies are constantly modelling what is around us. By developing the skill of being in our own body we can track our responses and begin to know what is happening around us more clearly.

Summary of Chapter 4

The chapter discussed the fundamental importance of stillness as the underlying health within all of us and how this is in fact a dynamic force that is the foundation for all changes in the body. There is a deep unfolding from this state through the form of the long tide. This conveys the animating force of the breath of life that nourishes and connects all living cells to a relational matrix. The relationship of tissues and fluids to potency is explored in some depth. Wider implications of spirit, consciousness and perception were explored in relation to biodynamic practice.

Notes

1. In particular, Chapter 2, 'Using the Stillness', of Becker (2000) is a wonderful piece of writing. Sills (2004, p.8) also lays out the territory exceptionally well.
2. Health is not just about how wealthy you are, though that helps, but the fairness of the society you live in. According to Wilkinson and Pickett (2009), in more unequal societies everybody is worse off.
    They also describe three transitions in improving the health of populations: (1) removing infections via clean water, sewage systems, food hygiene and rubbish collection; (2) accounting for lifestyle factors such as fat, exercise, smoking and alcohol; and (3) understanding the consequences of stress including low social status and poor social integration.
3. According to the World Health Organization, faith-based organizations provide as much as 70 per cent of healthcare in sub-Saharan Africa. This is amazing. (However, there can be huge ideological strings attached. For example, much of the faith-based funding of projects around HIV prevention is focused on sexual abstinence. This does not always meet the needs of groups strongly affected by the epidemic such as gay men, drug users and sex workers whose lifestyles conflict with religious doctrine. For the 70 per cent figure and a critique of abstinence-based programmes see Stearns 2008.)

4. See Herrigel (1953), Soho (1987) and Suzuki (1970) on Zen or Roth (2004) and the Addiss translation of the *Tao Te Ching* by Lao Tzu (1993) on the Tao. Jim Jealous describes *Zen Mind, Beginner's Mind* (Suzuki 1970) as the best book on biodynamic cranial work. *Zen in the Art of Archery* (Herrigel 1953) has a memorable passage on the perils of technique where the author goes outside his teacher's recommendation of letting the arrow shoot itself.

5. See Emerson (2009), Workshop on 'Healing the Wounds of Soul and Spirit': 'The deepest roots of spirit and soul wounding occur in the preconception and prenatal periods. Emerson Egressions© (spirit-based regressions), Spirit Experiencing©, and Soul Experiencing© will be used to resolve spirit and soul wounding, allowing spirit and soul to be expressed in daily life.'

    Also see Terry (2009), 'Embodiment Courses': 'The emphasis is on facilitating a direct connection to the soul, and the understanding and re-integration of the purpose of the soul in this life.'

6. Chapter 11, 'On the Value of Dissociation' of Shea (2008) discusses attunement and flexible attention. The chapter also has a good debate on society and dissociation. Shea (2007) has a good discussion on the soul in the glossary.

7. From an amazing talk on TED.com. For her, the right hemisphere is about connecting to the universal energy and the left hemisphere is about self and individual history.

8. *The Tao of Physics* by Fritjof Capra (1992) is classic book exploring links between physics and Taoism.

9. All quotes in this paragraph are from Pinker (2002, p.30).

10. The website www.craniosacral.co.uk has a research webpage listing the interesting research relevant to cranial work.

    There is no doubt that cranial bones move and that the cerebrospinal fluid flows around the CNS. Chaitow (1999) has a good review of the basic science. The debate is how significant the movements are for health and how the fluids and bones move. In cranial work our experience is that the movements are fundamental.

11. Many books have emerged over the last few years as a necessary counterpoint to some of the wilder claims made by some practitioners and approaches in alternative medicine. The blanket term is not useful as there are many approaches. Singh and Ernst (2008) are more virulent in their attacks.

12. Taleb describes the nerdy statistician Dr John who argues that if you are tossing a coin and it comes up tails 99 times in a row then the chance of the next toss coming up tails is still 50 per cent. He opposes Dr John to the real-world operator Fat Tony. Fat Tony knows that the coin is more likely to be fixed. Taleb argues that the Dr Johns have taken over the world and do not understand the real nature of risk as applied to human behaviour.

13. *The Spell of the Sensuous* is an amazing book on perception drawing on the phenomenology of Merleau Ponty.

14. Growing up in a green, flat, mild-weathered place in Warwickshire in England generates a very different set of expectations from an Eskimo in the snow or a nomad in a desert, for example. We are embedded in our history and that includes the physical landscape. To some extent I am Warwickshire, it defined my horizons and my expectation of what is around me. Being in an eclipse in Egypt and feeling an earth tremor in Turkey were deeply unsettling events. The sun really should not disappear like that and the earth really needs to be still.

15. *Tricks of the Mind* is a surprisingly wise and interesting book.

16. This view of consciousness makes it a uniquely human event. It excludes animals, the earth and the universe from being conscious in the way that humans are.

17. On p.260 Diamond describes becoming upright as a significant jump in human evolution, accelerating development: 'The first [jump], occurring between 100,000 and 50,000 years ago, probably was made possible by genetic changes in our bodies: namely by evolution of the modern anatomy permitting modern speech or modern brain function or both.'

18. *The Feeling of What Happens* is fabulous on understanding the importance of the body, emotions and feelings to how humans function.

19. They confirmed the illusion by holding a knife over the other person's arm within the visual field of the camera and then holding a knife over the participant's hand during the test. They measured the stress response in the participant's body and the participant reacted more strongly when the body opposite them was threatened – confirming the sense of inhabiting another body. See Petkova and Ehrsson (2008).

5

Whole Body Dynamics

5.1 RECIPROCAL TENSION MEMBRANE

If, as someone interested in bodywork, you are not excited by connective tissues then you are probably in the wrong profession. The science emerging from researchers into connective tissues is fascinating. It provides many clues as to how information moves between cells, how the body holds and maintains stories and how change can be facilitated that affects the whole system. This chapter will review some of the highlights of recent developments in the understanding of fascia and their application to cranial work. Amazingly, Sutherland intuited the importance of connective tissues very early in his thinking. The reciprocal tension membrane model he developed, linking the dural membranes to the bones, can be applied to all the relationships between soft tissues and bones. It is an early way of describing biotensegrity.

The core link

'The function of the reciprocal tension membrane' is a key feature of Sutherland's model for the craniosacral system. The connections provided by the dural tube, the tent and the falx, collectively called the reciprocal tension membrane or RTM,[1] provide a fundamental bridge between the bones of the skull, the spine and the pelvis. Sutherland also described the RTM as 'the core link' between the cranial bowl and the pelvic bowl (Sutherland 1998, p.224).

Nature has evolved a powerful infrastructure for the central nervous system that gives support and protection along with a controlled environment. The brain and spinal cord are wrapped by three layers of membrane: an innermost layer (the pia mater) which holds to the surface of the CNS; a second layer (the arachnoid) which contains the cerebrospinal fluid; and an outermost layer (the dura mater) which is a thick fibrous layer. In the cranium the dura are a double-layered system that projects into the central fissure between the hemispheres and horizontally divides the upper and lower parts of the brain. This is the falx and tent, and together they act like a membranous skeleton that holds the brain in situ.

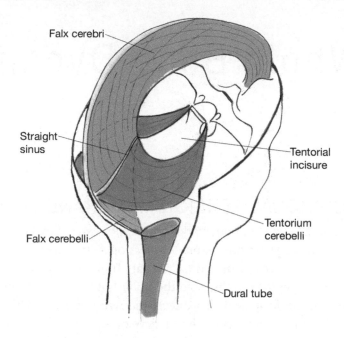

Figure 5.1.1 The reciprocal tension membranes in the skull

In the text the tentorium cerebelli is referred to as the tent and the falx cerebri and falx cerebelli collectively as the falx

The dura mater of the cranial and spinal cavities are a continuous structure made from one sheet of collagen fibre. This offers an intelligent system creating postural balance for the axis of the body and beyond. In health there is a reciprocal tension throughout the whole. For the craniosacral therapist this quality of the dura as a single sheet is very useful therapeutically. It enables you to be in relationship with the whole of the structure from any one point. Hence, from a contact at the temporals, for instance, you can be listening to the movement of the dura in the sacrum, and vice versa. Any reorganization in the dura as a result of a state of balance will affect the whole unit of function of the cranial and spinal dural enfoldment. Its holistic nature means that any trauma to part of the system will inevitably have an effect on the whole. For instance, a fall on the coccyx, if strong enough, can affect the whole of the dura and result in headaches as well as a sore coccyx. Over time this can result in a lowering of the potency at the core of the body.

Bone and membrane

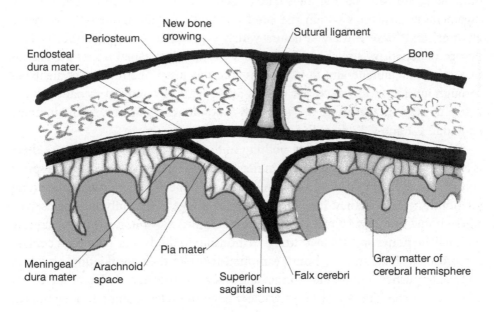

Figure 5.1.2 Schematic diagram of the superior sagittal suture

Note the bones growing within membrane, the firm attachment of the endosteal layer of dura at the bone margins and the double layer of meningeal dura that folds inwards to form the falx. The falx extends down between the two hemispheres (after Scarr 2008)

The outer layer of cranial dura is attached to the cranial bones, most firmly around the bone margins, the cranial base and the foramen magnum. Graham Scarr has written an excellent article on the cranial vault as a tensegrity structure:

> The tensegrity model is a novel approach for understanding how the cranial vault could retain its stability without relying on an expansive force from an underlying brain, a position currently unresolved. Tensional forces in the dura mater have the effect of pushing the bones apart, whilst at the same time integrating them into a single functional unit. Sutural potency depends on the separation of cranial bones throughout normal development, and the model describes how tension in the dura mater achieves this, and influences sutural phenotype. Cells of the dura mater respond to brain expansion and influence bone growth, allowing the cranium to match the spatial requirements of the developing brain, whilst remaining one step ahead and retaining a certain amount of autonomy. (Scarr 2008 and 2009)[2]

The sutures in health remain 'patent' or unfused. The external periosteum and dura mater are connected at the suture (Figure 5.1.2). According to Chaitow the 'ligamentous structures within the cranial sutures' contain 'numerous free nerve endings' and 'have a wavy structure which suggests that they are subject to a degree of repetitive stretching' (Chaitow 1999, p.19). Cranial bones are islands in a sea of membrane and fluid. This is true not just in early development but throughout life. In the spine, the dura is like a sleeve around the spinal cord and is free to move in the vertebral canal with major attachments only at the foramen magnum, C2 and C3 and at the sacrum.

Bones are never alone. In fact nothing in the body is ever alone because there is always connective tissue close by. In the case of the neurocranium and the spinal column it's the dura mater membrane. The vault bones have a particularly strong relationship to it as they have grown out of a layer of membrane themselves. These bones are literally part of the dura mater and move in a strong synchrony with it. The bones are also in a strong relationship to fluids. The meninges contain cerebrospinal fluid and the bones can often feel like they are floating on water, and being pushed around like flotsam and jetsam. A true experience of the bones of the neurocranium would be to acknowledge the relationships to membranes, fluids and nervous tissue.

As a practitioner it's important that these bony, membrane, fluid qualities become familiar. In addition the bones themselves are highly fluid and have internal space. There is a constant flow of blood. Their movements are fluid-like even though they are discrete structures that have motion around specific geometries. The dura mater has a more elastic quality and its nature is less discrete; it is a sheet-like structure that traverses the whole central nervous system and whole axial skeleton. You will naturally feel more holistic patterns in the dura mater whereas if you just orient to bones you may only feel their individual extent and local area.

5.2 ARRANGEMENTS OF FASCIA IN THE BODY
The transversal

Restrictions in the horizontal tissue fields have a particularly dramatic effect on the body. The most important horizontal tissue field is the respiratory diaphragm. The diaphragm's size and function makes it a powerful force in the body. Any reduction in its ability to move will not only affect the exchange of air, and therefore cell metabolism, but also movement of abdominal venous blood, liver function, digestive process and movement of the spinal column. The diaphragm is the natural fulcrum for the myofascial network of the body. Any restrictions in the diaphragm will be translated into the myofascial network and vice versa.

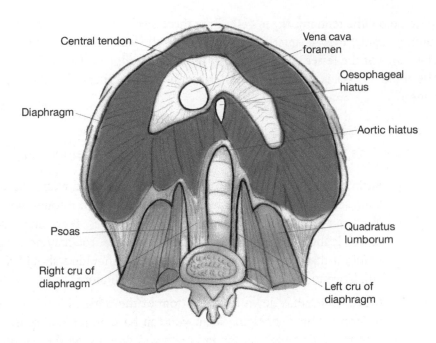

Central tendon

Vena cava foramen

Oesophageal hiatus

Diaphragm

Aortic hiatus

Psoas

Quadratus lumborum

Right cru of diaphragm

Left cru of diaphragm

Figure 5.2.1 Respiratory diaphragm: inferior view

The body operates as a reciprocal unit of function. This means that the whole is affected by the particular. Every structure is in relationship with the whole; therefore the whole will be affected by the parts and the parts by the whole. In health there is a reciprocal tension that is akin to a balanced tone. Tone describes the quality of tissue and reciprocal tension the movement of tissue. The holism of the body is a thing of beauty when there is health, but there is a tipping point when the holistic nature of the body apparently breaks down and restriction spreads throughout the system causing the body to fragment and lose its reciprocal nature. That's when fatigue and ill health start to express themselves.

The tent

The tentorium cerebelli (tent) is a relatively horizontal extension of dura mater in the skull. It resonates powerfully with all the horizontal diaphragms discussed below. The tent attaches to the squama of the occiput, the parietals at the region of the asterion (this is often forgotten), the petrous ridge of the temporal bones and into the clinoid processes of the sphenoid body. It joins the falx at the straight sinus, forming a tent-like structure. The tent separates the cerebellum below from the cerebrum above. The tentorial incisure is the space created by the anterior free borders of the tent; the brainstem passes through this space.

Looking down onto the bones of the cranial base, the curve of the petrous ridges is a very obvious feature. The posterior cranial fossa is the name for the space below the tent; it is the lowest of the three levels, or fossae, of the skull. The anterior cranial fossa is anterior and superior to the lesser wings of the sphenoid. The edges of the lesser wings are a very clear sharp ridge in the base of the skull. The middle fossa is between the lesser wings of the sphenoid and the petrous ridges.

Awareness Exercise: Reciprocal tension in the respiratory diaphragm

- Sitting still comfortably, allow yourself to settle and relax. Place your hands on the front of your chest. Follow your breath through your nose into your chest. Notice how your rib cage moves. How much does it move? It should rise and widen on the in breath. You may notice places within it that may be resistant to movement. Shoulders should rise and fall. Try and feel your ribs moving. Do they all move?

- Move your hands down to the bottom of the sternum – to the level of the top of the diaphragm. See if you can have an internal sense of the diaphragm flattening on the in breath and doming on the out breath – its natural movement. How much movement does it make? It's so big you can't miss it.

- Continue breathing and notice if the diaphragm softens and if that changes your breathing, your spine, your sense of your body or your mind. Encourage your diaphragm to soften by consciously letting go of it and relaxing as you breathe. Just bringing your hands to this part of the body is often enough to relax the muscles and connective tissues of the diaphragm along with the organs on either side of it.

- As you start to get more attuned to the movements of the diaphragm and your breathing, notice how much pressure on the in breath there is in your abdomen. When you are breathing well you can feel it in your pelvic floor! It feels as if the abdomen is inflating.

- Bring your other hand to the back of the diaphragm (behind the navel) and notice how much your lower spine moves in response to your breathing. Keep listening with your hands and you will notice the curves of the spine shift and change in response to your in and out breaths. If your breathing is healthy your whole spine joins in and all the curves deepen on the in breath. Move your hand from the lower back area and place it on the back of your neck. Notice how your neck responds to the movements of your diaphragm. There are muscles in your neck that assist with raising your rib cage on the in breath and you might feel muscles tensing under your hand. The curvature of the spine here also deepens on the in breath.

Respiratory diaphragm

The respiratory diaphragm is truly global in its effects and is often a place in the body that is critically involved in most health conditions. Learning how to relate to the diaphragm as a practitioner is vital. The diaphragm is so large that you can easily feel it from anywhere in the body. See the experiential and relational exercises below. The diaphragm is often a place of emotional expression. Strong trauma effects can be held in the diaphragm and the breathing mechanism. The shock response always involves the breath; commonly you start panting or holding your breath when you are in a state of fear. The celiac ganglion lies very close to the crura of the diaphragm and is often very active in the stress response. When the body fails to fully recover from shock there will still be shallow breathing or holding of the breath. You will notice this as a tension in the diaphragm that so often goes along with a hyper-arousal in the solar plexus area. Over time this will translate to a multitude of symptoms, commonly including digestive dysfunction.

When the diaphragm is healthy it moves like a bellows. It flattens on inhalation and domes on exhalation. In its craniosacral motion it widens on inhalation and narrows on exhalation. It also resonates with other horizontal structures in the body, in particular with the pelvic diaphragm and the tentorium.

The anatomy of the diaphragm is fascinating. In Figure 5.2.1 you can see how complete a division the diaphragm creates. It divides the thoracic and abdominal cavities. The outer parts of the diaphragm are muscle and the central white area is tendon. There are three leaves of the central tendon onto which sit the heart and both lungs. The central tendon is unique in that it acts as the attachment for the movement of diaphragmatic muscles. You can see there are a number of holes for important tubes to pass through: the oesophagus, the aorta, the vena cava and the thoracic duct. The diaphragm inserts into the ribs and the spine. You can see the crura of the diaphragm attaching to the anterior longitudinal ligament in the lumbar curve. You can also see the proximity of the psoas and the lumborum muscle groups.

Treatment Exercise: Relating to the respiratory diaphragm
as the natural fulcrum for the connective tissue field

1. Make contact at the diaphragm.

   • This exercise is for working in pairs. Set up the space you are in so that you are either both sat down on chairs next to each other or one of you is on a treatment couch.

   • Spend a while getting comfortable. Allow yourself to settle and relax.

   • Notice your breathing. Notice body sensation.

- Gently bring both hands into contact with your partner's diaphragm, one hand at the front and one hand at the back of the body. Try to position your hand at the front around the zyphoid sternum and the one at the back between T11 and L2. This should give you a sense of the diaphragm between your hands. Allow their system to get used to the contact.

2. Orient to the tissue field from the diaphragm.

- See if you can notice the tissue continuity of the diaphragm between your hands. It's a large transverse structure in motion. Be interested in the connection between the diaphragm and the fascial network through the body.

- The diaphragm is a muscle and has its own fascial covering which is in contact with the fascia of the whole body. Invite this relationship into your perceptual field. When this expresses itself it can feel like you are in touch with webs of connective tissue spreading out in all directions, or connecting into the diaphragm from all parts of the body.

3. Take your time to orient to the diaphragm as the natural fulcrum for connective tissues.

- It may be that you are unable to obtain such a global sense of the whole connective tissue matrix. Perhaps you are able to sense this connection in one direction or slightly beyond the diaphragm. The exercise is new and relating to this tissue layer might be unfamiliar to you. It may be however that your partner's system is not able to offer this relationship. Why might that be?

- All the fasciae of the body orient to the diaphragm as the natural fulcrum around which their health and motion is organized. This makes it a powerful place to work from. Any change here has a global reach. Any pattern of experience here also has a global reach.

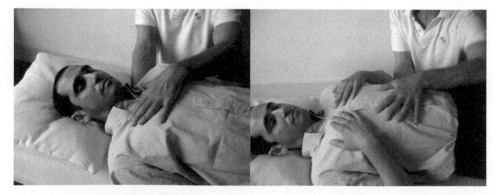

Figure 5.2.2 Contacting the thoracic inlet and the respiratory diaphragm

Pelvic diaphragm

The pelvic diaphragm is like a mirror image of the respiratory diaphragm. Essentially it is structured like a hammock with a set of muscles moving front/back (the levator ani) and a set moving across (the coccygeus). This is a very personal area of the body because of its connection with the sexual organs and functions of elimination and defecation. The body can hold patterns of experience here going back to early childhood and to early experiences as a baby. Many people who come to see you will have experienced some form of sexual abuse. Sadly this is not uncommon and can present as a frozen state in the pelvis; this can be felt as a profound lack of motion, tissue density, fluid turgidity and often a sense of a held charge. The whole system too will be showing signs of trauma around breathing, digestion, sleeping, energy levels, posture, nervous system effects and emotional imbalance. So there are lots of signs that will present to you, and of course there is the client's own story to alert you to this.

We can hold lots of tension in the pelvic floor muscles. There are many possible reasons, but often the tension is associated with fear and protection. We all do this from time to time when we react to threatening situations; however, sometimes when the event has been overwhelming the pelvic floor tension doesn't return to normal and it remains as a constant pattern. The body adjusts to it the best it can so that it becomes normal. Compensations will take place throughout the body to mitigate the effects. One of the commonest effects is the tightening of the respiratory diaphragm, as if it's coming out in sympathy. When the diaphragm tightens up then the whole system will be affected through the deep fascia and through reduced breathing.

In treatments it might well become necessary to treat the pelvic floor directly. Sometimes tissues need direct attention to enable them to reorganize. As you become more skilled at relating to tissues it may be that you can orient your contact to the pelvic floor by simply touching the sacrum. Perhaps though it might need you to contact the sacrum and the pubic bone. With this double contact it's as if the pelvic floor is between your hands. Now the muscles can begin to orient to the breath of life more powerfully.

Verbal negotiation is absolutely essential for making contact with the pelvic floor in this way. Make sure you discuss this with your client first before making contact. Let your client know the reasons you are making this contact. Explore if they are comfortable with the idea; don't be too cursory about it but also try to avoid making it a huge issue. Let your client know that you will stay in communication with them during the contact and they can at any time ask you to disengage. Get them to locate the pubic bone for you, using their fingers, so you can make contact precisely. Explain to them too that the contact may bring up difficult feelings and this is the body's way of processing and you will help them move through this in a paced and resourced way. It can be very difficult to know a client's reaction the first time you make this contact. However, the approach you need to take will become quickly apparent. Other reasons why you might contact the pelvic floor are due to issues of childbirth or surgery.

Thoracic inlet

The thoracic inlet is another key place in the health of the body. There is a lot of traffic here. Blood in particular is moving around in a small space up and down from the head and in and out from the arms. Anatomically there are many blood vessels packed into a small space. There are also many nerves moving down from the neck into the upper thorax and the brachial plexus. There is a complex array of muscles in the neck and shoulders with strong attachments into the clavicle, sternum, jaw, occiput and acromion. Many people react to stress by becoming tense in this area. Often there are structural imbalances between the head and chest that produce tension patterns and compensations. Hypertension can create pressure here from both shallow breathing and high blood pressure. In practice you will notice how often this area presents itself as a priority for treatment. This may involve exploring relationships between the jaw, the cranial base, the spine and the upper chest. For the moment let's concentrate on the area around the upper chest and shoulders and the segment from approximately T3 to C5.

When making contact with this area it is important that you negotiate the holds clearly and make sure your client knows what you are going to do and that they are comfortable with it. This area is a delicate place in us and we can feel vulnerable from contact into the upper chest and anywhere near the throat. This is a strongly emotional area and can often lead to strong emotional expressions as tissues reorganize. If you think this might be the case, be clear about this with your client. Let them know that when you put your hands there the body may have a strong response and work at an appropriate pace and in relationship to resources.

Other transverse diaphragms

It is possible to relate to the foramen magnum, the roof of the mouth and the planes of the major joints as transverse diaphragms. The dome of the roof of the mouth is discussed in more detail under the facial complex in Chapter 10. Any transverse arrangement of connective tissue is a useful staging place to relate to when treating.

Awareness Exercise: Feeling your deep fascia

- This exercise is a self-exploration, using experiential anatomy guidance.

- Sitting calmly, place your hands on your thighs.

- Come into an awareness of sensations from the palms of your hands. Have an intention of feeling the tissue layers under your hands. First there is the skin. Can you feel the unique quality of the integumentary system? Do you get a sense of continuity?

- Underneath the skin is a superficial layer of fascia. This is a different kind of tissue structure. Can you sense how different it is?

- Underneath this are muscles with their individual fascial wrappings. This is deep fascia and has much more collagen fibres packed into it to give it strength. It's denser than the superficial layer.

- Notice how much glide there is between the individual fascial wrappings of the quadricep muscles. Can you feel the tissue continuity of the fascia, surrounding of the muscles to the tendon and its attachment into the bones?

- If you widen your perceptual field to include the whole of the body's deep fascia, what happens? Do you get a sense of connectivity through the fascial framework to other areas of the body?

The longitudinal

Most of the body is organized longitudinally. The spine spends around 16 hours a day in a vertical position. When we stand upright many structures of the body orient to the long bones of the legs and the spinal column. Think of the flowing lines of muscles, and their associated fascial coverings, running along the spine and extending the length of the limbs. Craniosacral biodynamic expressions have a strong vertical component. When there is health, the spine is mobile and the connective tissues glide longitudinally with ease. When there are restrictions in the tissue field there will be a reduction into the amount of easy movement. Some specific longitudinal connective tissues are explored below. Sutherland used the term 'fascial drag' to name the quality that can be felt when orienting to fascia (Sutherland 1998, p.278).

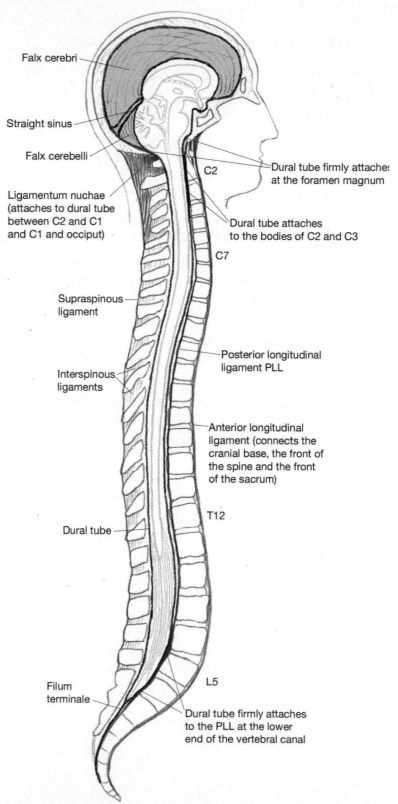

Figure 5.2.3 Sagittal section of the neural cavity showing spinal ligaments, the dural tube and its attachments and the falx

The falx

The falx cerebri and its little brother the falx cerebelli, underneath the tent, are frequently just referred to as the falx. The falx is a vertical extension of the dura lining the skull. It attaches to the occiput, the parietals (underneath the sagittal suture), the frontal bone and the crista galli of the ethmoid. It connects to the tent at the straight sinus. In the vault, the falx divides the two cerebral hemispheres and, inferior to the tent, divides the cerebellum into two.

The dural tube

The dural tube is an extension of the dural membranes of the skull. It surrounds the spinal cord as it passes through the vertebral canal. The dural tube narrows and closes around the filum terminale at around the second sacral segment. The filum terminale extends from the end of the spinal cord and attaches to the periosteum on the back of the coccyx, anchoring the spinal cord inferiorly. One of the dural tube's most interesting anatomical features is that it is only attached to bone at the top and bottom of the canal: at the foramen magnum, the posterior surfaces of the second and third cervical vertebra and at the lower end of the vertebral canal to the posterior longitudinal ligament. Relatively new dissections of the cervicocranial region have revealed that one of the suboccipital muscles (rectus capitus posterior minor) and the ligament nuchae also attach to the posterior surface of the dural tube between the occiput and the axis (Dean and Mitchell 2002; Standring 2005). The sleeves of dura that extend out along the spinal nerves and the fat in the epidural space around the dural tube provide some restrictions, but essentially the dural tube floats in the vertebral canal. The free movement of this longitudinal arrangement of fascia is a key awareness in cranial work. It can often feel irritated, sticky and restricted compared to a quality of fluidity and glide in health.

The spinal ligaments

One way of thinking about the spine is as a set of stacked cotton reels held together by ribbons running the length of the stack. The ribbons in reality are the spinal ligaments; they are described below working from front to back. Another useful image is of the plastic, segmented play snakes you can get in toy shops. The ligaments provide some continuity but allow lots of movement. The anterior longitudinal ligament is probably the easiest to feel in practice; however, all the spinal ligaments can help in making relationships to the vertebrae and can help orient to a connection between the occiput, spine and the sacrum.

- Anterior longitudinal ligament: connects the basiocciput to the anterior vertebral bodies and discs all the way down to the front of the upper sacrum.

- Posterior longitudinal ligament: lies posterior to the vertebral bodies. It connects more strongly to the discs rather than the vertebral bodies. It extends from C2 (at C2 it is continuous with the ligaments binding C1, C2 and the occiput) down to the sacrum.

- Ligamentum flava, interspinous and supraspinous ligaments, transverse ligaments: these are ligaments that connect between the lamina, spinous and transverse processes and facet joint capsules of the individual vertebrae.

- Ligamentum nuchae: extends from the inion on the occiput along the spinous of the cervical vertebrae. It attaches into the dural tube, as described above, and helps maintain an upright neck.

The sock of ligaments around the sacrum

The sacrum is held in place between the ilia by a sock-like arrangement of ligaments. Muscles attach to the sacrum (going to the head of the femur and up the spine) but there are no muscles directly connecting between the sacrum and the ilia. The ligaments of the spine blend into the ligaments of the sacrum. The sacrotuberous ligament between the inferior part of the sacrum and the ischial tuberosity is an important stabilizing ligament. This can be palpated as a solid band deep to the buttock muscles. The sacrospinous ligament attaches the sacrum to the ischial spine. The ischial spine is one of the lumps in the pelvic outlet that the baby's head has to negotiate during birth. There are strong ligaments bonding the sacroiliac joint.

Muscle sheaths

Muscle cells, muscle fascicles and muscles are all sheathed in layers of fascia. These blend together to form tendons attaching to bones or sheets of aponeurosis as found over the head, abdomen, lower back and between some long bones. These sheaths, tendons and sheets often have a clear longitudinal arrangement.

Treatment Exercise: Fascial drag and glide from the feet

1. Make contact at the feet.
   - You can either stand with a wide stable posture and place your hands on the dorsum of the feet or sit and place your hands over or under the feet. It is important to be comfortable so be careful standing with a stooped posture for a long time.
   - Take time to set up the relational field, establish resources, wait for the holistic shift and orient to mid tide.
2. Orient to tissues.

- Allow the twists and pulls of connective tissues in the whole body to be part of your awareness.

- Explore the longitudinal lines of fascia. Is there a sense of continuity all the way up to the cranial base? How does the left side feel compared to the right and the front compared to the back?

- Give yourself permission to feel the fascial drag from inertial structures remote to your contact. In health there should be a sense of glide in the fascia.

3. Acknowledge the transverse diaphragms.

- The pelvic diaphragm, the respiratory diaphragm, the thoracic inlet and the cranial base are important transverse relay stations in the fascia matrix. Notice if there are different qualities above and below the transverse diaphragms.

4. Be precise.

- The continuity of the fascia can allow you to have very precise perceptions of the patterns of experience. Specific bones, joints, muscles, ligaments and organs can all present their story in exquisite detail.

5. Move to the shoulders.

- Explore the fascial drag or glide from the other end of the body with a light contact on the shoulders.

6. Negotiate ending.

Spirals and diagonals

A simple but powerful differentiation between transverse and longitudinal fascia is made above. It is important to remember that fascia is everywhere and connects everything. There are spirals of fascia and diagonal relationships. Myers (2001) describes a pair of 'spiral lines'. Each spiral line loops around the body in a helix, from the back of one side of the skull to the opposite shoulders, round the front of the body across the abdomen, curling across and down the same side on the hip and leg as the original skull attachment and then returning up the back of the leg and the spine, back to the skull. (You need to see the picture in his book.) A clear impression of the diagonal lines of myofascia comes from watching female hurdlers or heptathletes in the Olympics. They often have bare midriffs with incredible tone; the diagonal lines of force are impossible to miss as they move their bodies over the hurdles or when throwing. The myofascia of the heart is arranged in spirals.

There is a spiral inherent in the transformation from the early gut tube to the mature organs. Held (2009) relates this 'visceral asymmetry' back to molecular chirality. Chirality describes how molecules are the same but are mirror images; think of a pair of gloves. Our DNA is a right-handed helix; proteins such as collagen typically fold into right-handed helices. The cilia (moving, beating 'oars' of cells) all turn clockwise. In an early embryo the beating of the cilia waft certain signalling molecules from right to left. Held argues that this is a causative factor in creating the twists and asymmetries in the gut tube.

Membranes, cavities and bags

Another way of appreciating connective tissue is to understand its role in creating compartments in the body. The physical barriers prevent infection and inflammation spreading around the body. We are very keen on orienting to the cavities in clinical practice; exploring how the spaces of the body are filled often leads us to interesting places. Section 8.1 outlines the cavities in detail.

Myers (2001) points out how structures are enfolded in bags of fascia. In the embryo the organs bud and invaginate, surrounding themselves in mesoderm. The heart is contained in the pericardium, the lungs in the double-layered pleura and the abdominal organs in the peritoneum. Some of these layers blend or adhere together as they grow. The CNS is contained in the bag of the meninges. The identity of a bag is a useful perception in the work. We are compartmentalized, hairy, salty bags of fluid.

5.3 THE FASCIAL MATRIX

Fascia anatomy

Connective tissue is a collective term that includes bone, cartilage, fat and blood and lymph as well as fascia. The essential elements of all connective tissues are specialized cells (fibroblasts and immune cells), protein fibres (collagen, reticular and elastic) and the fluidic ground substance (sticky, gel-like and made from proteoglycans and glycoproteins). The mix of solid fibres versus gel-like fluids determines the properties of connective tissues, the 'sol-gel continuum'. Fascia can be divided into two broad categories: loose connective tissues or dense connective tissues. Loose connective tissues help form epithelial layers and adipose tissues. The anatomical classification of fascia is 'the connective tissue fibres, primarily collagenous, that form sheets or bands beneath the skin to attach, stabilize, enclose and separate muscles and other internal organs[9] (Martini 1998) Fascia can also be divided into superficial and deep. Superficial fascia lies immediately beneath the skin. It is the hypodermis and is composed of loose connective tissue. It enables the dermis of the skin to be freely mobile over its surface. Deep fascia is dense connective tissue, such as tendons, myofascia, aponeuroses and the periosteum of bones. It surrounds and protects muscles and organs.

These components are interwoven so that the myofascia around a muscle blends into the tendon which intermingles into the periosteum creating a strong fibrous network for the body. This means that the whole of the deep fascia creates a relationship throughout the body, one set of deep fascia ultimately being in touch with others, so that in a healthy individual a deep reciprocal tension fascial system exists. This is a whole body matrix that can be felt by the sensitive hands of a craniosacral therapist and used for the assessment of health and to bring about a new order.

When fascia is healthy there is a natural hydration to the structure through the ground substance. On the surface there is a moistness that allows different surfaces of fascia to move easily against each other. Muscles and viscera of the abdomen also need this property otherwise there are adhesions and restriction between structures. As a craniosacral therapist you are looking for this property of glide. When it is present it is as if the fascial matrix is bathed in a fluid film, the fascia feels mobile and expresses primary respiration as a whole. When this is not present you will feel it as a point or area that does not express motion or fluid exchange. If it is extensive enough, and if it has been in this state long-term, you will notice that this can have a dragging effect on the whole system.

If you can imagine the whole body as a series of encapsulated spaces with all the individual structures having a covering or skin, this would be an accurate picture of the body. Membrane and fascia invest organs, nerves, blood vessels, bones, muscles and joints. Each part is separate but, because of the interconnected nature of fascia, part of a whole lattice work of coverings. If you can imagine taking out all the contents of these individually wrapped spaces you will be left with the connective tissue framework of the body. This living tissue system is highly intelligent and very responsive to both the internal and external environment. All nerve, blood and lymph vessels move within this network. The fascia seems very sensitive to touch and will engage powerfully to a relational touch. Some authors believe that the fascia is also a tissue that responds to chi in and around the body and is the interface for body/energy effects.

The most common extracellular substance in the body is collagen. This is a protein-based structure that makes up bones, ligaments, tendons, fascia and membranes, so when you relate to fascia you are making a relationship in particular to collagen. You are feeling the qualities of collagen: strong but bendy. Collagen fibres are long, spiral-shaped and hollow. The fluid inside has a similar chemical composition to CSF, making the fibres mini-spines with a special potency invested in the fluid. The spiral fibre mimics a copper coil and perhaps the fluid charges up with potency because of the fibre's electrical nature. In healthy fascia there is a quality of shimmering electric-fluid potency that is unique.

Awareness Exercise: The living matrix

- Sitting calmly, let your mind settle and your body relax.

- Take some time to feel the outline of your body. Begin to notice the cavities and compartments of your body. The inside versus the outside. The torso versus the head and limbs. The neural, abdominal and thoracic cavities. Notice the transitions and connections between the different areas.

- Begin to orient to the tissues of your body. Can you get a sense of fascia interlaced throughout your whole body? Enveloping, surrounding and connecting everything.

- Gently bring an image of the collagen fibres into your mind. Allow the image to fill your mind. As this is happening notice any new sensations coming from your body. Appreciate that you are using the image as a way to make a direct relationship to collagen fibres throughout your body. Notice in particular where you are drawn to in your body.

- See if you can allow a sense of connective tissue matrix connecting all the way down to the cellular level. There is a continuum between our genetic material at the core of the cell and the connective tissues. James Oschman (2000) termed this system the 'living matrix'. Do you get any sense of this within your body? Sit with it for a while and stay with the intention of noticing what arises.

Cells talking to cells via the living matrix
Integrins

> ...molecules, cells, tissues, organs, and our entire bodies use 'tensegrity' architecture to mechanically stabilize their shape, and to seamlessly integrate structure and function at all size scales. Through the use of this tension-dependent building system, mechanical forces applied at the macroscale produce changes in biochemistry and gene expression within individual living cells. (Ingber 2008, p.198)

The science is now very clear that the DNA expression of cells is affected by tensions in the connective tissue matrix. Ingber uses the term mechanotransduction. Integrins form bridges between the cell's membranes, the internal cytoskeleton of the cell and the extracellular matrix of connective tissue. Integrins embed the cells in the whole fascial matrix.

> Thus, tensegrity is used to stabilize the shape of living cells, tissues and organs, as well as our whole bodies. (Ingber 2008, p.198)

Liquid crystallinity

> There is a dynamic, liquid crystalline continuum of connective tissues and extracellular matrix linking directly into the equally liquid crystalline cytoplasm in the interior of every single cell in the body. (Mae Wan Ho 1999)

Mae Wan Ho is a biophysicist who describes her experiments which show that living things are so dynamically coherent at the molecular level that they appear to be crystalline. Water and collagen are the essential molecules that form a 'rapid, noiseless intercommunication' system between cells.

Fascia as a sense organ

Schleip states that fascia is densely innervated by mechanoreceptors, which are intimately connected with the central nervous system and especially with the autonomic nervous system.

> Our richest and largest sensory system is not the eyes, ears, skin, or vestibular system but is in fact our muscles with their related fascia. Our nervous system receives its greatest amount of sensory input from our myofascial tissues. Yet the majority of these sensory neurones are so small that until recently little has been known about them. (Schleip 2003a, p.15)

The majority of the receptors are the poorly researched 'interstitial muscle receptors'. The interstitial receptors function as pain receptors and mechanoreceptors and futhermore, they:

> have been shown to have autonomic functions, i.e. stimulation of their sensory endings leads to a change in heart rate, blood pressure, respiration, etc... It seems that a major function of this intricate network of interstitial tissue receptors is to tune the nervous system's regulation of blood flow to local demands, and this is done via very close connections with the autonomic nervous system. (Schleip 2003a, p.17)

This feedback from myofascial tissues to the autonomic nervous system, leading to local regulation of blood flow, would seem to provide a sensitive mechanism by which the autonomic nervous system could influence muscle tone. He describes three possible mechanisms: changes in local fluid dynamics, changes in intrafascial smooth muscle cells and global muscle tonus change due to 'hypothalamic tuning'. His article states that it now appears that fascial tonus might be influenced and regulated by the state of the autonomic nervous system, and that 'any intervention on the fascia is an intervention on the autonomic nervous system' Schleip 2003b, p.108).

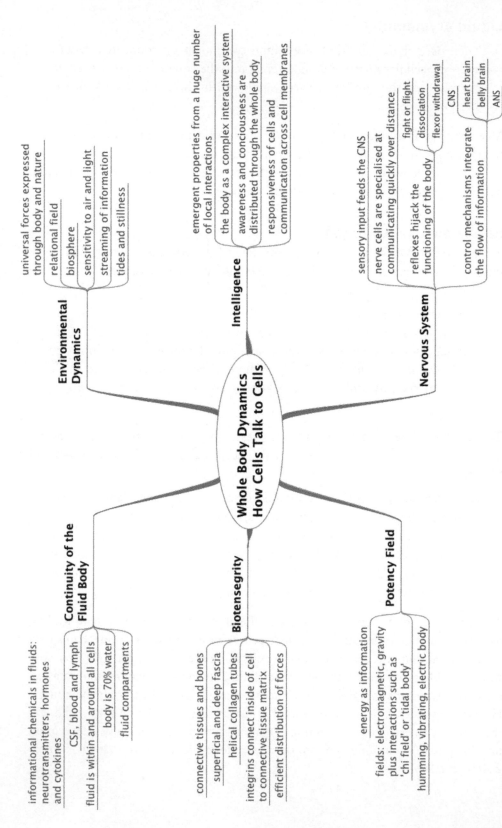

Figure 5.3.1 Mindmap showing different models of how cells talk to cells

This chapter has focused on biotensegrity. Previous chapters have explored intelligence, environmental dynamics, fluid continuity and the potency field. The nervous system will be discussed in Chapter 9.

Summary of Chapter 5

This chapter will deepen your skills of assessment of health by relating to superficial and deep myofascia with anatomical knowledge and precision of touch. Relating to the body as longitudinal and transverse structures creates a deep connecting to its wholeness. Exploring the integrity of motion and tension reveals how structure and force are held in a natural tensile field throughout the healthy body.

Developing touch and relational field skills from the material in this chapter will help you to recognize how the health of the connective tissue matrix can affect the health of the whole system. This may be achieved by:

- becoming familiar with assessing connective tissue health

- feeling whole body patterns

- differentiating between longitudinal and transverse strains in the body; appreciating their convergence and inter-relationships

- relating to transverse diaphragms, including practical and psycho-emotional considerations

- recognizing the qualities of the dural membrane, being able to relate to the falx and tent as key structures for health

- learning to listen to the dural tube, observing dural glide as a way of assessing mobility.

Notes

1. The RTM is one of the five phenomena (see Sutherland 1990, Chapter 2).
2. The brain of the early embryo is covered by an outer membrane called the ectomeninx. At about 8 weeks, the vault bones start to condense and grow within the membrane, separating it into an outer periosteum (firmly attached to the bone) and the dura mater. Thus the external periosteum and dura mater are connected at the suture, there is no periosteum internally; this is the endosteal layer of the dura mater. The endosteal layer is most firmly attached to the bone near the sutures.

6

Craniopelvic Resonance

6.1 THE VAULT
Origin of tissues

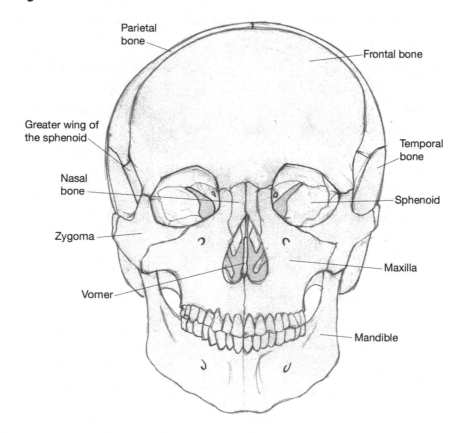

Figure 6.1.1 Skull: anterior view

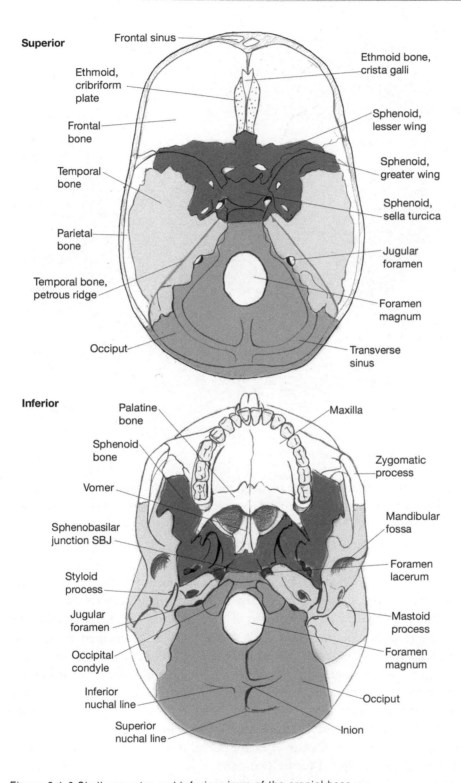

Figure 6.1.2 Skull: superior and inferior views of the cranial base

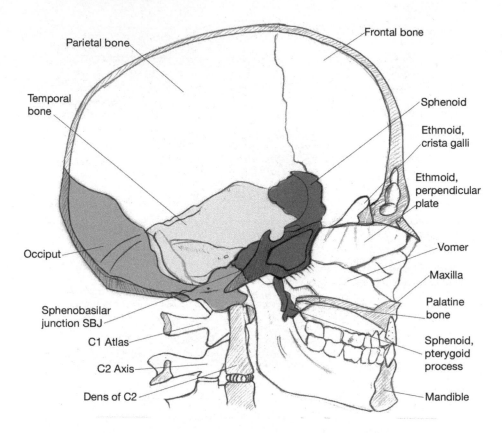

Figure 6.1.3 Skull: mid sagittal section

The cranial vault refers to the crown of the head. The vault is formed by the parietal bones, the squamous part of the temporal bones, the frontal bone and the squamous part of the occiput.[1] The parietal bones and the temporal bones are paired bones, the frontal bone acts like a paired bone (this will be explained later) and the occiput is a single midline bone.

The cranial vault is formed from ossified membrane. In the early embryo the central nervous system grows very quickly. 'A 7mm human embryo is mostly head' (Blechschmidt 2005, p.139). The origin of the vault bones occurs in relationship to the development of the brain. This relationship is maintained throughout life, making the vault bones a powerful handle into the dynamics of the brain. The bulging of the hemispheres stretches the embryonic connective tissue, the mesenchyme. As the mesenchyme is stretched it forms a series of anchoring bands, the dural bands or dural girdles. These go on to form the tent, the falx, and the region of the coronal suture. These anchoring bands form window-frames around the bulging cerebellum and parts of each cerebral hemisphere. The five windows formed roughly correspond to the two parts of the frontal bone, the combined parietals and squamous temporal bones and the squamous occiput. The windows become foci for ossification in the connective tissue of the developing cranial vault. Ossification starts due to the dehydration and subsequent densification of the stretched membranes.[2]

The rest of the neurocranium is called the cranial base and is characterized by bone formed in cartilage. The growing brain compresses the mesenchyme of the cranial base. The different metabolic field[3] gives rise to cartilage as an intermediate step. The brain leaves a footprint in the base of the skull. For example, the ram's horn curling growth pattern of the temporal lobes creates the middle cranial fossa. Ukleja (2005) likens the mesenchyme to snow that is being pushed around that later dries and hardens.

Awareness Exercise: Differentiating the vault and the cranial base

1. In sitting position place your hands on your cranial vault.

   - This is a short exercise so it is usually alright to lift your hands on to your head so your hands are draped over your parietal bones. You can use the parietal eminences as a guide.

   - Alternatively you can lean forward and rest your elbows on your knees.

2. Tune into the movements of the vault bones.

   - Slow your awareness down. Let your hands make a feather-light contact.

   - Explore the head as a fluid membrane bag. Orient to primary respiration. See if you can get a sense of the vault bones as islands of bone in a sea of membrane. Which words are applicable to the vault bones?

3. Change the hand hold so that you are closer to the cranial base.

   - You can place two hands over the occiput and mastoid processes of the temporal bones, or one hand over the inferior part of the occiput and one hand over the inferior part of the frontal bone.

   - Orient to the cranial base. Take your time to tune into the characteristics of the bones. Which words are applicable to the cranial base?

   - Typically people report words such as 'feels lighter, airy, softer at the vault' and 'the cranial base feels more dense, compressed, solid, complex'. The different qualities are very obvious with a little practice. You are tuning into the whole history of the formation of the bones; how they feel reflects their underlying biodynamic development as well as layers of conditional experience.

At the time of birth the vault needs to be soft to pass through the birth canal. Incomplete ossification of the vault bones creates fibrous areas called fontanelles. At birth there are six: the anterior and posterior fontanelles, the sphenoidal fontanelles and the mastoid fontanelles. All of these close up within two months of birth, apart from the anterior fontanelle, which persists until the child is nearly two years old.

Each bone contains a number of ossification centres. Some of the bones of the cranium can have many centres. The temporals for instance are formed from eight centres. These centres start to function from week 6 after fertilization. At birth the temporal bones consist of four parts: squamosal/zygomatic, petrous/mastoid, tympanic ring, and styloid process. This is why the temporal bone looks as if it has been stuck together from a number of parts. It also may explain why the temporal bone has such an unusual primary respiratory motion – a wobbly wheel motion.

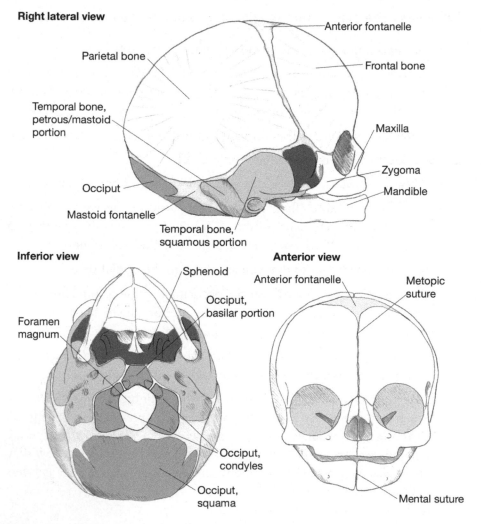

Figure 6.1.4 Foetal skull
Note the tiny two-part jaw, the four-part occiput and the membranes between the bones

The parietal bones in comparison are much simpler and each is formed from one centre. These centres become two of the five eminences of the cranium. The inion of the occiput and the two frontal eminences are the others. They are useful landmarks on the skull. The temporals and the parietals contribute to the widening side to side of the cranium on inhale.

The frontal bone developed from two centres above the orbits which radiate upwards into the forehead and backwards over the orbit. At birth the bone consists of two pieces which become united along the centre by a suture called the metopic suture. The suture normally closes between 3 and 9 months (Vu *et al.* 2001). In some people the suture never closes (metopism) or there is only partial closure. Estimates on the incidence of metopism vary and it depends on ethnicity. Castilho, Oda and Santana (2006) discuss figures of between 2 and 10 per cent for metopism and around 30 per cent for incomplete closure; they indicate normal closure is any time between 1 year and 10 years. In any case, the primary respiratory motion of the frontal bone exhibits motion around this suture line, acting as a paired bone.

The occiput consists of four parts at birth and like the temporal bones is a mix of endochondral and intermembranous bone. Considering the occiput's many attachments and articulations and its pivotal nature in the body between the cranial base, vault and spine, it has a simple respiratory motion of a midline bone.

The formation of the bones is still revealed in their craniosacral motion, so an understanding of the history of the bones will help the practitioner appreciate the nuances that are being revealed in the bones' expression of the breath of life. The fully formed bones expresses discrete motions; however, it is also possible to feel their composite parts. As you increase your skills, you can begin to appreciate the intraosseous motions that take place within the bones. This has the effect of deepening the contact and opening up the dialogue to new levels of health.

Awareness Exercise: Formation of the occiput

- Sitting still comfortably, allow yourself to settle and relax. Bring your awareness to the back of your head. Notice how the bone feels. This is the squamosal area of the occiput and is formed from membrane. This area extends from the lambdoid suture to the superior nuchal line. This is the uppermost of the two transverse ridges on the occiput. Below this line the bone transitions into bone formed from cartilage.

- Then put your hands on the occipital ridge; this is an area of transition where the occiput becomes internalized. See if you can get a sense of the rest of the occiput curving and moving anteriorly to the centre of the cranial base.

- Let your awareness enter the internal part of the occiput as it shifts from a structure that bounds the back of the cranium to the base of the inferior fossa of the interior of the cranium.

- You should be able to sense the foramen magnum (which means 'big hole') and is exactly what it feels like. A hole through a bone is an unusual structure in the body and you can feel how pivotal it is in the make up of the whole bone. It feels like the centre of the bone even though there is no bone there. From here you can get a sense posterior to the occipital ridge and beyond, laterally to the condyles and anteriorly to the sphenobasilar junction.

- Let your awareness rest on the occipital condyles. These are the articulating facets for the atlas and therefore the place where the spinal column meets the head. These parts of the bone have formed independently.

- Move your awareness to the basilar part. This should feel as if it is right at the centre of the cranial base. It's in relationship to the sphenoid and petrous portions of the temporal bones. This area of the bone has formed as a separate ossification centre and has a feeling of wholeness in it.

Mobility and motility of vault bones

Motility is a word defining how a structure moves from within itself, rather than motion between structures which is mobility. Each structure in the body has both of these movements in its biodynamic expression of life. The occiput for instance will widen across its whole structure, but mostly in the squamosal area, in inhalation. That is a movement within the structure as if the bone itself expands as it is filled with the breath of life. The occiput also moves in relationship to other structures around it. Typically this is a rocking movement that can feel as if the occiput is tucking into the cranial base so that the basilar portion actually rises superiorly and the squamosal portion descends inferiorly. The occiput is the only true midline vault bone.

The frontal bone exhibits some similar tendencies to the occiput in its expression. It also rotates in the same way to the occiput but expresses movements as if it is a paired bone. This is often a combined motion; however, some people's systems will exhibit a stronger paired expression and some a stronger midline expression. The frontal bone expands laterally across the forehead on inhalation and seems to have a paradoxical movement as the frontal bone rises upwards and backwards towards the top of the head. As the lateral parts of the frontal bone flare out and widen side to side, there is a dipping in at the metopic suture, particularly close to the eyes.

When healthy the temporal bones can express lots of motion as the squama roll out on inhalation. This can feel like the bones are dropping into your hands. The axis of motion is traditionally along the line of the petrous ridge which is angled into the centre of the cranial base. This means that the mastoid portion of the temporal actually rotates posteromedially while the squama rotates anterolaterally giving the movement a wobble. As if this wasn't complex enough, the motility of the bone is even more complicated as its original eight ossification centres try to express themselves. Perhaps the temporal bone expresses the complexity of the vestibular cochlear system which is housed within it.

The parietal bones are the quintessential paired bones. They express a strong widening and flaring around the lower border of the bone at the squamosal suture. The squamous portion of the temporal bone ('beveled like the gills of a fish')[4] overlaps the inferior margin of the parietal bone and they also flare outwards on inhale. The motion in inhalation shows a deepening into the sagittal suture that can feel like your hands are gliding into the central fissure of the brain.

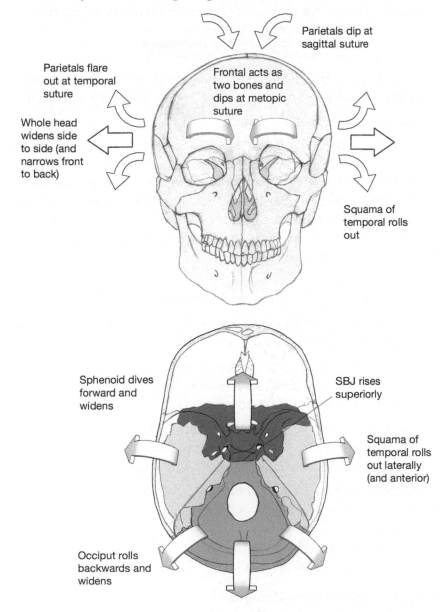

Figure 6.1.5 Skull on inhale

Top: The whole head widens side to side and narrows front to back. Bottom: The cranial base opens like a flower around the SBJ

Treatment Exercise: Motion dynamics of the frontal bone

1. Make contact at the frontal bone.

   - Start at the shoulders. Establish resources, negotiate contact and wait for the holistic shift. Orient to mid tide.

   - Move to the frontal hold (see Figure 6.1.6). Your finger tips can rest over the eyebrows. Make sure your elbows are supported so you can rest lightly over the frontal bone. It can help to keep your awareness in the back of your body to prevent you leaning in.

2. Orient to primary respiration of the whole head.

   - Slow your awareness down and within mid tide see if you can get a sense of the whole head expanding and contracting, emptying and filling.

3. Orient to the frontal bone.

   - Let the detail of the frontal bones come into your awareness. It is important not to narrow down or grab hold of the bone. Keep a wide perceptual field and within the space allow the motion dynamics of the frontal bone to begin to express themselves. The history of the frontal bone is all there; the challenge is, can we slow down enough and develop our perceptual skills enough to be able to experience how the pattern of experience is held in present time?

   - Can the frontal bone express its inner motility? Can you feel the two sides flaring out and dipping into the metopic suture?

4. Explore the relationship between the frontal bone and the falx and the reciprocal tension membrane (RTM).

   - Allow the falx to become part of your awareness. Can you feel the relationship of the frontal bone to the RTM? Feel how any distortions in the whole head and the whole body are reflected in the RTM and the frontal bone.

   - Allow the potency to work as you deepen your awareness. Support any states of balance and Becker's three-stage process. If the frontal bone is restricted can you help create space and a disengagement?

   - Negotiate ending, maybe at shoulders or sacrum.

Awareness Exercise: Relating to the primary respiration of the temporal bones – 'gills of the fish'

   - This exercise is for working on your own. Spend a while getting comfortable. Allow yourself to settle and relax. Notice your breathing. Notice body sensation.

- Gently bring both hands into contact with the sides of your head. Make a light contact onto the temporal bones. Listen for primary respiration. As the temporal bone goes into inhalation it feels like it is expanding and falling into your hands. Notice how the temporal bones open out in their relationship with the parietals along the squamosal suture. This feels like your gills opening.

- Let your hands down and follow the temporal bone motion with your awareness. As the tide surges upwards into the head see if you can follow the movement of the whole bone from its basal portion to the external mastoid area, the part around the external auditory meatus and the squama. Try to locate the axis of rotation which is traditionally along the line of the petrous portion.

- Notice how each of the temporal bones vary in their motion with each other. Often one of them has more freedom of movement. Deepen your awareness into the tentorium. How is the motion of the tentorial leaves in primary respiration? Commonly the temporal bone and the tentorium on that side share similar patterns.

- The temporal bone has lots of different relationships. Notice if your attention is drawn forwards towards the face via the zygomatic arch or posteriorly towards the mastoid and its connection to the sternocleidomastoid muscle, or internally into the inner ear. Often the body will show you its priorities by literally drawing your attention to it.

- If you bring an intention of stillness to your temporal bones, watch what happens as they take this up and drop into stillpoint. This can be a powerful way of calming the vestibulo-cochlear complex and resetting the central nervous system.

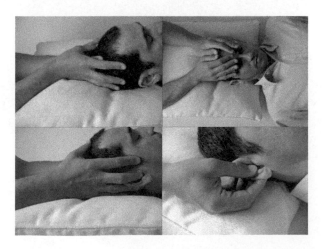

Figure 6.1.6 Various cranial holds
Clockwise from the top left: parietal hold, frontal hold, temporal ear lobe hold, temporal ear hole hold

6.2 THE PELVIS

Anterior

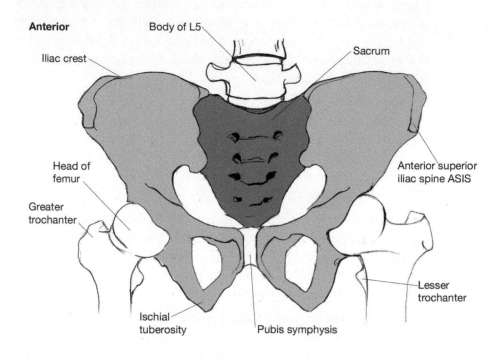

Posterior

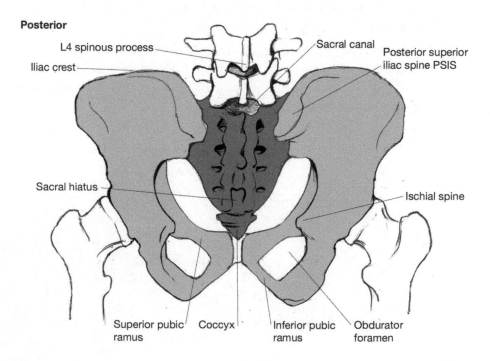

Figure 6.2.1 Pelvis: anterior and posterior views

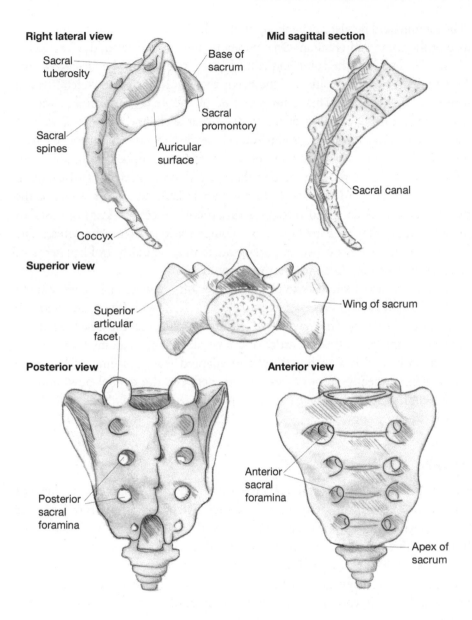

Figure 6.2.2 Sacrum: various views

As above, so below

'The involuntary movement of the sacrum between the ilia' was one of Sutherland's early five phenomena. The recognition of a fundamental connection – 'the core link' – between the cranium and the pelvis is an early and important framing within the work. One of the major insights of A.T. Stills (the founder of osteopathy) was that the sacrum moved with changes in posture and that optimum alignment of the pelvis is extremely important to the function of the whole body.

The sacrum (and pelvis) can be thought of as the foundation stone for the whole edifice of the spine and cranium. On a purely biomechanical level, dysfunction in the base will feed into the spine and cranial base. It can easily be visualized that if there is change in the position of the pelvis the whole muscular skeletal system will need to compensate. This is not just true of the pelvis; a profound way of understanding the functioning of the body is that a change anywhere causes a ripple of change in the whole system. You can never just move a big toe, or more graphically have your big toe stood upon, without a response throughout. This is the core of the biotensegrity model; the body is very efficient at distributing stresses in the totality of the body. No one part is isolated from the rest of the body. However, it is useful to recognize that there are certain staging posts, or transition points, that tend to hold more compensations than other areas. The pelvis and cranial base are two important areas that regularly hold patterns of experience to accommodate the stresses on the system.

Resonance is also a key feature of the relationship between the pelvis and the cranium. The potency field is very information rich. Randolph Stone, an osteopath who developed Polarity Therapy and whose ideas influenced the development of biodynamic craniosacral therapy, articulated a whole energy anatomy for the body. 'As above, so below' is a wonderful phrase adapted from a saying of Dr Stone (Stone 2009).[5] It neatly encapsulates the link between the cranial bowl and the pelvic bowl, the top of the spine and the bottom of the spine, and between higher and lower in many contexts.

Origin of the tissues

The pelvis is formed from the sacrum and coccyx and the two large innominate or pelvic bones. At the front the innominate bones articulate with each other at the pubis symphysis. At the rear each articulates with the sacrum at the sacroiliac joints (S/I joints – these will be covered in more detail in Chapter 11). The innominate bones are formed in cartilage. There are three main ossification centres – ilium, pubis and ischium. They meet within the acetabulum. At birth the innominate bones are still mostly cartilage. They do not fully ossify until the late teens/early twenties.

The sacrum ossifies from five vertebrae, formed from somites in the embryo. Again it is largely cartilage at birth and is not fully ossified until the twenties. According to *Gray's Anatomy* the remains of the intervertebral discs can be unossified up to or beyond middle life (Standring 2005). The origin of the tissues shows that the pelvic bones have an inner framework and that they are not fixed, static things.

Awareness Exercise: Tuning into your pelvis

- Lying on your back with your knees raised, it is a very natural contact to let your hands rest over each anterior superior iliac spine (ASIS). This can be a late-night cranial, something for a sleepless night that can often help you settle.

- Slow your awareness down and begin to orient to your whole pelvis. What are your first impressions? Can you get a sense of your base? How does it feel to acknowledge your reproductive organs? How does it feel to acknowledge your organs of elimination?

- See if you can get a sense of the space bounded by the bones and tissues, the pelvic bowl. Which words come to you as you deepen your awareness of this area? Sometimes it can feel stagnant, hidden, blocked, uneven left to right, tight, painful, many possibilities. Or can you get a sense of health, vitality, drive, flow – a relationship to the power of the potency held in our base. The lower two chakras from the yoga tradition are in this region and are often associated with drive and security.

- Once you have found some resources, orient to the tissue more explicitly. Begin to get a sense of the huge innominate bones slowly rolling out and widening across the front of the body on inhale. It is a wonderful feeling when you get it. It can be much more grounding than self-palpating the head. Enjoy.

- Play with the hold. Drop your hands towards the floor/table/bed and place your palms over your iliac crests. See if you can feel the flaring out of the iliac crest, more of a widening side to side.

- Finish by acknowledging the whole body. How does the pelvis reflect the whole of you, right now? Can you feel any resonance between the pelvis and the cranium?

Motility and mobility of the pelvic bones

Figures 6.2.3 gives some sense of the movement of the pelvic bones on inhale. There is a widening across the top of the pelvis and a rolling out across the front of the pelvic bones. These movements are most easily felt with your hands over the ASIS. The pelvic bones mobility is much bigger than the movements in the cranium. The motility can be felt as a softening within the bones, a sense of inner breathing and expansion.

It is common to feel twists across the pelvis; one ASIS feels superior and inferior to the other as it rotates posteriorly backwards on the sacrum. This often is due to postural habits of standing with more weight on one leg. As patterns of experience change the whole pelvis can shift and you can get a clear sense of one side dropping towards the feet or towards the table.

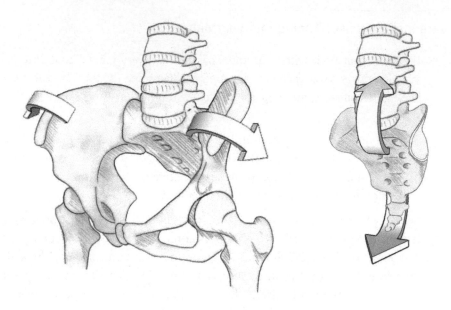

Figure 6.2.3 Pelvis: mobility of the sacrum and innominate bones on inhale

Treatment Exercise: Motion of the ilia

1. Start at the feet.

    • Establish resources, negotiate contact and wait for the holistic shift. Orient to mid tide. The legs roll out on inhale. Small movements at the top of the femur, due to primary respiration in the sacrum and pelvis, are amplified and can be much easier to feel at the feet. It can be very obvious that one leg is not rolling out as much as the other, or that one leg is drawn up and the hip is contracted. This is valuable information.

2. Bilateral contact across the pelvis.

    • Move to a bilateral contact across the pelvis with your hands resting over the ASIS on each side. You can use a cushion to support the arm that reaches over. (It is also possible to stand and make this contact; you can lean against the side of the table for support. Make sure you widen your legs rather than bend your back.)

    • Slow your awareness down and begin to orient to the whole pelvis. What are your first impressions? Acknowledge that there can be many stories coupled to the dynamics of the pelvic bowl. Take your time, allow the relational field to deepen, verbally check in with the client.

3. Orient to the primary respiration of the ilia.

- Once you have found some resources, orient to the tissues and bones more explicitly. Begin to get a sense of the innominate bones slowly rolling out and widening across the front of the body on inhale. See if you can feel the flaring out of the iliac crest, more of a widening side to side. Does it correspond to what you felt from the feet?

- With phases of the tide, notice any shapes and patterns that emerge as part of the inherent treatment plan. What organizes this? Can you support Becker's three-stage process through your contact at the pelvis? Can the innominate bones come back into relationship with the midline and the original matrix?

- Finish at the feet. Make sure you register if there are any changes in how the whole body moves. Can you describe the changes to yourself and in simple language for the client?

6.3 FEELING CRANIOPELVIC RESONANCE
Craniopelvic resonance in treatment

Making contact at the feet or at the sacrum or the two-handed contact on the spine or contact at the cranium via the occiput or vault are the bread and butter holds for craniosacral therapists. From these holds you will be able to perceive clear reorganizations along the midline and at the two poles of the midline. Often there is sense of toing and froing between the two poles. You can sense this in the whole system from whatever contact you are making. The clinical highlight box on craniopelvic reorganization covers some of the ways you can appreciate the dynamic between above and below.

There are some extra holds that can be very useful to help you learn to appreciate craniopelvic resonance, namely holding the sacrum and occiput together in side position, holding the ethmoid and coccyx together, also in side position (see Figure 2.3.3), or with the client in supine coming from one side and contacting a temporal bone and a pelvic bone together. With any two-handed hold, coherent movement under both hands is a clear sign of health. Often when you first put both hands on there is a sense of fragmentation and a loss of synchronicity. Orienting to the whole body, the reciprocal tension membranes, the fluid midline and craniopelvic resonance are particularly good ways of improving communication and facilitating primary respiration. We can deepen into the experience of resonance between the cranium and the pelvis by appreciating them as opposite ends of the midline. Healthy motility in the cranium and in the pelvis facilitates smooth communication along the midline.

Treating the occiput and sacrum in side position is a wonderful way of learning to feel the fluid tide and fluid drive. Practically it can help to get the client to move away from you to the other side of the table; use cushions and bolsters to support your arms and wrists. Your fingers can point along the midline or you can make a general contact with your hands resting over the occiput and sacrum and your fingers pointing to the ceiling. It takes a little practice to get comfortable working in side position, but it is time well spent. Sometimes, in late pregnancy or acute back pain, it is the only position that is safe or comfortable for your client. Holding the occiput and sacrum in side position is a very integrating hold at the end of a session, useful to help you appreciate the reorganization phase of Becker's three-stage process.

Holding the ethmoid and coccyx in side position is a classic way of orienting to the anterior midline and the notochord and the movements of the central nervous system. From behind the body, the upper hand reaches around the front of the head and the middle finger rests over the glabella (between the eyebrows); the palm of the lower hand contacts the sacrum with the fingers pointing towards the feet and the middle finger resting over the coccyx. The contact needs to be delicate to pick up the nuances of the movements. This hold frequently shows you quite a different quality to craniopelvic resonance from the sacrum/occiput hold. It tends to be more about the primal midline and the CNS rather than the fluid midline. It can also give a clear sense of the falx and dural tube connecting between the crista galli of the ethmoid and the posterior surface of the coccyx.

As you learn to deepen your awareness in side position you can feel many things. When orienting to inhale and exhale in the bones you can feel the bones rocking together. When orienting to fluids you can feel surges in the fluid drive; often you can get a sense of something like mercury rising in a thermometer or warm, runny honey flowing up the spine. When orienting to the dura or the CNS you can get a sense of a rising upwards and a curling forward. In this orientation both hands on the sacrum and coccyx can feel as though they shift upwards on inhale; this can be slightly confusing if you are used to feeling the rocking motion of the sacrum on inhale. As you slow down further and orient to long tide and the deeper forces of health, a further confusion can arise. Sometimes there is just a sense of the whole midline lengthening and the whole body curling forward. In this case you may perceive your hands as moving apart. Do not worry, you are getting in touch with embryology and early shapes and forces; over time you will learn to differentiate and name these different expressions (see Figure 10.1.4).

Holding one temporal bone and one pelvic bone is a more unusual hold, but can be surprisingly effective. The temporal bones resonate strongly with the pelvic bones. The articulations with the coronoid process of the mandible and with the head of the femur mimic each other to some extent. The flaring outwards of the temporal bones is similar to the opening and rolling outwards of the pelvic bones. We have often observed in practice hip pain and patterns of experience in the pelvis resolving with shifts in the temporal bones or the temporal mandibular joint.

Clinical Highlight: Noticing craniopelvic reorganization in practice

It is very common for the body to reorganize itself by making an adjustment in the cranium, then in the pelvis, before a further change can take place in the cranium. This can go back and forth a few times before there is a general reorganization towards the midline.

How do you notice this?

Quite simply the treatment priority moves away from where you are in contact with in the body. This can feel like the process has stopped, but if you widen your field of perception to the rest of the body you will notice that it's the priority that has changed and potency is now actively bringing about tissue and fluid changes at the other pole of the body.

- *Being clear.* As you get to know the synchrony between the pelvis and the cranium you can learn to expect these shifts. It may well explain what is happening in the system when you thought things had ground to a halt, or the process of change had simply disengaged. This can be a useful clarification of sections of your treatment that you thought you had not understood or that you thought you didn't have the skills to follow.

- *Changing your expectations.* Be open to the inherent treatment plan weaving back and forth between the head and pelvis. Commonly the shifts are with structures that have particular resonances with each other, like the sacrum and occiput, though often it is more complex than this. A good way to follow this is to work in a pair with one practitioner at the head and the other at the pelvis.

- *Don't get too caught up in local events.* Adjustments around the immediate area of your handhold or the region of the body where changes are taking place are just part of the whole reorganization event. The more you can always be in relationship to the whole body as well as the local field the more you will enable craniopelvic adjustments.

Awareness Exercise: Surface anatomy of the cranium

Some descriptions of the essential lumps and bumps of the skull, and how to find them, are given below. Figure 6.3.1 shows all the landmarks described. Practise finding them on a partner.

Cranium

- *Mastoid process.* This is the big lump behind the ear lobe. Part of the temporal bone, it moves medially on inhale. Palpate posterior to the mastoid process and you can feel the occipital mastoid suture. This is a very useful landmark.

- *Temporal squama.* Note the position of the squama relative to the ear. It is mostly anterior of the ear. The external meatus is just inferior to the line of the tentorium.

- *Greater wing of the sphenoid.* If you find the lateral corner of your eye and move more laterally (away from the eye) there is a bony ridge; this is where the frontal bone meets the zygoma. As you move even more laterally, going over the ridge, it will feel relatively soft. Go gently; under your finger is the greater wing of the sphenoid. It is covered by the temporalis muscle. This is a classic piece of anatomical awareness in cranial work. Just superior is the pterion. Which four bones meet here?

- *Coronal suture, sagittal suture and the bregma.* The coronal suture is between the frontal bone and the two parietal bones. The sagittal suture is between the two parietal bones. The bregma is the meeting place of the sagittal and coronal sutures, the site of the old anterior fontanelle. Moving posteriorly from the eminences you can often feel an indentation along the coronal suture.

- *Frontal and parietal eminences.* If you imagine a Frankenstein, square head, the frontal eminences are the two lumps on frontal bone that roughly correspond to the anterior 'corners' of the head and the parietal eminences are the posterior 'corners' of the head.

- *External occipital protuberance.* Also called the inion, this is a very useful midline landmark on the occiput. Directly in front, on the internal surface of the occiput, is the end of the straight sinus at the internal occipital protuberance.

- *Angle of the mandible.* The most posterior inferior part of the jaw, very easy to find.

- *Zygomatic arch.* This can be felt as a ridge in the anterior posterior plane just in front of the ear. You can palpate the upper and lower margins of the arch and feel the temporalis muscle above and the masseter muscle below.

- *Temporal mandibular joint (TMJ).* Anterior to the tragus of the ear. It can easily be verified by opening and closing the jaw. The TMJ can also be felt by placing a finger in the ear canal and opening the jaw.

- *Sphenobasilar junction (SBJ).* A good guide to the position of SBJ, deep in the centre of the skull, is a point midway along a line between the lateral canthus of the eye and the tragus of the ear.

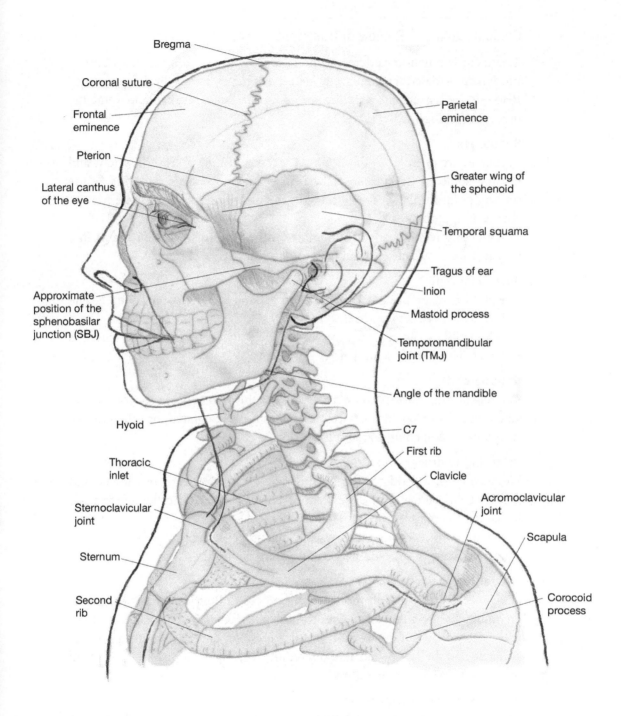

Figure 6.3.1 Surface anatomy of the skull and thoracic inlet

Clinical Highlight: Review of treatment process and skills

Treatment is a non-linear, creative process. However, healing is not arbitrary. Biodynamics describes commonly perceived stages in the healing process.[6] Below is the sequence of unfoldments and treatment skills that help frame the process of change.

Resources

Resources are essential to the healing process. Creating a sense of safety, and helping someone develop an embodied awareness of their resources, is the starting point for the work. This allows the practitioner to ensure the pace of change is appropriate.

Orienting to stillness and stillpoints can be very useful if someone is in a very low potency state and can help to develop resources.

Relational field

The skills here are bringing awareness to making contact, establishing a state of balanced awareness, and being present.

The ability to match your perceptual field to the needs of the client is essential. This is a constant dance.

Holistic shift

The relationship clarifies and the resources of the system begin to work. It can take a number of sessions before it becomes fully integrated into the process. It signifies a deepening of the session work.

Orienting to primary respiration

We encourage mid tide as the starting orientation. Can you feel inhale and exhale? Can you feel how the system organizes in relation to the midline and its natural fulcrums?

As the work develops, can you widen your perception to support the emergence of long tide and deepen into dynamic stillness?

Inherent treatment plan

Let the breath of life lead the treatment process. Often the priorities emerge on an inhale surge. Potency moves towards the organizing centre of a pattern of experience. The primary fulcrum that presents depends on the resources available and the clarity and skill offered through the relational field. A useful question is, 'What organizes this?'

Becker's three-stage process

Seeking, settling and reorganization. States of balance occur within the settling phase. Can you support a state of balance in relationship to the primary fulcrum?

Augmentation/conversation skills

It is possible to augment the natural movements of potency to facilitate a state of balance. Useful skills are:

- Supporting space and disengagement.

- Orienting to stillness, slowing things down.

- Resonance with the intentions of the breath of life.

- Orienting to the midline and natural fulcrums.

- Spacious intentions.

- Differentiating tissues, fluids and potency.

- Orienting to the whole and a wide perceptual field.

Negotiate ending

Moving to a different handhold can help clarify the ending. Bring as much awareness to ending as you do to making contact. Stillpoints can be helpful.

Summary of Chapter 6

Relating to the pelvis and cranium as biodynamic reflections of health is a key concept of this chapter material. This chiefly involves relating to bony and membranous patterns as well as primary respiratory motion at the cranial vault and the pelvis. Observing the natural shift between the pelvis and cranium during a treatment is an important ingredient of the biodynamic craniosacral therapy treatment process.

A number of skills emerge from appreciating the body in this way:

- Starting to recognize how bones feel and express healthy motion.

- Recognizing how the health of the RTM affects the bones of the midline.

- Feeling whole body patterns through craniopelvic resonance.

- Recognizing how the falx and tent are key structures for healthy motion of the vault bones.

- Learning to listen to the dural tube as the core link between the pelvis and cranium.

Notes

1. The greater wings of the sphenoid can also be considered as part of the vault; for example, see Scarr (2008). For simplicity the sphenoid is discussed in Chapter 7.
2. This whole section is based on Blechschmidt (2005, pp.139–144). The vault bones are formed in 'detraction' metabolic fields in Blechschmidt's language.

3.   A densation field is formed. See Blechschmidt (2005, p.142).

4.   Whilst at osteopathic college at the age of 25, the suture between the temporal bone and the parietal bone reminded Sutherland of the gills of a fish and this was the first trigger for the idea that the cranium could breathe. See Sutherland (1990).

5.   The full phrase is: 'As above, so below; as within, so without.'

6.   'Healing is not arbitrary, it occurs in stages.' This phrase is from a lecture given by Franklyn Sills at Karuna in 2005. The review of treatment processes is based on the original work of Sills; there is a flowchart in Sills (2004).

7

Birth

7.1 BIRTH

Overview

Life is essentially mysterious right from the start. The body is formed through a remarkable series of growth events that is only partly comprehended even though it is one of the most common things in the world. We are a mystery to ourselves. Then there is birth. The uterus is like a portal into this world. It offers a unique environment before we fully enter the world of gravity and air.

Earlier in the book we paid lots of attention to the embryonic formation of the body and the laying down of biodynamic movements. In this chapter we will look at the process of birth and how that affects us. Craniosacral therapists take a lot of interest in birth as it moulds who we are. Birth leaves an imprint. The passage down the birth canal is so profound it leaves a trail in our tissue field. It programmes the neuroendocrine–immune system and quickens the life force in us to be ready for life's experiences. We all move through this in a unique way. It seems that it's part of how we are created as individuals. So, in the natural order of things, we all have birth patterns. Our character as individuals is influenced by these patterns and sets up the particular orientation to the world around us. The patterning affects us on all levels, psycho-emotionally, perceptually, structurally and physiologically. Figures 7.1.1 to 7.1.4 give a simple overview of the birth process and some typical forces on the skull.

Difficulties arise when birth has been experienced as a traumatic event and the newborn's system cannot recover. The trauma energy and memory then becomes embedded within the birth patterns. The unresolved trauma then starts to affect the healthy development of the newborn, and commonly feeding and sleeping issues emerge, and difficulties in bonding. These may influence us throughout our lives from the body unconscious. Therefore, becoming skilled and relating to birth patterns, and knowing how trauma feels and looks, will enable you to help resolve birth trauma in your clients.

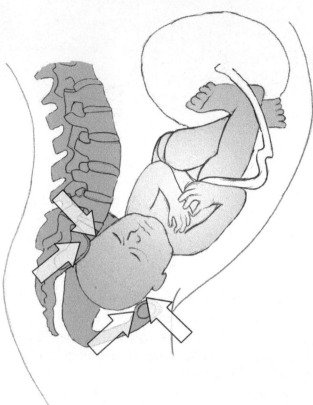

Figure 7.1.1 Birth: head at pelvic inlet

As the baby's head meets the sacral promontory and the pubis there can be medial compressive and/or shearing forces

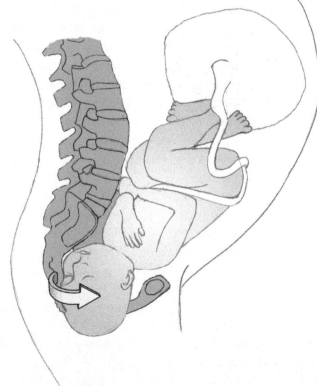

Figure 7.1.2 Birth: head at mid pelvis

The baby's face turns towards the sacrum and rotational forces are commonly imprinted on the skull. The arrow shows the direction of the force experienced by the baby's head as it drags across the sacrum

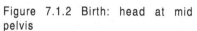

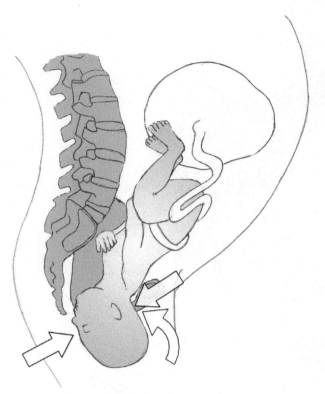

Figure 7.1.3 Birth: head at pelvic outlet

The baby's head initially flexes and then extends and arches backwards (extension shown) to pass under the pubis. Anterior posterior forces can be generated as shown

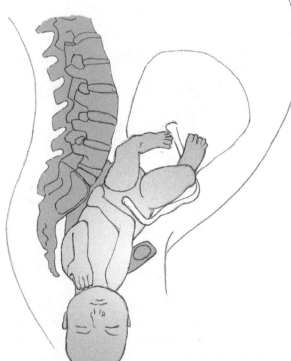

Figure 7.1.4 Birth: restitution and body birth

On leaving the pelvic outlet the head rotates to realign with the shoulders: restitution. The shoulders and then the body need to negotiate the pelvic outlet. Expulsion of the placenta follows as the final stage

Cranial base patterns

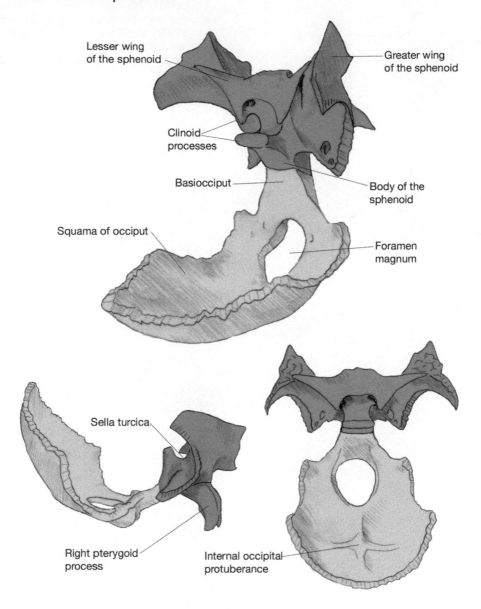

Figure 7.1.5 Various views of the sphenoid and occiput

The cranial base, the sphenobasilar junction (SBJ) and the sphenoid in particular hold an almost mythical significance for many cranial practitioners. When looking at the sphenoid bone in isolation it is easy to get lost in its beautifully complex form. Sutherland's book *Contributions of Thought* has a picture of the sphenoid (with the vomer and ethmoid) on its front cover.

The first cranial practitioner one of the authors saw would spend five minutes at the thoracic inlet and then only ever work with the SBJ. The author went with a chronically sore right ankle. Interestingly it got better. In the whole body shapes section we will explore some of the ways to understand how that might have happened. In this section we will cover some of the biodynamic approaches that can help create clarity when working with the cranial base.

In biodynamic craniosacral therapy there are a number of underlying principles and orientations that are very useful:

- Living bones are never found in isolation. They do not act like cogs. They are not fixed static entities; they have their own internal motility and the ability to bend and flex.

- The easiest way to model the motion of the cranial base is that it opens and closes like a flower. In health the SBJ is the natural centre of the flower, the natural fulcrum for the motions of the cranial base.

- The whole cranium is essentially a fluid membranous bag. Distortions from external (conditional) forces always affect the whole of the cranium.

One very powerful way of understanding the distortions in the fluid membrane skull is to be clear how conditional forces can be held at the SBJ. Sutherland (see Magoun 1951) described six basic types of patterns of the SBJ which he grouped in two ways:

- Physiological patterns (so called because Sutherland felt they were distortions of normal, non-traumatic movements of the SBJ, that is, they were exaggerated expressions of natural physiology). There are three types:

  ○ Inhale/exhale.

  ○ Torsion.

  ○ Sidebending.

- Non-physiological patterns (non-physiological as they were considered outside the normal possibilities of movement and were caused by very strong external forces). There are also three types:

  ○ Lateral shear.

  ○ Vertical shear.

  ○ Compression.

Name	Image of SBJ	Vault hand hold	How it feels	Comments
Side Bend Right side bend shown. Named for the side where the greater wing of the sphenoid moves anterior/towards the ceiling.	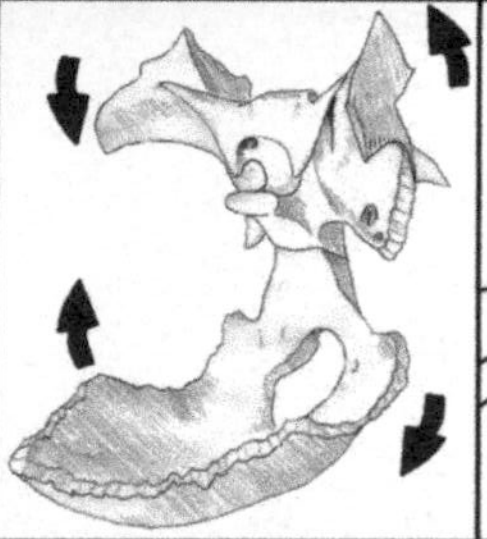	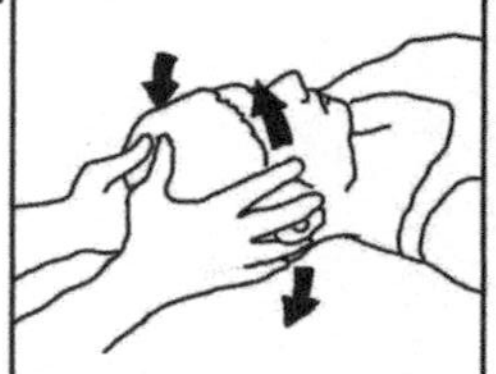	**One side of the head gets wider front to back, associated with sense of bulging outwards on the same side.** On the side bend side the contact at the greater wing of the sphenoid moves to the ceiling, the contact on the occiput moves to the table.	For a right side bend the right eye socket can often look bigger. The right side of the skull will look longer and more convex from the top. The temporal bone on the side bend side will tend to be in inhale/external rotation.
Torsion Right torsion shown. Named for the side where the greater wing of the sphenoid moves superior/ towards your body.	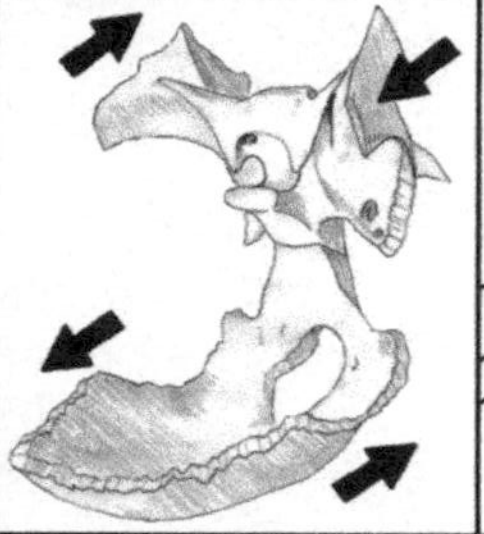	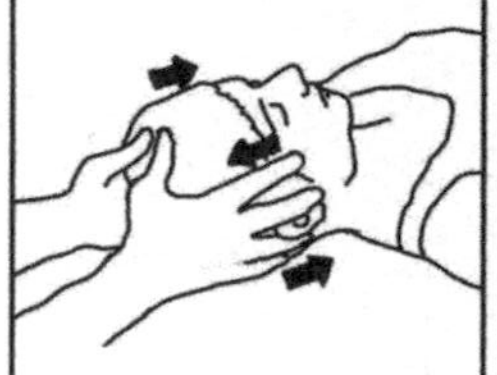	**One contact at the greater wing of the sphenoid moves towards your body, the contact on the other greater wing moves towards the feet.** On the same side of the head the contacts on the sphenoid and the occiput move in different directions, one towards your body, one towards the feet.	For a right torsion the right eye socket can often look bigger. The right side of the face can look longer from the front. The right temporal bone on the right torsion side will tend to be in inhale/external rotation.
Inhale/Exhale Inhale shown.	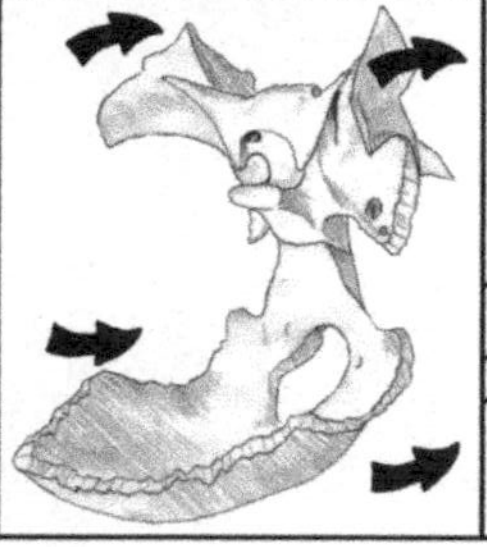	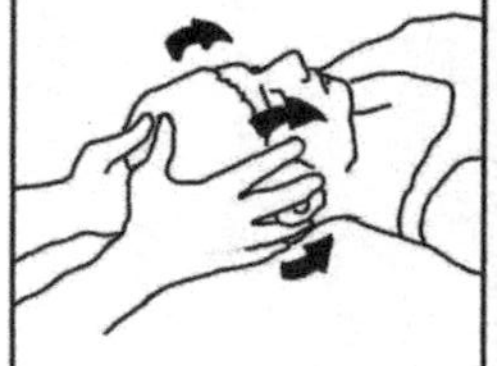	**In an inhale pattern you will feel the head widen side to side and narrow front to back but it will struggle to go into exhale. There is a sense of the sphenoid held diving forward.** On both sides the contact at the greater wing of the sphenoid moves towards the feet, the contact on the occiput also moves towards the feet.	In inhale the head will look wide across the front. The whole body shape can also be relatively short and wide side to side. Tall narrow body and narrow, long face can indicate relative exhale pattern.

Figure 7.1.6 Physiological patterns of the SBJ

Please note these tables are guides only, The bones are not things in isolation; the whole fluid membranous cranium will be distorted

Name	Image of SBJ	Vault hand hold	How it feels	Comments
Lateral Shear Right lateral shear shown. Named for the side where the greater wing of the sphenoid is most anterior and lateral.	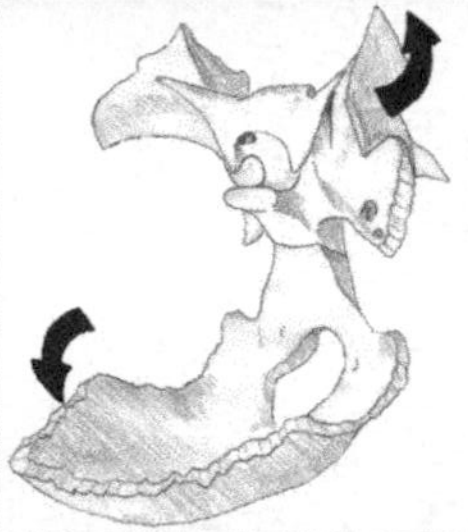	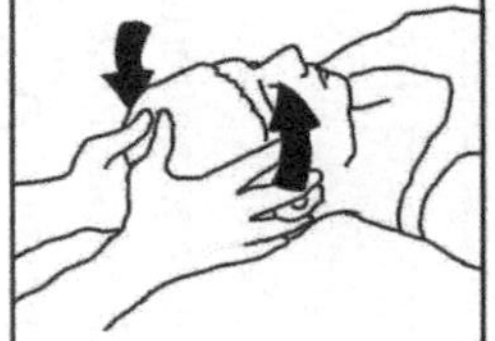	**In a lateral shear you will feel one hand move towards the ceiling and one hand move towards the table.** There is a lateral distortion of the sphenoid body relative to the basiocciput.	If looking at the top of the skull there is a rhomboid shape as one side of the skull is relatively anterior. It is also possible to feel a lateral shift of the sphenoid relative to the occiput. The shift is felt towards the side that is moving towards the ceiling. (The rotational element is shown in the images, rather than the lateral shift, as it is more commonly felt.)
Vertical Shear Superior vertical shear shown. Named for the position of the body of the sphenoid relative to the basiocciput.	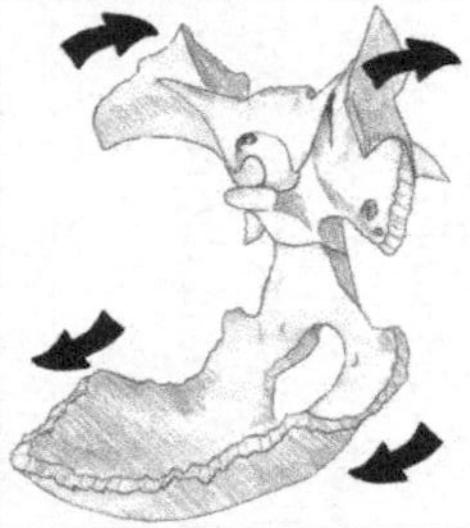	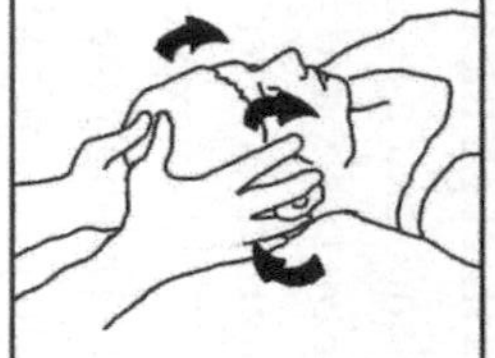	**In superior vertical shear you will feel, in both hands, the contact at the greater wings of the sphenoid move to the feet and widen, whilst the contact at the occiput moves towards you and narrows.** In superior vertical shear the sphenoid is in inhale whilst the occiput is in exhale. The opposite occurs in inferior vertical shear.	In superior vertical shear the front of the skull will be relatively wide, whilst the back of the skull will be relatively narrow. If looking at the top of the skull there can be a triangular shape, with the skull wide at the front. There can also be a sense of 'waggon wheel rolling forward' as the sphenoid rolls to the feet coupled with the contacts at the occiput moving superior. *
Compression	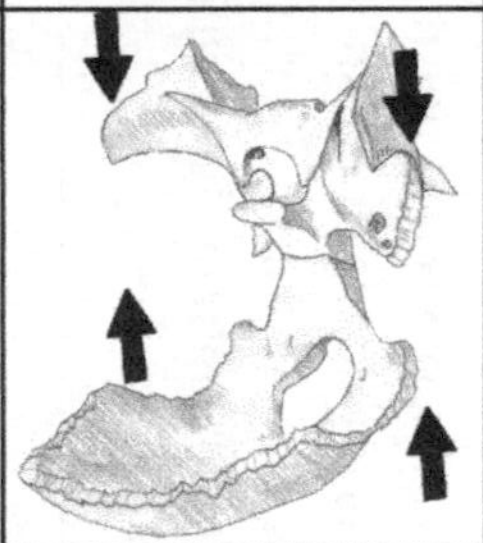	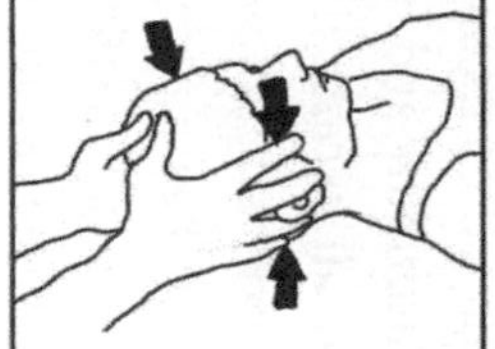	**There is a sense of density, inertia and compression front to back in the SBJ.**	The sphenoid and occiput feel jammed together.

Figure 7.1.7 Non-physiological patterns of the SBJ

In inferior vertical shear there can be a 'toboggan forehead' that slopes backward. The waggon wheel rolls backward. If looking at the top of the skull there can be a triangular shape wide at the back of the skull

The tables in Figures 7.1.6 and 7.1.7 describe the patterns in detail. It is worth spending some time studying them. In a training course, you will do lots of exercises to help gain a clear felt sense of the commonly experienced different shapes of the cranium (playing with water-filled balloons, working with boxes, looking at pictures, playing with bones, practising the movements just with your hands, and of course palpating on real heads).

Initially it may seem like a lot of new language and 3D images to hold; persevere as there is a huge payoff. Bringing clarity to your awareness of distortions of the cranium and appreciating how the patterns of experience are frequently organized around the SBJ is very important in clinic work. It is one of the unique features of cranial work to meet this area with skill. The SBJ is often involved in very early imprints; working there can often be the key to supporting healing in deep-rooted, hard-to-treat conditions.

Birth is one of the key conditional forces of the skull. Appreciating the patterns of experience at the SBJ nearly always involves engaging with forces generated at birth. As the conditional forces occurred at a very early and vulnerable period, meeting these forces in an adult requires very skilful negotiations around space and intentions. As birth involves a big head and a small hole, being born can involve moments of being overwhelmed and compressed. It is therefore common for the client to feel overwhelmed and compressed when working at the SBJ.

It is also important, however, to recognize that the impulse to be born and the ability of the human organism to meet obstacles and pass through them is essential to triggering normal development. There is a 'creative opposition' as the baby is shaped by its movements through the birth canal. It can be seen as the first step to autonomy and independence and a sense of being able to act powerfully.

We are all necessarily shaped by birth, and then life. The key differentiation in cranial work is to allow any imprints of overwhelm to become uncoupled from particular shapes and patterns, and not to expect the shapes and patterns to change to some external idealized norm. Through the therapeutic contact the practitioner can appreciate the early shapes and patterns and help the physiology generate more flexible responses and not repeat cycles of being overwhelmed in relationship to a particular fulcrum. It is hard work when there are lots of trauma energies bound up in a pattern. In clinical work these dynamics are frequently played out when meeting the fluid membrane head and the SBJ at the core of the head.

Treatment Exercise: The head as a fluid membrane bag

1. Start away from the head.
   - Start away from the SBJ. Take time to really establish resources, check in verbally, negotiate contact and wait for the holistic shift. Orient to mid tide and the fluid body.

2. Move to the vault.

   • Move to Sutherland's hold or Becker's hold (see Figure 7.1.8 and Clinical Highlight: Contact at the SBJ on p.186). Spend lots of time negotiating the space and making sure the contact is not compressive.

3. Orient to the head as a fluid membranous bag.

   • Can you feel the head expand and contract with phases of the tide? There may be a sense of filling and emptying as the tide surges and recedes.

   • Notice any distortions of the fluid membrane bag. Does one side feel more full than the other? Are your hands pushed and pulled differently on different sides of the head?

4. Can you be aware of conditional forces?

   • Can you get sense of the conditional forces acting on this fluid balloon in your hands? Orient to the biosphere and slow your awareness right down. Do not search for patterns, let the information come to you.

   • How are the conditional forces centred by the body? Allow the detail of the SBJ to come into your awareness. How do the sphenoid and occiput move in relationship to the forces present? Keep a wide perceptual field. Trust any impressions that come to you. In this session we are just being curious about how the fluid membranous head moves in relation to the SBJ.

   • Check in with the client and negotiate ending.

Treatment Exercise: Supporting space at the SBJ

1. Start away from the SBJ.

   • Take time to really establish resources, check in verbally, negotiate contact and wait for the holistic shift. Orient to mid tide and the fluid body.

2. Explore the cranial base opening like a flower.

   • Move to Sutherland's hold or Becker's hold (see Figure 7.1.8 and Clinical Highlight: Contact at the SBJ on p.186). Spend lots of time negotiating the space and making sure the contact is not compressive.

   • Explore the cranial base as a flower opening and closing. Can you feel a widening side to side and narrowing front to back on inhale and the opposite on exhale? You may also feel your contacts on the greater wings and the occiput move towards the feet on inhale as the sphenoid dives forward and the occiput expands and rocks posteriorly. Do not forget the head as a fluid membranous bag.

3. Explore the patterns at the SBJ.

- Orient to the SBJ and the relative positions of the sphenoid and occiput.

- Try to name the dominant pattern at the SBJ. The first few times you do this keep it simple. In class you will explore physiological patterns in one session then non-physiological patterns in a separate session. That is a good way to approach the SBJ when you first start to practise.

- Physiological patterns: the head may be stuck in inhale or exhale; one contact at the sphenoid may be relatively closer to your body – torsion; one side of the skull may bulge laterally outwards – sidebend.

- Non-physiological patterns: the SBJ feels very heavy and inert and there may be a strong sense of compression front to back at the SBJ; one whole side of the head moves to the ceiling and the other side to the table – lateral shear; your hands roll forward to the feet or on a different head backwards towards you – vertical shear.

- There may also be combinations of patterns. It's a living body – six options will never be enough, but they are a good starting place for your journey of enquiry in SBJ dynamics.

4. Just appreciate the patterns of experience.

- The main intentions are: Can you appreciate the dynamics of the SBJ and hold the whole field with a still consistent awareness? Can you help the natural agencies of the body create space at the SBJ? Can you be clear enough to respond to any early stories coupled to the pattern of experience that presents?

- It is always good to finish at the opposite end of the body after working at the head for a while. Negotiate the ending and check in with the client.

Sphenoid anatomy

Adult sphenoid

Figure 7.1.5 shows views of the sphenoid, together with the occiput, from various angles. Clearly the sphenoid is a very complex bone; however, the main parts are visible from Figure 7.1.5 and are a good starting point – the body, the lesser wings, the greater wings and the pterygoid processes.

You can directly palpate only two parts of the sphenoid:

- The hamulus of each of the medial pterygoid plates, the most inferior parts of the pterygoid processes, can be palpated as a definite lump approximately 1 cm medial and 1 cm posterior to the upper back tooth on either side.

- The lateral external parts of the greater wings can be contacted (sensing through the temporalis muscle) approximately 2 cm posterior to the corner of the eye, in the soft hollow posterior to the lateral border of the eye socket. (This is formed by the zygomatic process of the frontal bone and the frontal process of the zygoma. The suture between the frontal and zygoma can usually be felt.)

In the sagittal section of the skull in Figure 6.1.3 you can see the sphenoid air sinus. This will be lined with mucous membranes and connects into the other sinuses. It is amazing to think that at the centre of the head there is a pocket of air. One other feature of note from the sagittal section is the angle of the cranial base at the SBJ.

The sella turcica is also visible in Figure 7.1.5. This is the 'Turk's saddle' where the pituitary gland sits. This anatomical feature is thought to be one of the reasons why shifts in the sphenoid motion can have such wide-ranging effects – free movement of the sphenoid supports flow into and out of the pituitary gland.

Sphenobasilar junction

The sphenobasilar junction (SBJ), sometimes known as the sphenobasilar synchondrosis, is primarily a cartilaginous joint. It ossifies around 14 to 16 years of age and is fully ossified by 25 years.

This fact been used as an argument against the validity of Sutherland's cranial concept. The counter-argument is that the bones are not fixed static things, they are full of blood and connective tissue. Living bone is very different from dead bone where only the calcium matrix is left. The difference is similar to that between a living twig full of sap that bends and gives, and a dead, dry twig that snaps.

Another useful image is that if we have a piece of cardboard and bend it, for example in making the corner of a box, it is still one piece of completely joined cardboard. However, there is a give and flexibility where it was initially bent that will always be there. The SBJ retains flexibility, as do the greater wings in relation to the body of the sphenoid.

Whole body shapes

Often when touching someone with the skills learnt from the biodynamic approach you will become aware of shapes through the whole body. Some common perceptions are:

- One side shorter than the other – a sense of the body bent like a banana to one side.

- Twists through the midline – there can be diagonal pulls across the body, or the head seems to want to lead the body into a long spiral.

- There is a sense of arching backwards and tightness through the back of the body, often led by an arching quality in the neck.

- Curling around the umbilicus – there can be a sense of deep holding and contraction in the abdomen that you can trace back to the umbilicus.

- Long, thin body that orients to exhale more easily or short, wide body, with rolled-out feet, that orients to inhale more easily.

The shapes named above can all be traced back to pre- and perinatal experiences. They have consequences for the whole musculoskeletal system and are often bound up with life statements and patterns of neuroendocrine–immune expression. Please note that shapes such as the startle position or standing postures such as lordosis (sway back) in the lower back or collapse through the abdomen and anterior shift of the head are also strong body shapes that may be layered over or intertwined with the patterns named. Often these shapes have slightly different or additional aetiologies via postural habits or stress responses.

The shapes listed above are often correlates of SBJ patterns. The SBJ is the natural fulcrum for the spine as well as the cranium. Biodynamic awareness is founded on the ability to feel the whole body as a unified field of action. Healing occurs when you can feel a systemic neutral – a state of balance – as the whole body and whole field settles around a primary organizing fulcrum. Working at the SBJ, working with the fluid membranous body and working with the midline are very common pathways into the territory of whole body shapes.

Some possible explanations for pre- and perinatal whole body shapes:

- One side shorter than the other – this is often associated with the birth-lie side of the baby; the side of the baby (most often the left side) that was closest to the mother's spine in utero tends to feel relatively compressed and short.

- Twists through the midline – twists often echo the transition through the midpelvis as the head turns to face the sacrum. Birth involves a spiralling through the birth canal. Some babies, in the more uncommon birth lies, do big twists just to enter into the pelvis.

- Arching backwards – this can often be related to the movement of the head extending as it exits the pelvis. Some practitioners go even further back and relate the arching back as a primary tendency in the embryo reflecting implantation difficulties or resistance to engaging with the relationship to nutrients fed via the umbilicus in utero.

- Curling around the umbilicus – a very common pattern frequently due to shock from the cutting of the umbilical cord too quickly. Maybe also some opposite dynamics to the point above – a keenness to engage and move forward can be felt as a tendency to be at the front of the body.

- Long, thin body or short, wide body (see Figure 7.1.6). The system can be held in relative exhale or inhale, respectively, due to moulding of the cranium at birth.

Attachment

Attachment theory, originating in the work of John Bowlby, is a psychological, evolutionary and ethological theory that provides a descriptive and explanatory framework for understanding interpersonal relationship between human beings (Holmes 1993). In infants, behaviour associated with attachment is primarily a process of proximity seeking to an identified attachment figure in situations of perceived distress or alarm, for the purpose of survival. Infants become attached to adults who are sensitive and responsive in social interactions with the infant, and who remain as consistent caregivers for some months during the period from about six months to two years of age. During the latter part of this period, children begin to use attachment figures (familiar people) as a secure base to explore from and return to. Parental responses lead to the development of patterns of attachment which in turn lead to 'internal working models' which will guide the individual's feelings, thoughts and expectations in later relationships. Separation anxiety or grief following serious loss are normal and natural responses in an attached infant.

The human infant is considered by attachment theorists to have a need for a secure relationship with adult caregivers, without which normal social and emotional development will not occur. However, different relationship experiences can lead to different developmental outcomes. Mary Ainsworth developed a theory of a number of attachment patterns or 'styles' in infants in which distinct characteristics were identified known as secure attachment, avoidant attachment, anxious attachment and, later, disorganized attachment (Ainsworth and Bowlby 1965).

This is a very useful theory for biodynamic craniosacral therapists. The baby is innately interested in relationships above all other things, more than satisfying the basic physical needs. Birth trauma can have a strong influence on how babies relate and form secure attachments.

Pacing and containment

Things going too rapidly (heart rate, breathing, darting eyes, fast talking, potency rushing) in a session is normally a sign of sympathetic activity taking over. In fight or flight mode we mobilize our resources to escape. We go from a place where we are engaged with our environment and with other people, to a place where we are looking for an escape route. Instead of being aware of all our options we choose one option and focus our resources on that one option.

Alan Watkins describes how when the heart rate begins to race it inhibits the prefrontal cortex – part of the brain strongly associated with decision making and thinking (Watkins 2008). Watkins is very clear that the physiology of the body, particularly the neuroendocrine–immune system (in this case the nervous system of the heart), can inhibit the functioning of the higher brain centres. (He calls it a 'DIY lobotomy'.) We make bad decisions when we are stressed. Helping someone to regulate their physiology will help contain stress responses.

In our culture, ever since Freud, there is a long history of privileging approaches that focus on uncovering hidden stories in our past and in our unconscious. You often hear people talk about repression and denial and that the goal of therapy is to try to find reasons why we behave in certain ways. Frequently in biodynamic clinical practice it is useful to challenge the idea that we need to uncover and excavate the past. It is much more about relating to things as they emerge in present time. If the meaning of an event is important it will become clear as biodynamic craniosacral work unfolds. 'How' is often a more interesting enquiry than 'why'.

What most people call repression can actually often be framed as attempts at containing overwhelming physiological processes. Sometimes the attempts are more skilful than others (numbing ourselves through various uppers and downers provides short-term relief, but they often generate additional problems). It is very powerful to appreciate mind–body interactions as frequently being led by the physiology of being safe. Help the physiology downregulate and you will be amazed at the number of intractable issues that resolve.

Stephen Porges, in his polyvagal concept, identifies specific neural circuits that regulate attachment processes (Porges 2003, 2008). He calls it the social engagement system. The social engagement system is mediated by a set of brainstem nuclei he groups together as the ventral vagal complex or new vagus. In evolutionary terms they are a relatively new set of nuclei that are only present in mammals and are particularly well developed in humans. We are very good at communicating. The ventral vagal complex consists of the nuclei for cranial nerves V, VII, IX, X (Nu AM not DMX) and XI. They control sucking, swallowing, voice, breathing, middle ear muscles, heart rate, ingesting, facial expression and head movements.

If the mechanisms are not inhibited then our natural response is social engagement. We engage with our environment, we spontaneously talk, we share, we check out what other people are doing by scanning their faces. Porges is very keen on face-to-face contact and voice modulation for safe interaction. We learnt what is safe and not safe and ways of responding to get our needs met through early attachment processes as described above.

Porges identifies three successively older (in evolutionary terms) responses:

• Communication (social engagement – working with our head).

- Mobilization (fight or flight – working with our limbs).
- Immobilization (freeze, dissociation – working with our viscera).

In stress situations we default to the older strategies. Mobilization inhibits communication and in turn immobilization inhibits mobilization.

Pacing and containment describes the process of helping your client stay engaged in the present and in communication mode. This frequently involves staying in relationship to you as the practitioner, clients being able to track what is happening in their body and clients being aware of what is happening around them. The appropriate interaction will help someone come out of immobilization and then out of mobilization to communication.

Biodynamic cranial work is not about big cathartic expressions and releases. It is about skilfully paced and well-contained change. Slowly is the quickest way of facilitating lasting change. Little and often is far and away the easiest and safest way of supporting change in overwhelming processes.

A pulsatile way of working is often best; we move towards an embodied expression of an issue (whether that is a painful sensation, a difficult emotion, or a fixed idea) and then move away again to return later. It is like tip-toeing towards something, having a peek and then returning to our sense of safety. Next time we move towards the issue we may go a little closer or stay a little longer, but the goal is to approach our darkest stories in bite-sized chunks.

The relational field established by the practitioner is fundamental to establishing safety and pacing and containing the work. Sills (2009a) is clear that we can recreate a safe holding field, through our therapeutic presence, that meets the basic needs of the human being to be recognized, validated and accepted – a quality of 'being to being'. For some clients it may be the first time they have ever been met in that way; it can allow a profound repatterning of the physiology. One of the nicest things a client ever said to one of the authors was that she did not know that it was possible to be held in such a way.

As a practitioner, key skills are learning to establish resources, learning verbal skills to support people to safely explore their experience of their body, noticing the early signs of activation and being able to modulate through cranial and verbal skills an unfolding process.

Early signs of activation include: twitching legs, darting eyes, dry mouth, change to shallow chest breathing, sympathetic buzz coming into the system, parts of the body becoming absent and changes in temperature. As mentioned above it is useful to check in with the client about anything going too quickly.

If the resources are present, it is alright to facilitate discharge of held, frozen energies; shaking, crying and strong emotional expression are not things to be scared of, but neither are they necessary to change. In the longer, slower tides, change in our deepest suffering can be felt as a subtle shift in potency. A realization creeps up on the client that the old fixed story is no longer relevant.

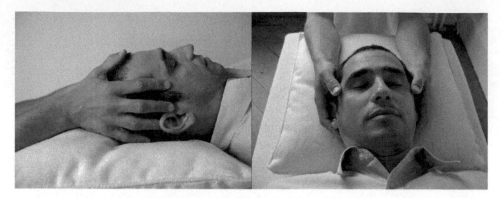

Figure 7.1.8 Vault holds for the cranial base
Left: Sutherland's hold. Right: Becker's hold

Clinical Highlight: Contact at the SBJ

Vault holds

The SBJ can be contacted via either Sutherland's vault hold or Becker's vault hold (see Figure 7.1.8). Over time it is good to become familiar with both holds. In Sutherland's hold the additional contact with the vault bones can really help you get a sense of the membranes and RTM dynamics as well as the SBJ (and, as we discuss later, the motions of the CNS). Becker's hold can be a little easier on your hands and, as you are just contacting the sphenoid and occiput, helps isolate the SBJ dynamics.

Support your forearms and hands

Having your forearms and your elbows supported will help with the contact. Often this means your client will need to go further down the table – it is rarely a problem for clients if their feet hang off the end. Try to keep your forearms at the same level as your hands. It is rare for a client not to need a pillow under their head and this also supports the underside of your hands.

Be precise in your contact

Precision in the contact is important. A very common mistake is to let the contact at the sphenoid slip towards the table. Frequently people wonder why it is hard to sense the sphenoid motion when they are palpating the squama of the temporal bone. The little fingers ideally make contact with the occipital mastoid, posterior to the occipital mastoid suture. With small hands and a big head this can sometimes be difficult. The sphenoid contact is the most important to establish first and then do your best, as your anatomy allows, to reach to the occiput.

Stay in physical contact with the body

There can be a huge temptation to let the contact at the greater wings float off the bone as we attempt to create space. It is possible to work in this way, and sometimes it is necessary to lift the contact off if it feels compressive, but there is a sacrifice in terms of the clarity of information that you will pick up. There is something very powerful about staying in contact with the form and working at the edge of where form and energy meet. Working off the body you give up the ability to interact with the form with precision.

Additional tips to help create space in the contact

- Soft hands, wrists and forearms – let your hands mould to the existing form of the skull with a butterfly touch.

- Staying in contact, imagine your hands flopping out.

- Imagine huge hands and a huge head – this can really amplify your perception of small movements.

- Staying in contact, imagine your hands progressively further from the body – they can be a few centimetres to many metres away.

7.2 INTRAOSSEOUS PATTERNS

Overview

The ability to appreciate bones as dynamic living structures instead of dead, hard lumps of calcium allows us to deepen into the internal dynamics of the bones. We have already described how in biodynamics we perceive the head as a fluid membrane bag. In Chapter 6 we discussed how the vault bones are formed in stretch and the cranial base is formed in compression. We also described that there are often numerous ossification centres in the foetal bone precursors and how at birth many of the bones are still in their composite parts within a cartilage matrix and not yet fully ossified. This is true not just of the cranial bones, but also the sacrum, pelvic bones and the long bones have large amounts of cartilage that persist for many years. In an adult there are typically 206 bones; in a baby it is more like 300.[1] In this section we will explore the bony parts of the skull at birth and discuss how orienting to the components of the adult bones allows a deeper relationship to the organizing forces of the body.

In the adult, the neurocranium surrounding the brain is made up of a total of eight bones: the sphenoid, the ethmoid, the occiput, the frontal bone, the two parietals and the two temporal bones. In the baby it is useful to think of the skull as having twice the amount of bones, a total of 16. The sphenoid is in three parts, the ethmoid is still considered a single bone, the occiput is in four parts, the frontal is in two parts, the parietals are still two single bones and we can simplify the temporal bones to think of them as each being in two major parts at birth.

You can easily see how this creates much more potential for complex shapes and patterns.

As the fluid membrane bag of the head moves through the birth canal the forces generated will imprint on the biotensegrity structure of the skull. If unresolved, the bones will ossify according to the conditional forces present. The parts of the bones will be distorted in their arrangements leading to non-optimum shapes and movements in the fused adult bones. These are intraosseous patterns. They affect the motility and the mobility of the bones and the whole system.

Birth is a major cause of intraosseous patterns. Early head trauma, positional deformation ('plagiocephaly' or flat head syndrome due to persistent lying on the back) and premature closing of the cranial sutures ('craniosynostosis', often corrected by surgery) are all extra conditional forces that can generate abnormal head shapes and intraosseous patterns.

Common patterns within the major cranial bones

The sphenoid develops from cartilage and has many ossification centres in utero. *Gray's Anatomy* states there are 14 ossification centres (Standring 2005).[2] It develops around the end of the notochord. The sphenoid is in three parts at birth. The body and the lesser wings form a central section with two side sections, each made of a greater wing and a pterygoid process. The intraosseous patterns of the sphenoid are very important. Often it feels as though one of the side sections is fixed and inert and this distorts the whole movement of the cranial base. There can be a sense of shearing or medial compression through the parts of the sphenoid.

The occiput is in four parts at birth: the squama, the two condylar parts and the basilar portion. The parts ossify around the foramen magnum. Frequently you can feel a sense of rotation within the squama and it feels jammed into one of the condyles. There can be a sense of telescoping anteriorly; all the occiput parts are compressed towards the sphenoid body. Medial compression and narrowing across the condyles is also possible. Resolution of intraosseous patterns in the occiput is often the key to patterns in the triad of the occiput, atlas and axis.

Each temporal bone is actually in four parts at birth: the squamous part (including the zygomatic process), the petrous portion (including the mastoid), the tympanic ring (around the external ear canal) and the styloid process. The latter two parts are so small compared to the sqauma and the petrous portion that their influence can be ignored. The petrous portion is a very dense bone; it often feels torsioned into the cranial base and medially compressed. The squama can feel as though it has been forced into an oblique angle in relationship to the petrous portion, a bit like the wall of a house tilting inwards.

The frontal bone is in two parts at birth. Its normal dynamic as a paired bone has already been covered in Section 6.1.

General approaches to intraosseous patterns

We are shaped by our experiences. The moulding of the head is an important process in development of the baby. Intraosseous patterns can be, but are not necessarily, coupled with overwhelm and major life statements. Because of the early nature of the experience, and because of the possibility of traumatic coupling, interacting with intraosseous patterns requires a high degree of skill.

Our experience is that intraosseous patterns often underlie many persistent issues. In biodynamics, how we deepen into the dynamics of the skull is not about examining the movement between bones more precisely, though that can be useful. Appreciating the internal dynamics and the restrictions to the inner breathing of the bones is often a much more successful clinical focus.

Even though the bones are fully ossified the internal junctions still represent relatively flexible areas. Think of a piece of cardboard that was once a box. The cardboard is one piece but the regions of the folds are more malleable.

The most important skills with intraosseous patterns are knowing the anatomy, going slowly, orienting to the fluids and membranes, orienting to space and disengagement, working with resources and emphatically not using techniques or strong intentions. Not that different from the normal biodynamic approach then, just a refinement and deepening of your perceptual processes.

7.3 IGNITION

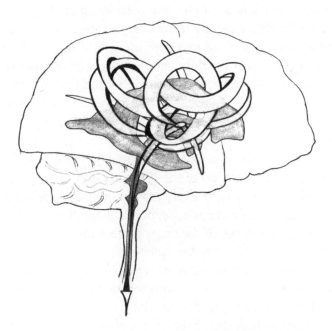

Figure 7.3.1 Artist's representation of ignition as potency spreading out from the third ventricle

Prenatal ignitions

There are a number of key events in the formation of the body that are not only highly significant in terms of the body's development but also are surges of physiological energy that determine the growth and life of the individual. The first big experience is conception. This unique fusion of two people's blueprints is like no other event in the course of the individual's life. Conception sets the stage for all subsequent growth, and acts like a sparking of life that starts a chain reaction. This is an igniting of health and potency to quicken and organize the formation of the body. A conception energy and intention is laid down from this event that runs through the uterine life and perhaps beyond into the rest of our lives. The authors have treated clients who have felt a resistance to embodiment and a low vitality that can be traced back to a difficult conception event. Spend a few minutes attesting to this life-changing event by sitting and thinking about your conception. Let any image come to mind. Obviously this event is not only preverbal and therefore pre-thought but also before the brain and its sensory system was even formed. Sit with the idea and see what manifests. Commonly people have strong experiences as if the cells within you are remembering the event. Most importantly acknowledge how it makes you feel. Interesting information about the beginning of your life, and perhaps an insight into how you are, is available here.

At the end of the third week of embryonic development a midline is formed between two membranous poles. The appearance of the membranes ignites cells to create a primitive streak which is like a furrowed line starting at the lower pole and rapidly arising to a node or pit about halfway up the length of the embryonic disc. Ectodermal cells are rapidly reproducing to create a flow of cells that moves like a sheet across the disc and into the furrow. This is part of the mechanism of gastrulation that produces the third germ cell layer of the mesoderm. This is the raw material for the creation of the notochord, the first midline tube to emerge on the centre of the disc. The whole of this movement looks like cells moving to an energetic imperative that involves not only a field effect but also a streaming action along the centre of the disc. The surge of energy from the primitive streak is a vital force that seems to catalyse the production of all the midline tubes that follow. This is a major ignition of the system that is as important and potent as conception. Things start to move very rapidly from this point onwards. Once the notochord is laid down there is a longitudinal fulcrum for the creation of the major physiological systems of the body, namely the central nervous system and the gut tube and viscera. Later the same week as the notochord is formed the neural tube is created and sealed as the embryo shifts into a curling movement. This is another key event in the formation of the body; this time there is an ignition for longitudinal fluctuation to start and the beginning of a fluid midline. The fluid fluctuation follows the movement of the curling embryo and rises and curves at the top of the neural tube bringing about a movement that will form the third ventricle and bring potency to the core of the growing brain. This is a further physical manifestation of the underlying organizing forces of health that allows laying down of the detailed anatomy and physiology of the body as the blueprint of life materializes.

The next key event to take place in the embryo is the igniting of the heart and the beginning of the heart beating and blood circulating around the growing vascular system. The body is never the same after this event. You can imagine how quiet things are without the heart beating and the brain neuralizing. The start of the heart beating takes place in the fifth week after conception. Suddenly blood becomes a potent fluid feature of the developing embryo as the heart starts beating in the fourth week.

The next key event is the formation of the umbilical cord and the movement of blood between the placenta and the growing vascular system of the embryo. This takes place in the fifth week after conception. This is a powerful potency movement that allows the embryo to move to a more physiologically potent state. Oxygenated blood is now flowing into the embryo and a new wave of growth can occur.

Birth ignition

There are key events in the formation and birth of the human body that promote new physical change and the emergence of potency. Once the embryonic period is over the foetal period is seven months of maturation. All structures are laid down in the first 50 days after conception. This is a huge surge of activity followed by growth and integration of systems. At birth the body gears up for more major transformations. The preparation in the uterus for birth stimulates the body cells and nervous system to be ready for passage down the birth canal and transition from water to air. The head is big compared to the body and is the major part of the body to pass through the birth canal. The vault is soft and the bony plates can be compressed. Why is birth such a tight squeeze? It's as if there's a programming of the brain and the body. The brain meets resistance and with effort and time successfully passes through. The squeezing sets things off. It tells the body about gravity and the neuroendocrine—immune system is engaged. There is a quickening. The third ventricle is stimulated again at this time and there is a further ignition that brings potency to the centre of the brain.

In chi kung and taoist mysticism the three dan tiens are created in utero. These are described as reservoirs of chi that balance the mind and the chi/body system. The dan tiens are located in the head, heart and gut. The first 'ignitions' occur in the embryo through enfoldment, through the heart sparking into life, and through the creation of the umbilicus. The second ignitions occur at birth. As the baby is born the umbilical flow reduces and stops and the pulmonary circuit is turned on. Suddenly there is a whole new circulatory system created and now oxygen/chi/potency is brought to the body through the lungs and the heart opens up to circulating blood around this circuit. Perhaps the biggest shift is the closing down of the umbilical flow, and the gut and hepatic portal systems are suddenly on line. That's a huge leap. The nervous system is stimulated, the third ventricle potentizes, the heart and lungs open up a new circuit and the umbilical connection is dissolved creating an activation of the gut. The baby often moves its bowels during or just after birth; opening and closing movements all in the space of a few minutes. An amazing design – the body is expecting this and waiting to do it. When this goes well there is a smooth transition into postnatal health and a readiness for life outside the uterus. The baby is present and perceptive, it settles into breathing well, the nervous system recovers in an orderly way and the baby bonds, suckles, feeds and digests well.

Awareness Exercise: Three ignitions

Third ventricle

Bring your awareness to the third ventricle. You can get to this in a number of ways. The best way is to have a wide field of awareness and recognize that the centre of the awareness field is the third ventricle which is at the very centre of your brain. Acknowledge it as a fluid space. Be very gentle with your awareness as it's a place of great sensitivity. Now let your awareness settle at the third ventricle. Imagine you are looking out from this place all around you. Notice how your body responds to this. If the third ventricle is ignited and potent it should feel like there is a powerful state of presence available here. There is a connection to a potency field of great magnitude that is in relationship to the space beyond the body. If the third ventricle does not feel like this then repeat the exercise. Accessing this space should start a chain reaction that will ignite or reignite the fluid potency here.

Heart

Bringing your awareness down to the heart, let your awareness settle into the centre of the chest and locate the structure of the heart. Be interested in the internal spaces of the heart, that is, the ventricles and atria. There is a potency here that is similar to the ventricles of the brain except the spaces are in much greater motion and filled with blood. Let your awareness rest in the heart spaces with a wide connective presence. This can feel like your whole system is being oriented to the heart and its potency field. Notice the effect on the body physiology and your mind.

Umbilicus

Bring your awareness down your umbilicus. Imagine the umbilical cord, imagine you are floating in the foetal fluid space. Notice the response in your system. Is there a sense of flow or streaming in or around or out from your umbilicus? Is there a sense of a connection to a potency field around the body?

This is often the most difficult of the ignition centres to connect with as there is often so much shock here from early clamping and cutting of the umbilicus after birth. Keep repeating the exercise to establish a healthy connection.

Three ignitions

Staying at the umbilicus, make an awareness connection to the two other centres at the heart and the third ventricle. Try to be with all three equally. Notice which one or ones you are drawn to more than the others. Stay with it and be open to all three places communicating smoothly with each other. Letting a balance arise between all three will deepen your relationship to the potency spaces and help invigorate and ignite an original state of health. See if you can support ignition as a permeation of order and coherence through the bodymind, spreading outwards from the ignition centres.

Ignition in treatment

As craniosacral therapists we can palpate these places and feel their health. They are primarily expressions of potency in the physiology of the body.

Potency ignition spaces

- Third ventricle potency – expresses as a longitudinal curling, circular motion.
- Heart as a potency field – expresses as expansion and contraction.
- Umbilicus – expresses as flow in and out.

All three of these need to be in place for full expression of potency in the body, a deepening into the primal midline and a connecting to original resources. These potency movements are as vital as primary respiratory motion.

Birth can be traumatic but we have a powerful ability to recover from it. However, sometimes events are too difficult and the ignition process is interrupted or disrupted so that the nervous system does not settle and there is then a whole series of effects that can create agitation:

- Overstimulation.
- Poor breathing and diffusion across alveolar membranes.
- Gut shut down and imploded/absorption issues.
- Immune system dysfunction.
- Difficulties bonding and forming relationships.
- General low potency and poor development.

Each ignition site needs to be able to express its potency for the body and mind to function optimally. Poor ignition can result in low potency effects, poor physiology and a lack of maturation at a psychoemotional level. So changes that occur in the potency expressions of these places can powerfully change the whole system. Orienting to the potency states at each of these sites will produce a natural regeneration of motion and potency that can restimulate the original ignition process. As part of this, trauma effects can manifest that involve the autonomic nervous system. These can be difficult effects to resolve especially if the original trauma is in utero as it will have been laid down during the development of the autonomic nervous system and so potentially become embedded within it. This is the importance of relating to biodynamic health rather than the trauma effects. Offering the right relational field can facilitate these forces to emerge and bring about states of balance that begin to resolve the early tissue, fluid and potency balance.

Summary of Chapter 7

The main themes of the chapter have been the understanding of the formation of the body in utero and the birth process along with key developments of biodynamic health and expressions, in particular the development of ignition sites. Also discussed was understanding the importance of imprinting and the consequences of early experiences on the development of the body. The process of birth was introduced and in particular how this relates to the cranial base and whole body patterns.

Here are some of the many skills that can emerge from working with these factors:

- Working with whole body shapes and patterns; exploring links to the cranial base and perinatal events.

- Orienting to the cranium as a fluid membrane bag; appreciating the effect of birth stages in distorting the fluid-filled bag.

- Recognizing ignition potencies as they emerge during treatment.

- Deepening skills around facilitating resources, presence and understanding pacing and containment.

Notes

1.   According to Wikipedia (accessed Oct 2009).
2.   *Gray's Anatomy* is the source for all information in these three paragraphs on ossification of the sphenoid and SBJ.

8

Visceral Intelligence

8.1 ORGANS OVERVIEW

Introduction

The organs are characterized by their fluid nature. Most of the organs have originated from the gut tube and are endodermal in origin. The heart of course is unique and derived from specialized mesoderm. The bladder, uterus, spleen and kidneys are also mesodermal in origin.

Treating organs is making a relationship with the physiology of the body; this is where most of it takes place. It is also about relating to the autonomic nervous system rather than the somatic nervous system which is oriented towards muscles and bones. The ANS anatomy is covered in Chapter 3.

The other major feature is the strong role that connective tissues play. Organ capsules, membranes and ligaments create an infrastructure for the stability and balance of the organs. These are the organizing structures for maintaining the position and biotensegrity of the organ system.

Of pivotal importance to the visceral cavities is the diaphragm. All the organs and connective tissues are strongly linked to the health of the diaphragm.

Principles of working with organs

We will introduce a fair amount of anatomy and embryology to help you work with the gut. Initially this can feel a little daunting. There are, however, some very clear principles to working with the organs that simplify the work and cut through some of the complexities.

- Never forget the motility of the organs. Orienting to the inner breathing of the organs will naturally take you into the slower tides. The mobility (how the organ moves in relationship to other structures) and patterns of experience will often clarify when you become aware of the inner breathing.

- The embryological growth directions of the organs determine the motility and directions of movement in the adult (Barral and Mercier 1988).[1]

- The abdominal organs open like a flower around the umbilicus (Ukleja 2009a). This can be a very beautiful awareness and really orients you to the umbilicus as the natural fulcrum for the endoderm. There can be many layers of experience layered around the umbilicus: ignition, early patterns of being nourished in utero and umbilical shock from the cord being cut too soon.

- The heart moves to some extent in the same way as the sphenoid. Simply, it rolls forward on inhale (there are other more complex expressions of the heart). The heart and the sphenoid are the main structures that move in this way. It is a nice way of connecting their central importance to the functioning of the body.[2]

- The organs are a messy, non-linear place (Ukleja 2009b). They can be strongly contrasted to the more linear spine and musculoskeletal system. The organs hold deep stories, often with a strong emotional context.

- Keep an awareness of the body cavities and spaces when you work with the organs (see below for more on this).

- Relating to ignition dynamics can be very important in working with organs. Acknowledging the history of how potency spread through the thoracic cavity from the heart and the abdominal cavity from the umbilicus often deepens the contact.

The gut as a tube

The gut tube forms from endoderm. It is essentially a long tube stretching from the mouth to the anus. The identity of the gut as a tube is very obvious when you look at its embryological development. Figure 8.1.1 gives some idea of the early gut tube.

The organs of the lungs, pancreas and liver develop as buds and invaginations of the gut tube. They develop from the upper section of the tube, known as the foregut. See Figure 8.1.1.

The oesophagus, stomach, small intestine and large intestine are all sections of the tube that twist and bulge. The embryology is fascinating but a little complex (for example, at one stage the developing small intestine bulges out through the umbilical orifice, rotates and then moves back into the abdominal cavity). Figure 8.1.1 gives an introduction to the gut tube and some of its twists.

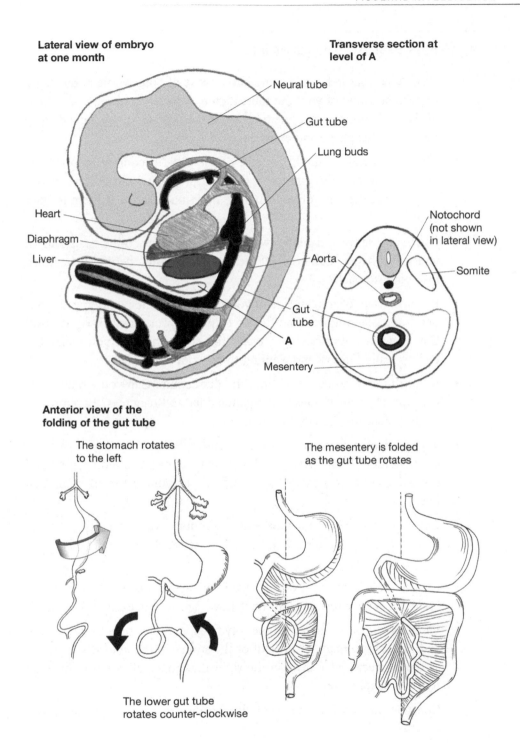

**Lateral view of embryo
at one month**

Neural tube

Gut tube

Lung buds

Heart

Diaphragm

Liver

**Transverse section at
level of A**

Notochord
(not shown
in lateral view)

Aorta

Somite

Gut
tube

A

Mesentery

**Anterior view of the
folding of the gut tube**

The stomach rotates
to the left

The mesentery is folded
as the gut tube rotates

The lower gut tube
rotates counter-clockwise

Figure 8.1.1 Development of the gut tube

Awareness Exercise: The gut as a tube

- Close your eyes, relax and come into a sense of your whole body. Begin to become aware of your gut tube. Picture the early embryo and a sense of the early gut as a midline tube at the front of the body. Spend some time with this image and experience.

- Allow the detail of the upper part of the tube to come through. How does your mouth feel right now? Is your jaw tight, can you relax your tongue into the base of your mouth, how much saliva is there in your mouth?

- Form some saliva and gently swallow. Track the wave of peristalsis down your oesophagus. Can you feel the wave pass down behind your heart, into your stomach?

- Become aware of the left side of your upper abdomen, underneath your heart and diaphragm. How full or empty is your stomach right now? Can you remember having a really full stomach? Can you remember feeling really hungry and wanting to fill your stomach?

- Move through your stomach into the duodenum. Can you visualize the C shape, the connections to the gallbladder and pancreas? Begin to get a sense of all the activity in this area.

- Take a detour into the right side under the diaphragm – feel the powerhouse of the liver. It's huge, maybe dense, fluid, warm, and humming with activity. Which words fit to your sense of your own liver?

- Come back into the gut tube and duodenum. Move through into the metres of twists and turns in the small intestine. How does it feel around your belly button?

- Picture the transition into the large intestine, go up, across and down. How full is your rectum right now, how tightly squeezed is your anus?

- Offer a sense of relaxation all the way from your jaw, to your diaphragm and cardiac sphincter, to the exit of the stomach (the pyloric sphincter), to the ileocecal valve deep in the right iliac fossa, all the way through to the anal sphincter.

- Can you finish with a sense of the whole gut tube and its accessory organs?

Cavities and membranes

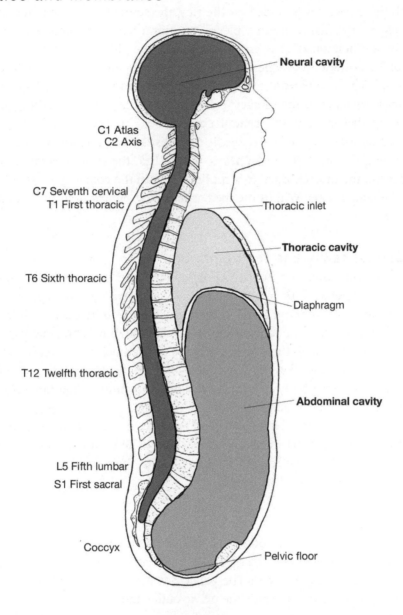

Figure 8.1.2 Neural cavity, thoracic cavity and abdominal cavity: right lateral view

It is a very useful orientation to be able to appreciate the body cavity spaces and their membranes. Tracking the fluctuation of CSF is much easier with a clear understanding of the neural cavity and the RTM. Similarly the organ dynamics are much easier to feel if an awareness of the thoracic or abdominal cavities and membranes are included. See Figures 8.1.2 and 8.1.3.

Thoracic cavity

The thoracic cavity is bounded by the ribs, the spine, the thoracic inlet and the diaphragm. It contains the two pleural cavities, each containing one lung. The bronchi and pulmonary arteries and veins enter the pleural cavities at around the level of T5 posterior to the heart. The pleural membranes are a double layer filled with fluid. The lower pressure in the pleural cavity (more a potential space) keeps the lungs expanded as the thoracic cavity increases its size on breathing air in.

The mediastinum is the central compartment of the thoracic cavity. It is bounded by loose connective tissue. It contains the heart, major vessels entering and leaving the heart, the oesophagus, the trachea, the thymus, some nerves and ganglia and the thoracic duct. It is continuous with the connective tissue hanging from the cranial base. Within the mediastinum the pericardium further envelops the heart.

Abdominal cavity and the diaphragm

With one hand over the epigastric region and the other hand on the back underneath, maybe a little lower, you are in contact with essential elements from all the major systems of the body. This hold will put you in touch with the spine, postural muscles, the lymphatic system, the end of the spinal cord, many important autonomic centres, major endocrine glands (liver, adrenals, pancreas) and nearly all the major organs (barring reproductive). The diaphragm is a wonderfully complex area of the body relating to walking, breathing, digestion, circulation and neuroendocrine–immune functions.

There is a front and a back to the abdominal cavity. The retroperitoneal space contains the kidneys, pancreas and duodenum. These structures tend to cause more referred pain to the back of the body due to their position in the posterior part of the abdominal cavity.

Pelvic cavity

The area within the pelvic bowl is continuous with the abdominal cavity but deserves a special mention. The organs of elimination and reproduction give the pelvic bowl a unique character. The pelvic bowl is much wider between the ilia and then narrows down towards the pelvic outlet and pelvic floor.

Awareness Exercise: Feeling the cavities

- Follow your breath into the thoracic cavity. See if you can have a sense of the cavity space and the organs within it.

- Follow your breathing into the abdominal cavity. Feel the different size and volume of the space and the different quality in the organs.

- Notice the difference between the upper abdomen and the pelvic cavity.

- The abdomen and the thorax are the ventral or anterior spaces of the body. Move backwards into the dorsal neural space bounded by the vertebral canal and cranium. How is this cavity, containing the central nervous system, different?

Membranes

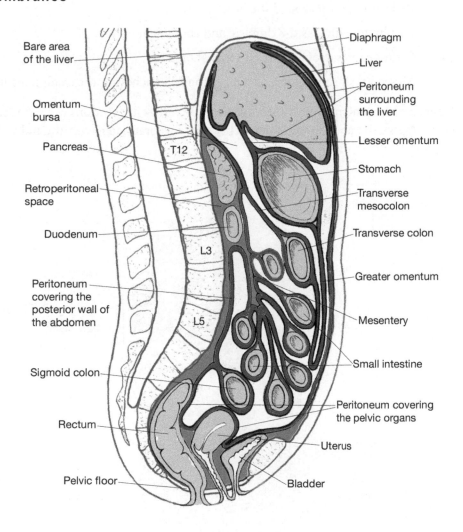

Figure 8.1.3 Peritoneum enfolding the organs of the abdomen: right lateral view

All the connective tissues of the body and the layers of fascia enveloping the organs are deeply interconnected.

A central argument for bodyworkers is that healthy organs are supported by healthy fascia – diseases of organs are associated with adhesions, scarring, dryness and compression in the enveloping connective tissue structures. Without a free flow of blood and lymph, which can be limited by fascial restrictions, organs do not work as effectively.

It is worth becoming familiar with the major connective tissue structures and membranes of the organs:

- Pleura: surround the lungs.

- Pericardium: bag around the heart.

- Diaphragm: divides the thoracic and abdominal cavities.

- Peritoneum: surrounds the abdominal organs.

- Mesentery: a subdivision of the peritoneum anchoring the small intestine.

There are also a number of named ligaments, in reality just sections of peritoneum, that support the abdominal organs. These are explored later with the individual organs.[3]

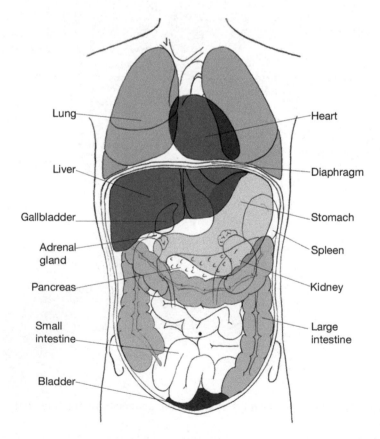

Figure 8.1.4 Topography of major organs above and below the diaphragm

Awareness Exercise: The cavities and the diaphragm

- The diaphragm is the partition between the upper and lower cavities of the torso and is in direct contact with almost all the organs of the body. Thus the health of the diaphragm has a profound effect on the health of the organs.

- The intention of this exercise is to bring you into an appreciation of the thoracic and abdominal cavities as spaces separated by the diaphragm.

- Sitting comfortably, bring your awareness to your breathing and see if you can feel the movements of the diaphragm.

- As you get a deeper connection to the diaphragm open up to the space on either side of it.

- Now invite the thoracic space into your perceptual field. Notice the size of the space and the containment of the rib cage.

- Then invite the abdominal space and notice how different the space is.

- Now be equally aware of both spaces coming together around the diaphragm. Sit with this for a few minutes and note the changes that take place.

Treatment Exercise: Biotensegrity of the peritoneum

The peritoneum is a double-layered connective tissue that wraps around most of the abdominal organs creating a supportive and nurturing environment for digestion. Its good health leads to a fluid and flexible movement that enables peristalsis and free movement of blood, lymph and nervous flow. As a communication device, the peritoneum is a wonderful structure to relate to for a craniosacral therapist. Just like the dura mater it is composed of one continuous sheet of membrane that contains the liver, stomach, small and large intestines and spleen. Any distortions in the membrane will reveal itself to the sensitive touch awareness.

1. Make contact at the abdomen.

- Organize your chair so that it is next to the abdominal area of the body of your client. Bring a hand into the lumbar arch and the other hand onto the surface of the abdominal wall. Try to avoid the umbilicus as there is a strong energy there.

2. Orient to the peritoneum.

- Invite the peritoneum into your hands. Sometimes imagining the anatomical structure can help. You are looking for a sense of continuity and biotensegrity across and throughout the whole abdominal space. The sense you get in the dura mater of a whole unit of function can be felt here too.

3. Orient to the attachments (Stone 2007).

   • The peritoneum is an organ bag and you will feel it enfolding around and into the organs of the gut. For the most part the peritoneum is free moving; however, it has major attachments into the diaphragm, particularly around the liver, the stomach and the hepatic and splenic flexures of the colon.

   • The colon has extensive attachments. The transverse colon attaches indirectly to the posterior wall of the abdomen via the fascia covering the pancreas at around L1. The ascending and descending colon are firmly attached, via the kidney fascia, to the posterior wall.

   • The root of the mesenteries of the small intestine is the other major attachment site. The root of the mesentery indirectly (the duodenum is in the way) attaches to the back wall of the abdomen into the lumbars, around L2 and L3.

   • The retroperitoneal structures are sealed to the back wall. These are the kidneys, the pancreas and the duodenum. The duodenum is the only section of the gut tube that loops posteriorly into the retroperitoneal space.

4. Orient to patterns of experience.

   • Any distortions in the peritoneum will show themselves as tensions or places of inertia in the connective tissue. These can be formed by adhesions, scar tissue or strain patterns. So relating to the peritoneum is both a way of assessing health and a treatment process.

   • Sit back and create the right contact for the inherent treatment plan to unfold.

8.2 ORGAN ANATOMY AND DYNAMICS
Thoracic cavity
Lungs

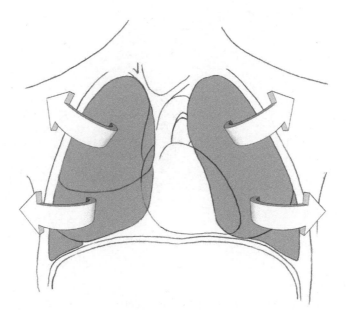

Figure 8.2.1 Lungs on inhale
The upper lobes roll out at a more oblique angle

Primary respiration: The lungs express internal and external rotation. The different lobes have different axes of rotation because the bronchial tube enters them at different angles. The upper lobes have a diagonal axis and the lower lobes a vertical one. The lobes (three on the right and two on the left) should slide over each other.

Anatomy: Movement is felt through the covering and supporting layer of the pleura. The upper lobes and pleura hang from C7, T1 and the first rib by the suspensory ligaments.

Embryology: Both the trachea and lungs develop from the foregut which itself becomes the oesophagus.

Clinical focus: Adhesions to pericardium or diaphragm, between the pleural layers, to the ribs or in connective tissues between lobes. Dynamics of the lungs are very tied into the transverse diaphragms of the thoracic inlet and the respiratory diaphragm, hyperventilation and upper chest breathing in activated states and the dynamics of the ribs and thoracic spine.

Heart and pericardium

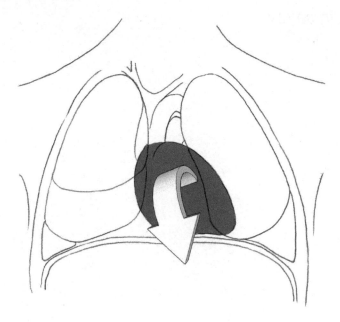

Figure 8.2.2 Heart on inhale
The heart rolls forward on inhale; see text for more detail

Primary respiration: There are many possibilities that reflect its complex embryological growth. Most simply the heart expresses inhalation around a transverse axis and follows the sphenoid. You can also feel the top of the heart drops slightly to the right as there is a slight twist in the roll forward. There can also be a sense of an uprising spiral through the heart following the formation of the vessels and chambers. Finally there can just be a sense of the motility of an expanding heart filling the thoracic cavity. A very pleasant feeling.

Anatomy: The pericardium is a major feature of the thorax and has strong ligamentous connections to the diaphragm, sternum, vertebrae at T2 and T5, the cranial base and the thyroid, hyoid and mandible.

Embryology: The heart and diaphragm have the same embryological origins in the cardiogenic area of the embryonic disc. The heart folds into the centre of the growing embryo at a very early stage and the growing brain leads the embryonic disc to curl around the heart. This is one part of the rolling-forward element that can be felt in the adult heart. Another similar embryological movement occurs as the heart tube folds over itself as the ventricles grow over and then up and behind the atrial chambers. This latter movement has a right to left element as well. Finally there is a complex uprising spiral movement within the heart as the vessels and chambers take up their final positions.

Clinical focus: A very important organ in terms of emotional context and ignition dynamics. The nature of the heart is very expansive; in the early embryo it is a relatively big structure occupying lots of space.

Abdominal cavity

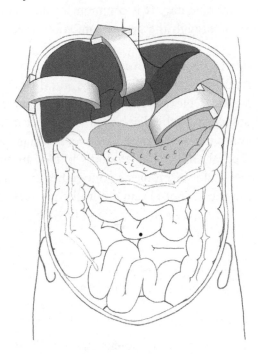

Figure 8.2.3 Liver and stomach on inhale

Liver

Primary respiration: The liver expresses internal and external rotation around an oblique axis. It rotates superiorly and laterally in inhalation, the lower border lifting diagonally away from the umbilicus.

Anatomy: The liver lies in a parietal enfoldment of the peritoneum underneath the diaphragm on the right side of the body. It is attached to the diaphragm by several large ligaments:

- The falciform ligament (a fold of the peritoneum) which attaches to the diaphragm and anteriorly to the abdominal wall then continues on as the round ligament (of Teres) to the umbilicus. This is the remnant of the umbilical vein.

- The coronary ligament and the right and left triangular ligaments connect the diaphragm to the liver.

- The liver is connected to the stomach via the lesser omentum. Enervation comes from T7–10 and the vagus nerve.

Clinical focus: The area around the liver should feel warm as the liver contains large amounts of blood and is very active in its physiology. The back of the liver curls round the vena cava. The liver should feel mobile and move freely, enabled by the serous fluids in its membrane bag. It is common for adhesions to occur around any of the ligaments or through the peritoneum when there is dehydration and stagnation.

From the right side in supine, it is easiest to contact the liver with one hand on the side of the ribs or one hand under the ribs and the other along the margin of the ribs up to the solar plexus. The liver is intimately associated with the diaphragm. Any dysfunction of the diaphragm will affect it. If the diaphragm is tight and fixed the liver will feel the same. The liver is a huge factory for the body, a filter and waste disposal unit, and it produces bile as an aid for the digestion of fats. Digestive issues and liver problems go together. It is also important in the immune response. The hepatic portal vein drains the products of the gut tube into the liver. Congestion in the liver will limit blood flow from the gut and can cause a wide range of digestive issues.

Treatment Exercise: Working with the liver

1. Overview of working with the liver.

   - The liver is an enormously potent structure in the body that is both physiologically and anatomically significant. The liver is a factory of activity that regulates most chemical levels in the blood, stores vital substances and in the process creates lots of heat that helps keep the body warm. Along with the kidneys and the heart, it is one of the essential organs to learn to treat.

   - Its size makes it the largest single organ in the body and its juxtaposition with the diaphragm provides a strong relationship to the breath.

   - In Chinese medicine it is considered the General and its healthy function allows all chi to move through all the other organs freely. Liver stagnation is a very common condition and craniosacral therapy can help free up the liver.

   - Often you will be drawn to the liver through priorities set by the inherent treatment plan. The liver can have a big effect on the connective tissue matrix, major blood vessels and the digestive system.

2. Making contact at the liver.

- Bring your hands to your practice client's liver. The liver is so big it's useful to make contact with the whole of it, one hand above and one on the side or below.

- Upper hand: Place one hand across the anterior part of the liver so your fingers make contact with the solar plexus area.

- Deep to this part of the body is the left lobe of the liver. The bigger right lobe is housed under the whole of the right lung and diaphragm down as far as the margin of the rib cage. (If you bring your hands to the inferior margin of the ribs on the right you should be able to feel the edge of the liver protrude on inhalation.)

- Lower hand: Place your other hand on the side of or underneath the lower rib cage.

3. Orient to primary respiration.

- You should be able to get a sense of the density of the liver between your hands; notice where you are drawn to in or around the liver. Perhaps you are drawn more towards one lobe, or perhaps to the diaphragm or to the gut. Patterns of experience will often involve the liver.

- Try to tune into the primary respiratory motion of the liver. You should feel a rolling movement around an angled transverse axis. Adjustment in the liver will lead to systemic changes.

Stomach

Primary respiration: The stomach expresses an external and internal rotation around an oblique axis; it rotates up and diagonally away from the umbilicus in inhalation. It also expresses a slight rotation around an anterior posterior axis.

Anatomy: The stomach is a J-shaped organ suspended under the diaphragm and the liver by folds of mesentery. According to Stone (2007, p.156), 'The stomach swings like a hammock under the liver and diaphragm.'[4] Essentially the stomach ligaments are part of one extended structure, though various ligaments are named. It is connected to the liver via the hepatogastric ligament (part of the lesser omentum). The greater omentum attaches to the lower border of the stomach like an apron trailing down in front of the peritoneum. The position and tone of the stomach is highly variable; the lower border can sag downwards. Obviously it also fills and empties and changes shape during digestion.

Pancreas

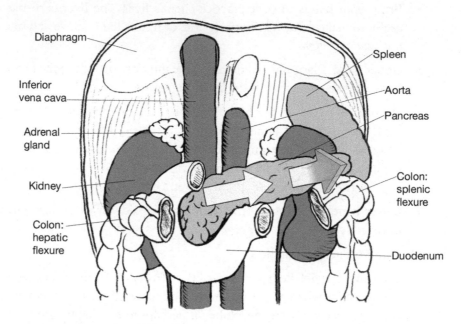

Figure 8.2.4 Pancreas on inhale
The pancreas lengthens towards its tail and curls anteriorly

Primary respiration: It lengthens towards its tail in inhalation with a slight anterior rotation of the tail (Sills 2009b).

Anatomy: The pancreas lies at a slight angle posterior to the greater curve of the stomach. The head of the pancreas rests in the duodenum and the tail points towards the spleen. The body of the pancreas is anterior to the vertebral body of L1.[5]

The organ is a key endocrine and exocrine organ. At its head, the pancreatic duct joins with the bile duct, draining digestive enzymes into the duodenum via the sphincter of Oddi. The tail of the pancreas rests anteriorly to the spleen.

Clinical focus: The pancreas is commonly a major influence on digestive issues and tiredness. It is retroperitoneal and can be felt by orienting towards the back of the abdominal cavity on the left.

Spleen

Primary respiration: The spleen expresses internal and external rotation around a vertical axis and descends in inhalation.

Anatomy: It acts as a super-charged lymph node for the blood circulation and it acts as a blood reservoir. It lies under the left leaf of the diaphragm. It is attached to the stomach via the gastrosplenic ligament and to the posterior wall of the peritoneum via the splenorenal ligament. Stone describes the spleen as tucked into a pocket of peritoneum that is part of the greater omentum (Stone 2007, pp.115 and 117).

Small intestine

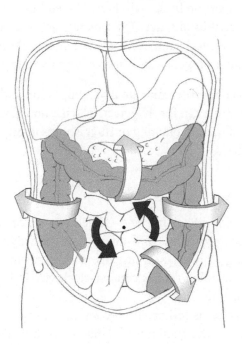

Figure 8.2.5 Large intestine and small intestine on inhale
The large intestine rolls out, opening like a flower from the umbilicus. The small intestine (and large intestine as a whole) rotates counter-clockwise

Primary respiration: It expresses its primary respiration motion following its embryological spiralling. It rotates/uncurls counter-clockwise in inhalation and rotates/curls in a clockwise direction in exhalation. It expresses a strong motility when healthy which feels like an expansion on inhalation throughout. Stone (2007, pp.116–123) describes the coils of the intestine as subtly swinging and wafting as they hang from the root of the mesentery.

Anatomy: The small intestine is invested in its mesentery. The loose connective layer of the mesentery supports the nerve and blood supply. It is part of the gastrointestinal tract engaged in absorbing nutrients from food and is about 6 m long. It is held in the middle and lower abdomen and is surrounded above and on its sides by the colon, in the front by the greater omentum and connected to the spine at L3 by the root of the mesentery, attaching over the transverse duodenum.

The duodenum is a part of the small intestine of special interest. As the end of the stomach becomes the duodenum the tube loops backwards into the retroperitoneal space. It forms a 3D shape like the letter C. It is firmly attached to the posterior wall via the renal fascia, the psoas and right arcuate ligament of the diaphragm. The end of the C, the duo-jejunum junction, is suspended by the ligament of Treitz from the back wall. From the end of the C the rest of the gut tube returns to the peritoneal space. The pancreas and the bile duct discharge into the mid portion of the duodenum. A lot of hormones are secreted and produced in this region of the gut to regulate stomach activity and digestive enzymes.

Clinical focus: Commonly there may be fluid congestion and toxic build up in the lymphatics. The intestine can feel hyperactive, tense and hard if there are IBS-type symptoms or static if there is bloating or sluggishness in digestion. It can also hold umbilical shock effects.

Large intestine

Primary respiration: The ascending and descending colon can act like a paired organ and show some external and internal rotation dynamics. They can also express a shortening in inhalation just like the deepening of the curves of the spine. As a whole the colon rotates counter-clockwise in inhalation following its embryological formation.

The transverse colon is intimately in contact with the stomach, liver, kidneys and spleen and follows the craniosacral dynamics of the mid organs.

Anatomy: The large intestine rises on the right side of the body, traverses across the body just under the liver and stomach and descends into the right side of the pelvis where it flexes into the sigmoid colon and rectum. It is attached by a complex mesentery carrying blood and nerve supplies. It touches all the other organs of the abdomen. This is a hollow digestive organ. You may well notice slow rhythmic peristaltic movements as the organ goes about its digestive functions.

The transverse large intestine is attached posteriorly to the abdominal wall via the mesocolon attaching to the pancreas, and is suspended from the diaphragm via the suspensory ligaments at the hepatic and splenic flexures. The ascending colon and descending colon are firmly attached, over the kidneys via Toldt's fascia, to the posterior abdominal wall. Stone describes three relatively fixed sections of the colon – the ascending colon, descending colon and rectum – and three mobile sections – the caecum, transverse colon and sigmoid colon (Stone 2007, p.123). The size and arrangements of the mobile sections can be very varied. Barium X-rays of the large intestine show that it is rarely the neat-ordered shape shown in textbooks.

Clinical focus: Adhesions to the diaphragm, contractions in the suspensory ligaments and toxicity within the colon. The iliocaecal valve is commonly the cause of many colon symptoms.

Kidneys

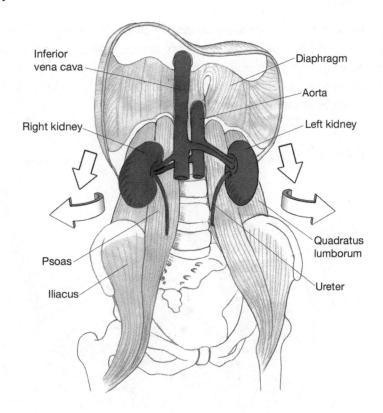

Figure 8.2.6 Kidneys on inhale
The kidneys drop down along the psoas muscle and externally rotate over the belly of the psoas

Primary respiration: In inhalation, the motility of the kidneys can be felt as an expanding away from the umbilicus and a dropping down and out; on exhale they gather into the centre and rise up. The mobility of the kidneys is a descent and rotation outwards over the belly of psoas muscle.

Anatomy: The right kidney is slightly lower than the left due to the presence of the liver. The kidneys are surrounded by a fibrous capsule, perirenal and pararenal fat and two layers of renal fascia. The kidneys slide inferior and superior (between the anterior and posterior layers of fascia) and roll out over the psoas due to movements of the diaphragm. The kidneys are retroperitoneal and so lie behind the peritoneum, out of the digestive environment. The blood pressure from the aorta plays a role in supporting the tone of the kidneys. There is a very strong relationship between the kidneys and the psoas muscle.[6]

Embryology: Embryologically the kidneys began life in the pelvis and then rose up through the body.

Clinical focus: Renal fascia connects superiorly to the diaphragmatic fascia and also connects to the fascia around the psoas muscles bringing the kidneys into strong relationship with breathing and walking. The kidneys are one of the most common and responsive organs to treat. The adrenal glands are located above the kidneys and can be strongly felt when they are active.

Pelvic cavity

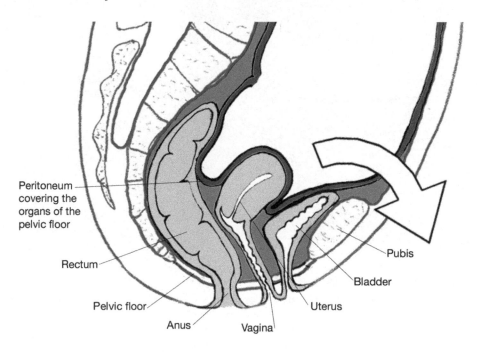

Figure 8.2.7 Uterus and bladder on inhale
In a male the prostate inhales in the same way as the bladder

Bladder

Primary respiration: The bladder in inhalation moves the same as the sphenoid.

Anatomy: It is a hollow muscular organ located posterior to the pubic symphysis and connected to it via the pubovesical ligament. It is surrounded by vesical fascia, which becomes the median umbilical ligament and connects to the umbilicus. In males the bladder is directly anterior to the rectum and in females the vagina is between the rectum and bladder.

Clinical focus: Common issues are fascial adhesions to surrounding structures, pressure from surrounding organs, hypotonicity of bladder sphincter muscles and laxity of pelvic floor.

Uterus, ovaries and prostate

Primary respiration: The uterus follows the movement of the sphenoid. Ovaries express internal and external rotation around an oblique axis. The prostate follows the bladder.

Anatomy: The uterus is supported by the broad ligaments and suspensory ligaments. It is continuous with the fascia of the psoas muscle. The ovaries are connected to the superior border of the uterus by the round ligaments. Structurally the broad ligament is the key structure for stabilizing and supporting the uterus and ovaries.

Clinical focus: Commonly there is a sense of stagnation or absence in the pelvic bowl associated with menstrual and fertility issues.

Clinical Highlight: Working with organs

Relating to organs is quite different than to any other tissues. The main feature is the lack of bony structure and the predominance of connective tissues. Like the central nervous system the action of organs is highly fluid-like. The membranes and ligaments that create the framework for the integrity of the organs in both the thoracic and particularly the abdominal cavities are very mobile and allow for a high degree of freedom of movement. In a healthy system primary respiration can be felt very clearly.

Another strong sense is the movement of blood as it courses down through the aorta; fresh blood courses out into all the organs. The major blood vessels are much more palpable here.

The organs can be divided into organs derived from the endodermal gut tube which includes the lungs and trachea, the liver and gallbladder, the pancreas and of course the stomach, duodenum, small intestine, large intestine and rectum. The kidneys, spleen and heart are all formed from mesoderm. The most distinctive organ is the heart, which is a specialized muscle. Things to remember when treating organs:

- Always listen to the membranes, in particular the pericardium and peritoneum, as they are attached to many other structures and therefore create connections across different tissue fields. The pericardium brings the cranial base, the rib cage, the spine, the heart and the diaphragm into mechanical relationships. The peritoneum brings the diaphragm, the spine and most of the organs of the abdomen into direct relationship.

• Be open to the autonomic nervous system expressing itself. This is the visceral nervous system and has a strong presence through the front cavities. If someone's system is emotionally charged or there is sympathetic activation you will need to relate to the nervous system directly. Getting to know the plexi and the sympathetic chains will help immeasurably.

• You might become aware of a change in the chemical balance within an organ or across organs as the body adjusts both mechanically and physiologically. Changes in the tissues create a new biochemical environment, which affects both the endocrine and the nervous system.

• A sensation of a gut midline may reveal itself to you. This is one of the original midlines to form in the first few weeks of life and, even though the gut has undergone dramatic transformation in size and complexity, the original midline is still there as an energetic quality.

Summary of Chapter 8

We treat the organs all the time and are endlessly excited by the changes that can manifest by being skilful with the viscera. This chapter explored the primary respiratory expressions of the organs. A key aspect was understanding how the embryology underpins the mobility and motility of the organs. We also stressed the importance of the membranes connecting and surrounding the organs and orienting to the cavities that contain the organs. A very simple approach is to appreciate the abdominal organs opening like a flower around the umbilicus and the heart expanding to fill the thoracic cavity.

Key skills from this chapter:

• Ability to work precisely with the pericardium and its connection to other structures, especially the link between the cranial base and the diaphragm.

• Ability to relate to the peritoneum as a visceral reciprocal tension membrane system.

• Orienting to the fluid nature of organs and the physiology of the body.

- Starting to get a sense of the gut tube and its particular potency and movement expressions.

- Ability to orientate to body cavities as internal spaces.

- Understanding the holistic nature of viscera, fluids, nervous system and potency and their interaction.

- Learning to differentiate the motility and mobility of the major organs and appreciating their different personalities.

Notes

1. This was one of the early, defining insights that emerged from Jean Pierre Barral's extensive investigations of treating organs osteopathically.
2. Strictly speaking the bladder, uterus and prostate also move the same way as the sphenoid, but it is easier to orient to their movements as an opening around the umbilicus.
3. Barral and Mercier (1988) and Stone (2007) are excellent resources for detailed anatomy of the organs and osteopathic approaches to organ dynamics.
4. This is a great quote from Stone. All other ligamentous relationships described in this paragraph can also be found in Stone (2007).
5. Acland (2004) states the head of the pancreas is over the body of L1. Stone (2007) describes the pancreas as being 'draped' over the upper lumbar spine.
6. 'The relationship between the kidneys and the psoas is one of the most marked within whole-body mechanics and kidney tensions can therefore spread up to the cranial base or down into the sacroiliac joints, hip and lower limbs to the feet, as a result of compromised psoas function' (Stone 2007, p.159).

9

Neural Matrix

9.1 NEURAL MATRIX OVERVIEW

Treating the brain

It is interesting that you have probably by now put your hands on someone's head many times, and for the most part you are noticing fluids, bones and membranes but perhaps you are not so aware of the natural movements of the brain. The brain fills most of the intracranial cavity and is the single biggest structure under your hands. It is also the oldest thing under your hands in terms of the order of embryological formation.

The neurons have been with you all your life as they do not undergo cell division. There is a strong potency in the central nervous system. Nerve tissue is unique in how it feels and as you get used to feeling the detail of the brain you will notice how each part of it has distinct properties. One of the most obvious differences is between the dense and solid cerebellum compared to lighter, spongier, ventricle-filled cerebral hemispheres.

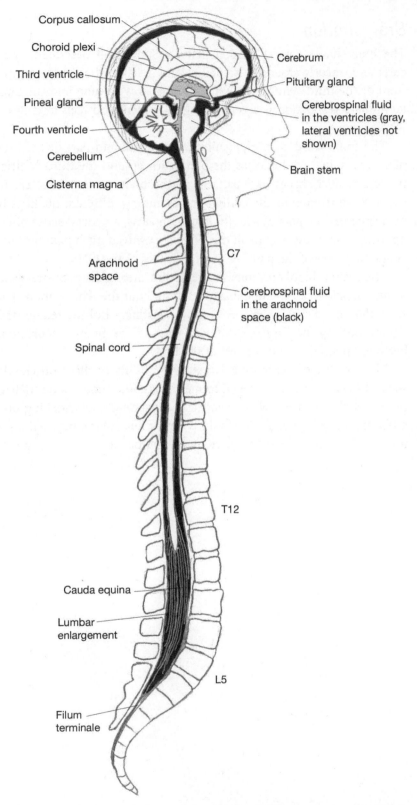

Figure 9.1.1 Overview of the central nervous system showing spaces occupied by cerebrospinal fluid

Brain motion

The brain has a natural motion that Dr Sutherland described as a motility. It curls and uncurls around a natural fulcrum, called the lamina terminalis, at the front of the third ventricle. When you learn how to tune into the brain's motion, its primary respiration is a very strong movement and feels as if it underpins the whole system.

The spinal cord is an elongation of the brain and part of the original neural tube. The spinal cord rises as the brain curls around the third ventricle. You will be able to feel shapes and patterns in the brain as quite distinct features. For example, restriction of the curling and uncurling, different qualities between the hemispheres, hotspots of activity in certain areas, a general sense of charge or the opposite, and a loss of tone in the CNS. Unresolved birth patterns and trauma are common causes of the patterns of experiences of the CNS.

The brain is highly responsive to emotion. Strong states of stress and emotional disorganization can create imbalance throughout the whole brain. The brain acts as an integrated unit when it is healthy. Creating a holistic relational field can be deeply healing, helping the different parts of the brain to communicate better between themselves and the rest of the body.

The motility of the brain is largely the motility of the ventricles. Figure 9.2.1 shows how the nervous system is formed as a tube around the ventricles. Sutherland gave us a classic image of the ventricles expanding and widening on inhale, like a bird opening its wings. The brain is a very fluid place, so orienting to both the flow of CSF and of blood are very useful approaches.

9.2 THE FLUID BRAIN

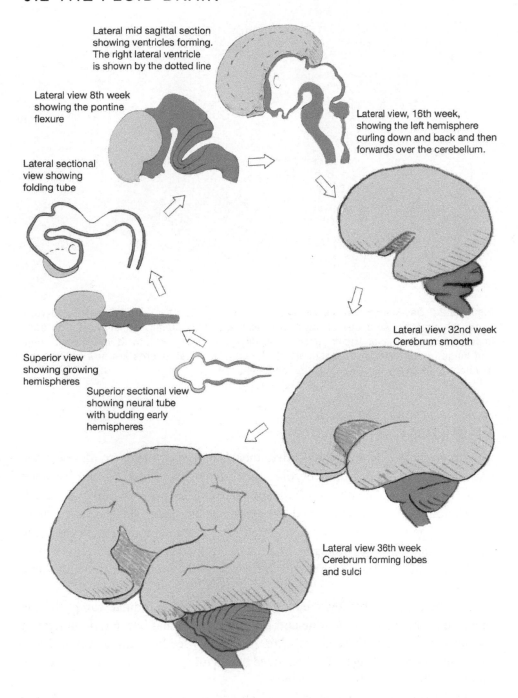

Lateral mid sagittal section showing ventricles forming. The right lateral ventricle is shown by the dotted line

Lateral view 8th week showing the pontine flexure

Lateral view, 16th week, showing the left hemisphere curling down and back and then forwards over the cerebellum.

Lateral sectional view showing folding tube

Superior view showing growing hemispheres

Superior sectional view showing neural tube with budding early hemispheres

Lateral view 32nd week Cerebrum smooth

Lateral view 36th week Cerebrum forming lobes and sulci

Figure 9.2.1 Development of the brain from the anterior neural tube

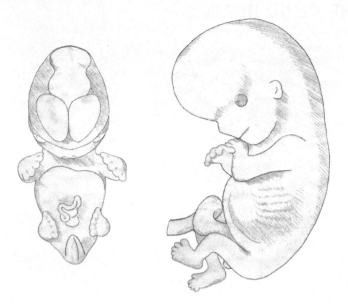

Figure 9.2.2 Development of the embryo. Left: At 51 to 53 days (8 weeks) the embryo is about 20 mm long. An image of the neural tube, with the bulging hemispheres, has been imposed over the head. Right: At 56 to 60 days the embryo is now about 30 mm long. The bulge in the abdomen is mostly liver. The organs and structures are now largely fully developed; from this time on, the term foetus is used

Embryology of the brain

The brain starts life as a fluid-filled tube but quickly starts to develop the characteristic bulges that will become the different parts of the brain by week three. The process of neuralation (formation of the CNS) occurs rapidly, producing huge amounts of neurons that need to be organized in space. This means the brain has to change shape in order to accommodate as many neurons as possible in the neurocranium, especially the large cerebral hemispheres which start to grow over the lower and mid brain sections from front to back throughout the embryonic period.

The brain does this by creating flexures, big longitudinal curves in the brainstem. These are the pontine and cervical flexures that become prominent in the second month of the embryo's life. As you can see from the embryonic and foetal development images, the fluid-filled neural tube is still intact throughout the process of brain growth and movement.

Neuralation takes place outside and around the original fluid space. As the brain takes on new shapes the fluid space changes shape to produce what are called the ventricles of the brain. These are distinct fluid spaces at the core of the cerebrum (lateral ventricles), mid brain (third ventricle) and brainstem (fourth ventricle) which are interconnected by thin canals. An interesting question to pose is whether the fluid space is being modified through brain growth and is therefore accommodating it, or whether the brain growth and shape is being originated by the fluid space.

The neural tube is the beginning of the fluid midline and is considered a powerful organizing midline. As you become more familiar with the ventricles you will notice how they act as reservoirs of potency which can be felt distinctly during stillpoints as they potentize themselves and bring health to the core of the body.

Awareness Exercise: Differentiating parts of the brain

- Place your hands on the top of your head so that each hand is over a hemisphere. Underneath the bones and membranes is the cerebrum, the upper brain. Keep your hands in place with a light touch and allow the bones and membranes to dissolve. You should be able to feel the cerebrum; it's got a particular consistency to it and its electrical flows vary from side to side. It's divided into particular lobes which have different functions so you should also be able to differentiate the lobes from each other. Move your hands around so that you can do that.

- Now if you move your hands to the back of your head, you should be able to sense the transition between the upper brain and the hind brain of the cerebellum. The tent divides them from each other. The cerebellum has a unique function and its activity and structure are quite distinct. It also has two hemispheres.

- Finally there is the brainstem which is deep to the cerebellum. Invite it into your hands. The brainstem is like an extension of the spinal cord, but also contains groups of nerve nuclei that control many of the basic functions of the autonomic nervous system.

- At the top of the brainstem is the thalamus which is the relay station of the brain. It distributes sensory information that comes in from all over the body to different regions of the brain. The other important parts of this area are the hypothalamus and the limbic system, both of which are strongly related to emotional states of being and to production of hormones.

Ventricles, CSF and deep potency

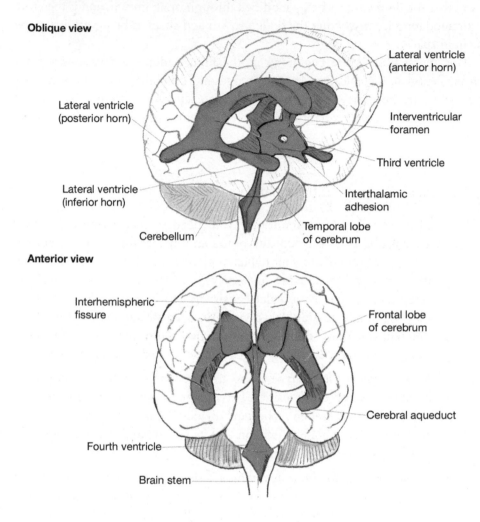

Oblique view

Lateral ventricle (anterior horn)

Lateral ventricle (posterior horn)

Interventricular foramen

Lateral ventricle (inferior horn)

Third ventricle

Interthalamic adhesion

Cerebellum

Temporal lobe of cerebrum

Anterior view

Interhemispheric fissure

Frontal lobe of cerebrum

Cerebral aqueduct

Fourth ventricle

Brain stem

Figure 9.2.3 Oblique and anterior views of the ventricles within the brain

> The fascia! Even the fascia is water, even the bony tissue is liquid… Fluid! A fundamental principle in our cranial concept. Fluctuation of the cerebrospinal fluid. A motion like that of the tide of the ocean. Something that is governed by the same Intelligence that governs the tide of ocean governs the rotation of the earth, the sun, the moon and all the planets. (Sutherland 1998, p.290)

In a healthy system the ventricles should be glowing with health and then the brain can function with greater energy and efficiency. You will notice too that some of the ventricles can feel depleted or indistinct and this can lead to a general lowering of the system energy and functional difficulties. Encouraging the ventricles to charge up is a key outcome in biodynamic craniosacral therapy.

The original neural tube is still present in the spinal cord as a thin central canal running down from the fourth ventricle through the centre of the cord emerging in the lumbosacral waterbed at L2. The spinal cord stops here as a unit and breaks up into fibre tracts called the cauda equinae (horse's tail). There is a lumbar enlargement of the vertebral canal that accommodates the fibre tracts. This means that there is a large amount of cerebrospinal fluid (CSF) around the lower part of the central nervous system (CNS). This is referred to as a waterbed.

Where there is CSF there is a powerful connection to potency. Potency particularly manifests within the CSF and in particular around the areas of the waterbeds and ventricles. The lumbar waterbed in some ways acts energetically as a lower fifth ventricle. The other significant waterbed is the cisterna magna around the cerebellum and behind the lower occiput.

CSF originates in the choroid plexi in all four ventricles. The plexi are like filter-beds which sieve the blood to allow the plasma and certain electrolytes to enter the ventricular spaces. Physiologically CSF provides support and protection for the brain; it protects against acute changes in arterial and venous blood pressure; it is a route of waste excretion, replacing in many ways the function of lymphatics (the brain has no lymphatics); it helps maintain the ionic homeostasis of the CNS.

CSF is produced at the rate of 500 ml/day and occupies a volume of 150 ml (adults). Consequently, CSF turns over every 8 hours (Martini 1998).[1] Two-thirds of the CSF is produced in the choroid plexuses of the cerebral ventricles. One-third of the CSF is formed via fluid shifts across the cerebral capillaries.

CSF is produced at the core of the brain and then fluctuates[2] around the surface of the brain and spinal cord exiting the ventricular system via small apertures in the brainstem. It then returns to the blood circulation via the arachnoid granulations into the venous sinus system. It is vital that this flow is unimpeded as it will lower the energy of the whole system if there is congestion. This can occur through constriction within the cranium or from back pressure into the head from poor venous blood return to the heart.

Tuning into longitudinal fluctuation will have the effect of creating better fluctuation of CSF. Sutherland (following A.T. Still) described CSF as containing the 'highest known element in the body' and as having a particularly strong relationship with the potency of the breath of life. He likened this to a fluid within the fluid. It is worth quoting Sutherland's own words:

> The cerebrospinal fluid, with its 'highest known element,' is considered as the *fundamental unit* in the functioning of the mechanism. I have frequently referred, during class instruction, to Dr Still's highest known element as a *primary* Breath of Life that was breathed into a form of clay, according to scriptural record, and emphasized the thought that it was *not* the breath

of material air utilized in man's walkabout on earth. In another symbolic illustration, this was likened to a 'liquid-within-a-liquid.' The element has also been symbolized in its function as like sheet-lightning which *lights up* the cloud in a brilliant array, though invisible as is the X-ray. (Sutherland 1998, p.299; italics as per original text)

9.3 THE BRAIN AND BLOOD
Blood supply to the brain

The heart and the brain live right next to each other in the early days of the body, and perhaps that early relationship forges an unforgettable bond between them. The heart's first priority is to supply blood to the brain. The heart will shut down blood to everywhere else in the body before stopping its supply to the brain.

The brain is thirsty. It needs gallons and gallons of blood each day to function properly, so it is of the utmost importance that the heart is healthy and strong and the bloodways are clear. As a craniosacral therapist you can help the passageway for blood in the neck and in the cranium.

The body in all its wisdom has created two arterial passageways to the brain. The main one is through the two carotid arteries and the other way is through the two vertebral arteries. The vertebral arteries come up through the neck inside a foramen within the transverse processes of the cervical vertebrae. The first artery to come off the aortic arch is the coronary artery which is the feed to the heart and the second one is the carotid artery. The third is the brachiocephalic artery and the vertebral artery comes off this.

Therefore, any tension in the neck and compressions or rotations in the cervical vertebrae will have a profound effect on blood flow to the head. Often during or after craniosacral therapy sessions you can feel shifts in the arterial flow as the neck lets go of tension patterns. Don't be surprised if you can think more clearly after a session. One of the reasons is probably because the brain is receiving unimpeded blood flow.

Lots of people carry deep tension in different sets of muscles in the neck, in particular the trapezius and the supra and infra hyoid muscles. Many people experience stiffness in their neck due to poor posture, injuries and emotional tension all resulting in reduced blood flow to the brain and perhaps more importantly poor blood return through the jugular veins.

Blood is pumped up the carotid arteries. The arteries are surrounded by the carotid sheath. This is part of the deep cervical fascia linking the diaphragm, heart, throat and cranial base. It also surrounds the jugular vein and the vagus nerve. The carotid sheath is an important structure that affects blood to the brain, blood return from the brain and the autonomic nervous system. The carotid sheath passes deep in the neck from the insertion of the SCM (sternocleidomastoid muscle) along the side of the thyroid and larynx and divides into the internal and external carotid arteries. The external carotids go to the face and the exterior of the head and the internal carotids pass through the cranial base into the circle of Willis.

The circle of Willis is like a blood 'ring mains' for the brain that is fed by the vertebral arteries and the internal carotids. It's literally a ring-like structure at the bottom of the brain that has a whole series of cerebral arteries moving out from it into all parts of the brain. The two vertebral arteries enter the neurocranium via the foramen magnum and converge to form the basilar artery passing over the SBJ. Via the basilar artery the vertebral arteries flow into the circle of Willis.

The two internal carotid arteries pass through the cranial base via oblique-running bony tunnels in the petrous portions of the temporal bones: the carotid canals. The internal carotids enter the neurocranium via the foramen lacerum,[3] at the medial superior end of the carotid canal. The foramen lacerum is situated between the tip of the petrous temporal bone and the basilar portion of the sphenoid. So the relationship of these bones could deeply affect the function of the carotid artery if there is compression in the joint or restriction in the primary respiration of the temporal bone.

Awareness Exercise: The carotid flow

- Come into a felt sense of your heart and feel how strongly blood is being pumped out of the left side of the heart into the aorta. This is where blood pressure is at its strongest.

- You can feel the aortic arch as a strong shape in your upper chest and off the arch extends the carotid arteries. Follow their passage up through the thoracic inlet, through the deep muscles of the throat, through the cranial base and into the circle of Willis.

- Notice how the left and right differ; one of them will feel more constricted. Notice too any places that feel they are having a particular effect on the flow; commonly this is around the thoracic inlet and the foramen lacerum, but strong contractions in the neck muscles can also affect things such as dural tensions around the arteries' entry into the subdural space.

- Now be with the power of the blood flow up from the aortic arch into the circle of Willis. This feels like a motorway, it's so strong and fast. Feel how potent arterial blood is.

Blood return

The dural enfoldments of the falx and tent act as the sites for most of the brain's venous return. Formed between the two dural layers, simple tube-like structures called sinuses form a network around the brain that drain into main collecting sinuses in the falx and tent. Unlike veins, these structures do not have a muscle layer and nor do they have valves.

The direction of blood flow is from the front of the head to the back of the head and to the confluence of sinuses. Then it flows into the transverse sinuses and into the jugular veins. The jugular veins exit the cranium through the jugular foramen in the suture between the occiput and the temporal bones. The vagus nerve exits with it and together they join the carotid sheath for passage through the neck. The jugular veins connect into the superior vena cava.

The health of the dura mater will have a profound effect on the ability of blood to return smoothly through the sinuses and back to the heart. Dural tension, adhesion and drag can exert a strong effect on the flow through the sinuses and can result in a back-pressure in the head. Craniosacral therapy can relieve these effects, thus freeing up the pathways to the heart by relating to key structures within this system, in particular the sagittal sinus, the transverse sinus, the straight sinus and the cavernous sinus along with the occipitomastoid suture.

Treatment Exercise: Relating to the venous sinuses[4]

1. Overview.

    • In order to get to know the sinus system better and to appreciate the critical nature of certain structures in the healthy flow back to the heart, it's useful to practise moving through the system from top to bottom so that you can feel the effects of the system releasing in sections.

2. Explore by working from front to back: sagittal sinus, transverse sinus, jugular foramen, carotid sheath and thoracic inlet.

    • Working from front to back in the head makes most sense as the blood return is in that direction. Start by contacting the superior sagittal sinus under the frontal bone by lining up your finger tips along the length of the metopic line. Stay with this for a few minutes and you should notice a softening in the falx and therefore the sinus. Continue this on along the whole of the sagittal suture.

    • Then bring your finger tips along the length of the transverse sinuses both left and right at the back of the head; make sure you have your small finger tips touching at the confluence. This should produce a strong effect of opening and flowing down into the cranial base.

    • Check the alignment of the occipitomastoid suture by contacting the occiput with one hand and the temporal with another. You should be able to feel the craniosacral motion of each of the bones around the suture.

- Then bring your finger tips to the back of the neck by lining up your finger tips along the length of the spine in the gully formed by the erector spinae muscles and the spinous processes. From here you should be able to get a sense of the carotid sheath carrying the jugular vein.

- Finally bring a hand in front of the back of the thoracic inlet in order to support a spaciousness in the tissues around the jugular veins. Take your time with this procedure. It is meant as a learning process so you can track the sinuses and veins and monitor the change in the tissues and the blood movement.

3. In clinic follow the inherent treatment plan.

- In a clinic situation, you are encouraged to work within the parameters of the inherent treatment plan. So avoid using a technique. The body will let you know if there are issues with the venous return if you are familiar with relating to these structures. It becomes more about knowing these relationships are revealing themselves during the treatment process, and sometimes when there are particularly strong patterns emerging you then need to relate to the tissues with specific hand holds.

9.4 EMOTIONS AND THE LIMBIC SYSTEM

Introduction to emotions

The experience of emotion is fundamental to the human condition. There are universal expressions of emotion that transcend culture. Darwin, one of the first systematic investigators of emotion, argued that emotions are even recognizable in animals. Facial features of primary emotions are quickly perceived. This universality of emotion argues for their very powerful role in evolution and in the interactions of humans.

The last decade or so has seen a radical reframing of emotion based on neurobiological research. Antonio Damasio is clear that it is not possible to make decisions without being able to experience emotion (Damasio 2006). Research into trauma has highlighted the unique processing of fear. If we do not feel safe, all the functions of the body are hijacked by the signals initiated from the amygdala in the limbic system (Porges 2003). Research into the neurological connections of the heart and heart rate variability shows that the functioning of the heart frequently determines our ability to think clearly.[5]

The body leads the mind as much as the mind leads the body. The body and mind speak and it is a two-way conversation. A large part of this conversation is transmitted via emotions. Candace Pert calls the informational chemicals of the neuroendocrine–immune system the 'molecules of emotion' (Pert 1999).

Emotions are an embodied phenomenon. The surge of energy you feel when adrenaline is secreted is frequently the emotion of anxiety. The connectedness and empathy you feel when oxytocin is secreted is frequently labelled joy. The different pieces of music played by the orchestra of cells secreting informational chemicals in our bodies are different emotions. Emotions emerge from the internal environment of the body. They are a particular pattern of secretions, musculoskeletal tone and behaviours; the complex reactions the body has to a stimulus

As we become more aware of our bodies we can interact with the process of emotion emerging from the internal environment. A physiological state becomes an emotion which becomes a feeling, which can trigger thoughts, reasoning, memories and actions. The feeling arises in awareness as the brain makes a neural map of the reactions of the body. Understanding this order of information processing leads to many clinical insights.

There is no hierarchy between mind, emotions and the body. Working with emotions is not different from or more important than working with the body. For every mental emotional event there is a correlate in the world of sensation; there is no separation between physiology and emotion and thought. Actually the sensation comes first; conscious awareness gets in on the act later. You can have physiological changes that are not coupled with emotions, but you cannot have emotions without a change in the body.

Biodynamic craniosacral therapy engages the whole body in as wide a field of perception as is possible. When working in this way the separations we can make between the body, emotions and thoughts become increasingly uneasy. There is just an organism responding to its environment. We do not exist as an emotional person or a physical person or as a thinking person; we exist as a whole unit of function. We respond with the whole of who we are. To meet a client at mid tide, and beyond, necessarily means starting from appreciating this wholeness.

Our responses are deeply entwined with our past history – what we have learnt to move towards or to move away from. When you meet someone in biodynamic craniosacral therapy you can access this whole field of action and perceive how their total experience is centred by the breath of life at that moment. However, this does not really work if you try to separate the organism's response into different levels, differentiating emotion from the body and from the mind. The depth comes from appreciating there is just one unit of function.

Clinical Highlight: Evidence for mind–body connection

- Depression produces the greatest decrement in health compared with the chronic diseases angina, arthritis, asthma and diabetes.

- This is a huge study from WHO (World Health Organization) published in the *Lancet*. It is about as reputable as you can get. It states that people with depression function worse and experience more ill health than some classic physical diseases of the heart, joints, lungs and metabolism. If you have the other diseases plus depression you also function worse than if you had the disease alone. This is quite startling evidence of interactions between the mind and body.

• Observations were available for 245,404 participants from 60 countries in all regions of the world. After adjustment for socioeconomic factors and health conditions, depression had the largest effect on worsening mean health scores compared with the other chronic conditions.

• Consistently across countries and different demographic characteristics, respondents with depression comorbid with one or more chronic diseases had the worst health scores of all the disease states.

(Moussavi *et al.* p.851)

Universal emotions

Emotions are about the life of an organism, its body to be precise, and their role is to assist the organism in maintaining life. (Damasio 2000, p.51)

Researchers into emotion, from Darwin onwards, classify emotions in different ways. The primary, or universal, emotions are considered to be:

• Happiness.

• Sadness.

• Fear.

• Anger.

• Surprise.

• Disgust.

Coupled with theses emotions are particular postures, facial expressions, biochemical profiles and patterns of neural activity – Damasio calls these somatic markers. An emotion is the bodily response before it becomes conscious. In neuroscience a feeling is the name given to the conscious experience of emotion (Damasio 2006).[6]

Additional classifications also exist:

• Secondary or social emotions: embarrassment, jealousy, guilt or pride.

• Background emotions: well-being, malaise, calm or tension.

The unique processing of fear

> There is no single brain center for processing emotions but rather discrete systems related to separate emotional patterns. (Damasio 2000, p.62)

Different parts of the brain are linked to the process of different emotions becoming conscious. Most emotions appear to be mapped initially in the cingulate gyrus (part of the limbic system). Fear, however, has its own unique processing in the amygdala. Figure 3.2.2 shows the amygdala and cingulate gyri. The autonomic nervous system coordinating centres are also essential – especially in acting on fear.

Damasio describes how damage to the amygdala results in people becoming fearless. This is not healthy. They do not recognize faces as untrustworthy. They do not learn from unpleasant situations. They are much more vulnerable and less independent in social situations (Damasio 2000, pp.64–67).

The brain can be thought of as a set of modules (or discrete systems to use Damasio's language) that interact to create the higher functions. These discrete systems work together in health. However, brain science increasingly shows that, when different modules of the brain are damaged, parts of the normal range of human consciousness also become lost. The damage to the amygdala described above is one such example. The patients Damasio worked with intellectually understood the idea of fear but could not experience the reality of fear.

The felt sense

> If there is no boundary, there is no body, and if there is no body, there is no organism. Life needs a boundary. (Damasio 2000, p.137)

The felt sense is a term coined by Gendlin (1981). It describes the possibility of a coherent experience of self emerging from skilful body awareness. The enquiry into our internal environment can often be unclear and fragmented. Gendlin offers that moments of clarity occur, and can be regularly accessed with practice, where we get a unified sense of how we feel at a given time. The felt sense is the perception that forms when our awareness of our muscle tone, the outline and boundary of our body, the insides of our torso and limbs and the metabolic processes coalesce into a distinct word, image, phrase or emotion.

Working with the felt sense is a very powerful adjunct to cranial work. We often start the process of enquiry by asking 'How does your body feel right now?' or 'How does your body feel as you talk about that?' This brings an immediate present-time awareness. It is also a useful question when people are lost in talking without a deepening of the process and the rational mind is working overtime.

Accessing the world of body sensations gives a whole new theatre in which we can play with our unfolding experience. It allows a host of other skills to be used to slow down and reframe our responses to particular stories. In the embodied realm we can move towards sensations or away from them; we can be in control by choosing what is centre stage and where the spotlight shines in a way that is not possible with mental processing alone.

This way of working is non-interpretive. Simple descriptive words work best. We do not need to fit stories and sensations into particular psychotherapeutic models. What emerges is not judged or explained. The responsibility of the therapist is to ensure appropriate pacing and an ongoing relationship to resources. The skills that deepen the process are reflecting back the essence of what people are articulating and keeping the focus on the shifting patterns of sensation.

There are a host of other useful questions and interventions. 'How did you respond to that?' can be very helpful, particularly when difficult stories emerge. 'What tells you you are OK in the midst of all this?' often reminds people of their resources. 'Can you deepen into that awareness?' or 'Is there anything underneath or alongside that quality?' often helps to draw out more essential issues. Frequently just acknowledging it is unclear or complex slows the process and allows an opening to a deeper relationship.

Sometimes the skill of helping someone access the felt sense is to add in the emotional context of a particular story. For example, a client might have a very painful shoulder and you could ask 'Are there are particular emotions that emerge when you feel your shoulder?' or 'What is your response to having a painful shoulder?' Sometimes the goal is to enhance the awareness of body sensations when the client is expressing strong emotions. These are both steps that lead you and the client into a sense of wholeness. The felt sense transcends the differences between physical sensations and emotion feelings and mental processes.

Clinical Highlight: The empathetic practitioner

Being empathetic is a key quality as a therapeutic practitioner. In the biodynamic approach to craniosacral therapy there is an emphasis on empathy at a body level. The body's story is being heard with empathy when you acknowledge it through your hands and through your felt sense. Felt sense is an enormous thing. It's using the general senses of your body in a heightened way to create a homogeneous sensing that includes pressure and fine-touch receptors, not just in your hands but also throughout your body. Often it feels as if you are feeling through the network of receptors, not only in your skin but also deeper interoreceptors, as if the receptors don't need immediate or local contact to sense. Your brain mirrors what you are perceiving on the inside of your body. Some of the major receptors in the body like Raffinian and Pacinian receptors might be far more sensitive than is currently understood.

Can these receptors respond to contact with other people? Can proprioceptors in you detect movement in others? It certainly feels like it. As your touch sense deepens, your ability to feel movements in someone else's system seems to go way beyond your hands.

How else do we feel? Can our very tissues sense another person's tissues and be empathetic towards them so that there is cell-to-cell recognition and a knowing that is cellular and more primitive than the nervous system? Certainly connective tissues have been shown to be highly sensitive to environmental factors, so why not the whole tissue field?

How else do we feel? Sometimes in the contact space it's as if we can feel through the space around us. It's like our potency field itself is highly sensitive and provides a responsiveness to our environment and our relationships in a way we do not recognize. Is instinct made up of this and cellular recognition? And perhaps not just cells but the chemical nature of the body. Neuropeptides have been shown to exhibit qualities of consciousness, so why not all chemicals in the body along with the matrix they all reside in – water? Do chemicals respond to each other body to body in ways we do not understand? Is the fluid electric nature of water a much greater force than is scientifically recognized? Do we connect with these information sources within us when we set up the relational field?

How else do we feel? Is presence itself sensory? Creating the right presence for your clients seems to generate so much connection and knowingness as if presence is a force. A force that is not only creative but also receptive, so you hear through your presence. Is presence itself the true empathy?

Treatment Exercise: Ventricles and limbic system

1. Start at feet.

   - Establish resources, wait for holistic shift and orient to mid tide.

2. Move to Sutherland's vault.

   - Awareness of motility of whole CNS – are the hemispheres moving together?

   - Awareness of ventricles – 'motility of CNS is actually motility of ventricles' (Ukleja 2007).

   - Use Sutherland's image of a bird spreading its wings on inhale.

   - Awareness of potency within CSF – 'liquid light'; 'the highest known element'.

3. Can you feel the structures around the ventricles?

   - Explore the possibility of potency spreading from the ventricles to surrounding limbic structures – structures highly involved in emotional processing, stress and memory formation.

- Can you feel the amygdalae – bilateral almond-sized areas, medial to the horns of the lateral ventricles in the temporal lobes?

- Can you feel the autonomic centres around the fourth ventricle in the brainstem?

- Often there is a characteristic sympathetic buzz in stress-fearful states.

4. Orient to the whole field.

- Deepen your awareness and widen your perceptual field.

- Can you feel the motility of the ventricles come back into relationship to the midline?

- Can you feel a sense of stillness permeate the field?

5. Negotiate ending – maybe return to feet.

9.5 STRESS AND NEUROENDOCRINE–IMMUNE RESPONSES

The brainstem and activation

The brainstem contains nuclei that coordinate the autonomic nervous system (ANS). Sutherland talked of a 'magic inch' just anterior to the fourth ventricle.[7] In this region are found nuclei that control the heart rate, levels of brain activity, breathing and digestion. The reticular system strongly connects the brainstem to the limbic system.

There is a direct neural signal from the brainstem down to the medulla of the adrenal glands. Sympathetic nerves connect directly into the adrenal medulla. This causes adrenaline and noradrenaline to be released into the blood stream within fractions of a second in response to a stressor. This surge of adrenaline gears the body up for activity, it sharpens our senses, and we may go into fight or flight mode.

Parasympathetic activity is also mediated through the brainstem. In overwhelming stress, brainstem nuclei, in response to limbic system signals, will trigger the release of endorphins. The endorphins flood the CNS inhibiting incoming signals. This is the freeze or dissociation response.

The brainstem can be perceived like the stalk of a cauliflower, below and deep to the hemispheres. It can be perceived as a dense, active core to the brain connecting the fluid ventricles and the lighter, more spongy, diffuse hemispheres into the information superhighway of the spinal cord.

The classic way of working with the brainstem is via compression of the fourth ventricle (CV4). In the early days Sutherland used to recommend physically compressing the squama of the occiput until there was sweat on the brow of the client. When he first tried this on himself he described a warm fluid feeling coming into the skull after releasing the pressure, followed by a general feeling of well-being. Things have moved on in biodynamic craniosacral therapy. Simply by orienting to the brainstem, appreciating its connections to the whole body and supporting the intentions of the breath of life will allow profound change in the physiology.

The brainstem is a very powerful portal into working with facilitation of the whole central nervous system. Facilitation describes the process where parts of the nervous system become oversensitive and overactive. This is often due to aberrant incoming sensory information (for example, from traumatic events, joints being out of position, organ inflammation, tight connective tissues). The nervous system is not a dry, telephone exchange, it is a very fluid place. Neurotransmitters can spread outwards from different neuronal pools of the various nuclei and cause non-optimal firing of surrounding neurons. In this case the nervous system can be said to be activated or facilitated.

Recent research, published in a reputable peer-reviewed journal, backs up the experience of practitioners that the CV4 has wide-ranging benefits for the body. A group of osteopaths measured changes in blood flow oscillations after they performed a CV4 (Nelson, Sergueef and Glonek 2006). The measure is an indicator of activity in the ANS. They concluded:

> This study showed that CV-4 has an effect on the TH frequency component of blood flow velocity. The practitioners of cranial manipulation who participated in this study affected their subjects in a quantifiable manner with the application of the CV-4 procedure. (Nelson *et al.* 2006, p.626)

The hypothalamus pituitary adrenal axis releases cortisol

> Regardless of the stressor – injured, starving, too hot, too cold, or psychologically stressed – you turn on the same stress-response... The stress response can become more damaging than the stressor itself. (Sapolsky 2004)

Sapolsky is fantastic on the long-term effects of stress. Some of his insights are summarized below. He has done amazing research on wild baboons, assessing cortisol levels, behaviour and disease. One of the advantages of wild baboon studies is that many of the confounding factors that appear in human studies, such as diet and lifestyle (baboons do not smoke), are eliminated.

While adrenaline is secreted by the adrenal medulla within seconds of a stressor, cortisol is secreted after minutes and for much longer periods. The signal for cortisol release starts in the hypothalamus, goes via blood circulation to the pituitary and then via blood to the adrenal cortex.

Coritsol is a steroid hormone produced in the adrenal cortex and maintains an active stress response. Coritsol has been widely studied. There is very strong evidence linking prolonged cortisol secretion to many diseases, including heart disease, diabetes, poor immune function and growth disorders.

Sapolsky's basic model is very simple. Short-term the stress response is adaptive. There is a 'logic of delay': we shut down everything that is not essential to dealing with immediate danger. All resources are geared to fleeing the tiger. The problems come with continued activation of the stress response. The changes become maladaptive and cause widespread health issues. Reproduction, growth, immune activity and digestion are all switched off when we are running from the tiger. Our heart and lungs and big exercise muscles are working overtime. 'If you experience every day as an emergency, you will pay the price' (Sapolsky 2004, p.13).

Clinical Highlight: Causes of stress

As measured by high levels of cortisol according to Sapolsky:

No control
Perception of no control over events.

Instability
Continued exposure to stress events with no warning – an unstable environment and social context.

No outlets
Limited ability to process stressful events.

Isolation
Isolation and limited social support.

Previous exposure to stress
Limited ability to tell the difference between threat and neutral activity. Previous exposure to stressful events and inability to process stress makes you more likely to misperceive neutral events.

Clinical Highlight: Stress signs

According to a national survey released by the American Psychological Association (APA), one-third of Americans are living with extreme stress. In small doses, stress may be good for you when it gives you a burst of energy. But too much stress or stress that lasts for a long time can take its toll on your body.

Are you having these symptoms of stress?

- Feeling angry, irritable or easily frustrated.

- Feeling overwhelmed.

- Change in eating habits.

- Problems concentrating.

- Feeling nervous or anxious.

- Trouble sleeping.

- Problems with memory.

- Feeling burned out from work.

- Feeling that you can't overcome difficulties in your life.

- Having trouble functioning in your job or personal life.

If you're having any of these symptoms, it's important that you take care of yourself. There are healthy steps you can take to stay well when you're stressed, like connecting to people close to you, getting enough sleep or being physically active.

If you feel overwhelmed, unable to cope and feel as though your stress is affecting how you function every day, it could be something more, like depression or anxiety. Don't let it go unchecked. Contact your health care provider.

(Copyright © Mental Health America,
downloaded September 2008)

DHEA

DHEA has demonstrated efficacy in humans in the improvement of mood, energy, interest, confidence and activity. (Strous, Maayan and Weizman 2006)

DHEA (dehydroepiandrosterone) is a neurosteroid, produced in the gonads, adrenals and brain. It has been shown to be essential in neuron development and growth and in the development of the architecture of the CNS. The ratio of DHEA to cortisol can be measured from saliva swabs. Watkins describes this ratio as a major tool, alongside HRV, into research in performance and physiology. The DHEA-to-cortisol ratio is a good predictor of ageing and certain diseases. High DHEA to low cortisol is good in this model (Watkins 2008).

Performance does not need to be about stress and high cortisol. Activation (either sympathetic or parasympathetic) is very different if the underlying trigger is about pleasure, novelty and creativity – there is a much stronger secretion of DHEA. By becoming aware of our motivations to our actions we can shift our biochemical profile to higher levels of DHEA rather than cortisol. We can still perform at a high level without the damaging consequences of high cortisol levels. Watkins describes two types of arousal: passion and anger. They are often confused. Passion is the number one predictor of performance. He recommends being clear about your motivation and focusing on what makes you passionate.

Clinical Highlight: Cortisol effects

1. Mobilizes energy.
   - Shuts down sugar storage and uptake of sugar everywhere except exercising muscles.
   - Opposite action of insulin.
2. Increases tone of the cardiovascular system.
   - Shuts down peripheral blood.
   - Increases blood to exercising muscles, heart and brain.
3. Decreases digestion.
   - Turns off digestive processes.
4. Decreases growth.
   - Secretion of growth hormone inhibited.
5. Decreases reproduction.
   - Reproductive hormones are inhibited.
6. Decreases immune activity.
   - Inflammation is suppressed.
   - Ability to fight infections is downgraded.
   - Other complex effects on immune activity.
7. Sharpens cognition.
   - Senses are heightened.

9.6 PAIN

Pain is complex and always involves emotion

There is a myth that pain is an objective experience. It can be easy to fall into the trap of thinking that there is a pain scale that we can all, bravely or not so bravely, measure ourselves against. In fact the opposite is true; pain is a very subjective experience with many layers of meaning and subtleties of expression. There is no one part of the brain, no pain centre, that always lights up when humans feel pain. The holistic, personal nature of pain has long been recognized by researchers:

> There can be no pain without emotion, as the currently accepted definition of pain recognizes: 'an unpleasant sensory and emotional experience associated with actual or potential tissue damage'. (Jackson 2002, p.276)

Pain is a warning signal that we ignore at our peril. It is designed to make us change our behaviour. However, there are many factors that compete to control our behaviour. Pain has to be considered in terms of the needs, priorities and history of the individual. Pain signals:

> modify information transmission at almost every synaptic level of the somatosensory projection systems…inputs impinge on a continually active nervous system that is already the repository of the individual's past history, expectations and value systems. (Melzack and Wall 1996, p.145)[8]

Pain cannot be separated from meaning and the context in which it arises. There are some famous studies that demonstrate this. In one study, soldiers injured in a battle requested morphine far less than civilians did for similar injuries not acquired in battle. For a solider an injury may mean that, if he is not going to die, it is a successful outcome. In another study, using ten years of data, a hospital discovered that patients who could view trees from their window after gallbladder surgery requested significantly less pain medication than those who looked at blank walls.

If you continue to drop grains of sand onto a surface the pile will grow with shifts in shape and occasional avalanches. The timings and sizes of the avalanches are inherently unpredictable and are best modelled by the recently developed framework of complexity (chaos) theory. It is very hard to predict which grain of sand will cause a large avalanche. However, if there is enough sand dropped, a big, complex shift in the pile will occur at some stage.

The body, as a system of communicating cells, exhibits complex behaviour. It has emergent properties and degrees of stability within various conditions.[10] One of the key elements of complexity theory is that predicting the behaviour of the whole is not possible from considering the behaviour of the individual components. In complex systems what matters is how things are connected. Similar events can have very different outcomes. Finding the cause of an event in a complex system is fraught with difficulties.

In chaos theory there is a common example of a butterfly flapping its wings on one side of the world and causing a hurricane on the other side. (In a complex, chaotic system a small change in initial conditions can have huge consequences on the behaviour of the whole.) However, once you are in the middle of a hurricane, trying to work out which butterfly caused the storm is meaningless.

From complexity theory we can see that we need to be very careful in being too certain about identifying the cause of a particular pain. There are a vast number of experiences, events and connections that shape and form a human being.

Treatment Exercise: Nerve flow and spinal cord facilitation

1. Start at the vault hold.

    •   Establish resources, wait for holistic shift, orient to mid tide.

    •   Explore the motility of the CNS.

    •   Notice any activity around the ventricles.

2. Two-handed contact from the side.

    •   Use finger tips to contact the spinous processes of C6, C7 and T1 with the upper hand and T11, T12 and L1 with the lower hand.

    •   How do the sympathetic chains feel?

    •   Orient to the fluid midline and the spinal cord.

    •   Can you get a sense of motility and connection through the whole cord?

3. Explore nerve flow.

    •   Is there a peripheral structure that draws your attention? It can be an organ or a limb.

    •   Place one hand on the relevant spinal cord segment and one hand on an organ or limb.

    •   Orient to settling within the nociceptive loop. Play with orienting to the cord and the nerve roots. Can the periphery come back into relation to the midline?

    •   Deepen the contact by orienting to the anterior midline and the discs as the natural fulcrum of an embryological segment.

The anatomy of pain

There are staging posts in the processing of pain by the central nervous system

Pain is an interpretation within the central nervous system. Unfortunately, the mapping of the root of the pain is often confused. Phantom limb pain is the clearest demonstration of this. Given that pain is a complex process, we can, however, identify certain staging posts in the processing of pain. The level of the spinal cord that the pain signal enters, the brainstem and the limbic system are transition places in the passage of pain through the central nervous system. These staging posts are potential places where the experience of pain can be influenced.

A signal comes from a sensory receptor and synapses in the dorsal horn of the spinal cord. From the spinal cord segment a second order neuron carries the signal into the reticular formation of the brainstem, connecting into the thalamus and limbic system and cerebellum. From these old brain areas, deep in the centre of the brain, there are many connections. Third order neurons carry the information into the cortex. It is at this stage that we become conscious of the pain.

Pain, the stress response and overactivity in the sympathetics go hand in hand. Pain pathways are largely carried along with sympathetic sensory/afferent nerves. Also, within the CNS neurotransmitters from pain synapses can leak into the neuronal pools of the nearby sympathetic nerves.

Junk in equals junk out: The functioning of the nervous system depends on the quality of the incoming sensory information

For the CNS to provide accurate control/coordination of the body's processes there needs to be constant feedback from the sensory system. Nerve cells that are not constantly stimulated form weaker connections to other cells and can atrophy and die.[11] Lack of stimulation reduces the overall functioning of the CNS ('use it or lose it'). One of the largest components of sensory information is about movement. Proprioceptive information is essential to the functioning of the CNS (Carrick 1997; Redwood and Cleveland 2003; Seaman and Winterstein 1998). Movement feeds the brain in a very powerful way.

The inputs to the brain, such as movement, determine it outputs and its ability to control the body (junk in equals junk out). The latest science from spinal mechanics and fascia researchers is clear: changes in connective tissues such as myofascia occur primarily due to improved neural feedback, not from mechanically changing the properties of the tissues following direct massage (Schleip 2003a, 2003b).[12] Every time a joint becomes restricted there is a loss of stimulatory feedback from muscle, joint and fascia receptors. There is also an increase in noxious signals, reinforcing pain and inflammation pathways from the poorly aligned joints and tissues. The largest consequences of misalignment in joints and tissues are neurological. It is the disturbance to feedback mechanisms that causes weakness, tightness, loss of control and pain. Orienting to the neural control is a very quick way of effecting change. Pain is rarely due to compression of nerves (the classic manipulative model), or caused by tight muscles (the classic massage model). If the disturbance to the sensory feedback mechanisms is removed frequently the pain goes away. When a joint comes back into optimum alignment it provides a burst of afferent/ sensory signals that significantly improves the functioning of the associated spinal cord segment, the whole cord and the CNS.

Powerful primitive reflexes can hijack the functioning of the body: Flexor withdrawal is a whole cord response that will affect the whole musculoskeletal system

The nervous system is a bag of reflexes that provide unconscious control of the body. There are three main reflex responses that commonly interfere with the functioning of the whole body:

- Fight or flight.

- Freeze/dissociation.

- Flexor withdrawal response.

The flexor withdrawal response is the reflex engaged when you step on a pebble. The essential point to understand is that it affects the whole CNS. You never just lift your foot. All the muscles in the leg will be engaged, there will be signals sent to the opposite leg to compensate for the change in weight, the muscles of the trunk and spine will change to accommodate the pelvis and the tone in the neck will also change.

In technical language the flexor withdrawal response has multisegmental, suprasegmental and contralateral effects, that is, it affects the whole spinal cord, the whole CNS and the opposite side of the body to the initial trigger. Over 50 per cent of the tracts in the spinal cord are prospinal tracts, coordinating reflex responses (Guyton and Hall 2000). Most of the tracts in the spinal cord are about the cord speaking to itself.

The flexor withdrawal response can be triggered in the whole body by a painful, irritating, noxious input from anywhere in the whole system. It changes the proprioceptive picture in the whole body. It will also trigger stress responses. There is neurological inhibition of some skeletal muscles causing weakness and poor functioning of the musculoskeletal system. Following an initial trigger a vicious circle occurs:

- altered proprioception and loss of sensory information leads to

- flexor withdrawal and reflex inhibition, which lead to

- patterns of chronically weak and chronically tight muscles, leading to

- poor joint mechanics, causing

- pain and further aberrant proprioceptive input.[13]

The inherent treatment plan frequently shows areas of the body that seem remote from the site of the pain. Understanding the whole body consequences of flexor withdrawal is the neurological way of explaining why a joint being out of alignment, anywhere in the body, can cause pain and poor functioning at a remote site. Supporting the system to come out of flexor withdrawal, often by being able to be aware of spinal and cranial joint restrictions, is a fantastic, effective and very quick model for supporting change.

Pain gate theory describes how fast fibre nerve signals inhibit slow fibre nerve signals

There are two types of incoming pain signals: (1) fast, large diameter, mylinated, A fibres carry sharp pain signals; (2) slow, small diameter, C fibres carry aching, dull, throbbing pain. The dedicated receptors for pain are called nociceptors.

Mechanoreceptors (fast fibres) carry non-pain information, but in intense bursts they can trigger pain perception. For example, rubbing gently can be very pleasant; rubbing too hard becomes painful. The receptor is the same, but the intensity of the signal is interpreted differently.[14]

Gate theory describes how fast fibres always trigger an inhibitory interneuron that after a period of time switches off the pain signal. Fast fibre pain is self-limiting; there is a short sharp burst, then the signal to the brain is inhibited by the pain gate interneuron.

In contrast pain signals on slow fibres actually stop the inhibitory interneuron from working. In slow pain the signal keeps going to the brain.

If slow pain is present then gate theory predicts that a burst of sharp pain will trigger the interneuron that stops the signal going to the brain. If you rub a pain vigorously, the pain will disappear. If you scratch an itch (fast pain), then the itch itself (slow pain) fades from awareness.

Fast fibre pain can be seen as adaptive to short-term, acute stress. The pain causes a quick reaction that is not maintained, allowing you to keep running or fighting – in evolutionary terms this is very useful if running from a tiger. The slow pain takes longer to arrive but tells you to slow down and recuperate.

The inhibitory interneuron that stops the pain signal can also be triggered by descending signals from the cortex. Pain has to compete with the other priorities of the organism. Varying behavioural priorities can inhibit the slow pain signal from becoming conscious.

If we do not slow down, recuperate and resolve the cause then problems occur. The nociceptors are still firing, adversely affecting the functioning of the body. Nociceptors are unusual receptors in that they keep firing, all the time, until the noxious stimulus is removed. In contrast normal mechanoreceptors are attenuated over time – the rate of firing decreases (for example, you stop being aware of the contact with the chair after first sitting on it). The pain signals, now largely unconscious, act as a constant internal stressor if the trigger is not removed.

Pain changes how the nervous system works

There are many consequences to unresolved nociceptive signals. Persistent nociceptive input causes facilitation within the central nervous system. Facilitation describes how groups of neurons are constantly primed to reach their firing threshold too quickly. Constant stimulation of pain neurons makes the connections between neurons along the pain pathways stronger. We become better at feeling our pain.

Pro-inflammatory chemicals are secreted in the peripheral tissues (partly by the nerves themselves via axonal transport) maintaining inflammatory states. Sills describes this as a nociceptive loop.

Synapses in the CNS are bathed in fluid. Neurotransmitters associated with pain and inflammation begin to leak into the surrounding neuronal pools of non-pain pathways. Via this mechanism, constant pain stimulation will affect the functioning of other reflexes (somatic, such as posture and abnormal contractions of muscles, and autonomic, such as abnormal signals to organs) within the CNS.

Low-level nociceptive input always triggers the flexor withdrawal response. Even if the noxious signal is no longer being consciously processed, it can still upset the proprioceptive mechanisms.

Sills (2004) states that low-level chronic nociception/pain and inflammation can cause higher-level facilitation – overwhelm responses in the autonomic nervous system.[15] This model develops the idea of a facilitated segment to include the brainstem and limbic system and a central sensitized state.

> It now seems as if pain carves a path through us in the same way that water creates a route down the side of a mountain. It flows where it must. Chronic pain is the result of flooding on that pathway, until it erodes a deeper channel, or creates new ones... The longer and deeper pain flows the more it lays down a sensitized trail for future pain. And this can become a conduit for other kinds of pain – divorce angst will head straight for that channel, until body pain and life pain become indistinguishable... Pain creates a language for wordless events like loss. Sometimes I think pain is just the body thinking out loud. (Jackson 2002, p.150)

Clinical Highlight: Treatment strategies based on understanding inhibition

Remember pain is complex. There is no one way to treat pain. Rather than just working at the site of the pain, use your creativity and trust what the inherent treatment plan shows you.

How often have you heard something similar to 'My back went when I bent down to tie my shoelaces?' You dig deeper and your client tells you that they are under pressure at work, their relationship is not going well, they have an old sports injury, they slouch at the computer and who knows what else. Which is the cause? They all are. The following strategies can help.

Inhibition to be supported

Mechanoreceptors inhibit nociceptors. Freeing up restricted joints will help prevent pain and is a wonderful way of supporting health. Movement information (especially spinal joints) provides afferent input (sensory information) to the nervous system that improves the functioning of the whole body and brain. Fast fibre input from mechanoreceptors can trigger the inhibitory interneuron that stops the ascending pain signal. Feed the brain movement information.

Treatment aimed at improving nerve flow can inhibit pain pathways. Resolving inertia in and around staging posts in the processing of pain presents an opportunity to influence the experience of pain. The sympathetic nervous system, the spinal cord segments, the brainstem and the limbic system and nerve flow between the periphery and the cord are all useful tools in treating pain.

Descending pathways inhibit nociceptors. We can think and feel our way out of pain. There are descending analgesia pathways from the cortex and reticular formation that can be consciously influenced. It is essential to not try and isolate pain from the whole of someone's life and previous experiences. Trauma, stress and life statements are intimately bound up in the experience of pain.

Parasympathetics inhibit sympathetics. The dynamic balance between the two arms of the autonomic nervous system is largely maintained by inhibition of the sympathetics by the parasympathetics. Any inputs that allow the parasympathetic nervous system to function more effectively will inhibit the sympathetic nervous system and pain. One of the most powerful ways of doing this is to offer stillness and space. Allow the system to orient to resources and the environment in present time. The extra information from the whole body and the whole field will allow contextualization of cycling and speedy stories and slow down the stress response. In addition, in terms of movement, the extensor muscles are associated with the parasympathetics. Inputs that stimulate extensors, allowing us to come into a softer, upright and receptive posture, generally improve pain. Feed the brain parasympathetic information.

Inhibition to be removed

Flexor withdrawal inhibits some muscles. Removing things that irritate the nervous system stops muscle inhibition and will prevent pain. Our clinical experience has particularly demonstrated that supporting free movement in the joints of the skull, the spine and peripheral joints of the limbs as well as free movement of organs is very effective at switching off flexor withdrawal. (Removing piercings, metal in the mouth, jewellery and environmental toxicity can work in the same way.)

Dissociation inhibits our ability to feel. As a short-term strategy, this can be essential and life giving. As a long-term strategy we would encourage the ability to have choice and skill in the ability to be present. The pathways of the analgesia system are triggered in dissociation. Dissociation often confuses the treatment of pain. In our experience helping resolve dissociative processes is often the first priority in treating chronic pain.[16]

Summary of Chapter 9

This chapter has looked at the central nervous system from a experiential viewpoint. As well as understanding the anatomy and physiology, getting to know how nervous tissue feels and expresses the breath of life is essential. It is important to recognize how different parts of the brain feel so that these can be identified in treatment sessions. Appreciating the natural fulcrum of the lamina terminalis and the strong organizing force of the third ventricle and how this can affect the potency of the whole nervous system is a key aspect. In addition, we explored relating to the venous sinus system and appreciating the crucial nature of the blood return from the brain. We looked at the neurology, and some endocrine physiology, of stress, emotion and pain and the importance of the orienting to structures around the ventricles, such as the hypothalamus, the pituitary, the amygdala and the brain stem nuclei.

Here are some of the key skills from this chapter:

- Feeling the ventricles of the brain and the deep potency that resides there. Following the potentization in the ventricles during stillpoint.

- Recognizing how the health and motility of the ventricles can affect the health of the whole system.

- Becoming familiar with nervous tissue expressions of health. Learning to recognize states of balance and work with different parts of the brain.

- Relating to venous sinuses. Assessing their freedom of movement and encouraging greater mobility, flow, potency, and movement expressions.

- Learning to identify brainstem activation and how to support a toning down of the nervous system.

- Understanding the reflexes, such as fight or flight, freeze and flexor withdrawal, and interacting with staging posts in the processing of incoming information.

Notes

1. Some books quote 135 ml and a turnover of 6 hours.
2. Sutherland was keen to use the word fluctuate in relation to the movement of CSF: 'The fluid does not circulate like the blood stream but fluctuates in its activity' (Sutherland 1998, p.300).

Gintis (2007) argues convincingly that fluctuation is a more efficient way of distributing the trophic contents of CSF than would happen if it was a circulation.

3.   The appearance of the foramen lacerum is quite misleading on a dry skull. In life it is packed with dense cartilage and fibrous tissue. The fibrous tissue forms a clean hole at the end of the oblique, bony tunnel of the carotid canal within the petrous temporal bone. The foramen lacerum does not open inferiorly. See Acland (2004, DVD4).

4.   Classically the approach is to start from the bottom and work towards the top of the venous sinus system. We find awareness of the anatomy, and orienting to the health of the whole drainage system is enough to facilitate change rather than applying a step-by-step mechanical approach.

5.   Armour (2008) is very clear on the extensive neurology of the heart. Watkins (2008) is doing fantastic research using heart rate variability.

6.   Technically, emotion is the bodily response before the conscious feeling.

7.   Sutherland goes further than just highlighting the influence of the nuclei around the fourth ventricle on basic physiological processes. He also strongly links primary respiration to the ventricles: '"All the physiological centers, including that of respiration, are located within the floor of the fourth ventricle." This statement specifically calls attention to primary respiration as commencing in the central nervous system, and, in our interpretation, indicates both primary and secondary respiration in the human mechanism.' (Sutherland 1998, p.298). (N.B. Lung breathing is secondary respiration in Sutherland's framework.)

8.   Melzack and Wall (1996) is a classic book on the physiology of pain.

9.   Both examples taken from Sapolsky (2004).

10.   Newell (2003) has written a whole article devoted to the spine as a complex phenomenon with emergent properties. Here we are extending his insights to the whole body. Johnson (2001) is also very good on emergence.

11.   Kandel (2007) is a wonderful guide to memory and how neurons work. Development and maintenance of the nervous system relies on exchange across synapses; this has a 'trophic and regulatory influence' and 'prevents cell death of the presynaptic and postsynaptic neuron' (Gilman and Newman 1996).

12.   Schleip is one of the defining authors on fascia and bodywork. Also see his Youtube lecture of 2007.

13.   This model of using flexor withdrawal and proprioception comes from the work of Dr Simon King (2008). For some great videos see www.live-without-pain.com.

14.   Descriptions taken from Sapolsky (2004).

15.   Sills is very good on nociceptive loops. We add in the importance of treating the whole cord due to flexor withdrawal and that mechanoreceptors inhibit the nociceptors.

16.   'We have begun to realise that there could be a link between pain perception and the feeling of ownership of the body' (Petkova and Ehrsson 2008). This quote is from the body swap illusion research described in Chapter 4.

10

The Facial Complex

10.1 THE FACE

The complexities of the face and the maxillae

Physiology of the face

The human face is the most-looked-at object in the world. We spend most of the day looking at each other's faces and its expressions. Subtle shifts of the many facial muscles convey a complex array of emotions and meanings. However, most people do not see the expression of primary respiration in the face, at least not consciously. The underlying movement of the face on the inhale phase of primary respiration is a widening side to side.

The face is a remarkably unexpected structure, dominated by the maxillae bones. They act as the mainframe of the face. The maxillae are the largest bones of the face. The other bones of the face join with them and are powerfully affected by their form and movement. To understand the face you must appreciate the motion dynamics of the maxillae.

Typically, the maxillae externally and internally rotate around their common suture – the intermaxillary suture – in the midline of the face. With your hands resting over the front of the face, finger tips just superior to the lips, you will feel a flaring outwards (external rotation) of your little finger on inhale. The maxillae are often said to hang off the frontal bones and the frontomaxillary suture acts as a pivot for the craniosacral motion of the bones. The hold of your fingers resting over the maxilla is a very common and easy hold. In practice try engaging with the tissues first from an external contact onto the face; frequently this is enough to allow the resolution of many patterns of experience organized around the facial complex. Sometimes tissues need immediate contact, so from time to time you may need to make contact into the mouth. An introduction to intraoral contact is described in a treatment exercise below.

Dental issues can create havoc in their health expressions.[1] According to Weston Price the development of the maxillae is also sensitive to early nutritional influences (Price 2008).[2] For Price, a broad face with a wide, even dental arch formed by the maxillae and non-crowded teeth was much more common in cultures that ate traditional, non-processed food. The maxillae are not only most of the face structure, but they are also part of the lower orbit of the eyes, part of the bridge of the nose, the first part of the airway creating the nasopharynx and the sinuses, and attachments for the conchae. They also form the upper jaw and the roof of the mouth. That's a lot of different functions for two bones in an area where there is a lot of movement from breathing, speaking, eating and eyeball movement as well.

Understandably the maxillae can become affected, and restrictions commonly occur that lead to shape in their craniosacral motion and a lowering of potency. Sutherland described common patterns of compression, sidebending and torsion (Magoun 1951). Compression describes patterns of experience where the maxillae are restricted on an anterior–posterior axis; the face feels squashed towards the back of the skull and/or up into the frontal bones or they are compressed medially into the intermaxillary suture. Sidebending and torsion in the maxillary complex follow the naming convention for sidebending and torsion of the sphenoid. Imagine you are looking at your client lying on the table from behind the head – the normal treatment position. A right sidebend through the maxillary complex would mean the right side of the face is closer to the ceiling (right maxilla is more anterior). A right torsion of the maxillary complex would mean that the right side of the face feels closer to your body (right maxilla is more superior).

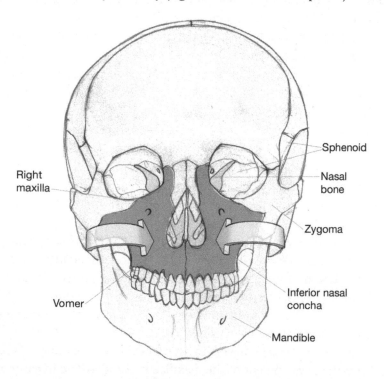

Figure 10.1.1 Maxillae on inhale

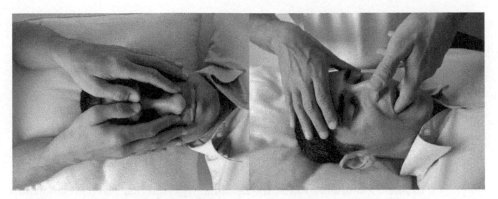

Figure 10.1.2 Contacting the maxillae

Treatment Exercise: Intraoral contact on the maxillae

1. Introduction to intraoral contacts.

    • In order to fully appreciate the craniosacral expressions of the maxillae you can make contact on the external surface of the bones, but you can also make an intraoral contact. Sometimes to be more precise it may be necessary to treat within the mouth, especially if there has been dental trauma, damage to the tissues or strong compressions.

2. Clearly explain the reasons and process.

    • You will need to explain why intraoral contact is necessary to your client, along with a clear explanation of how you intend to make the contact.

    • Make sure your client has a signal that you recognize if they want you to remove your fingers. Practise the signal.

3. Use two fingers to contact the inferior surfaces of the upper teeth.

    • Using finger cots, place a finger cot onto the first and second fingers of one of your hands. Finger cots are latex covers for individual fingers; you can also use latex gloves.

    • Make sure you are physically positioned so that you can drop your fingers onto the surface of your client's teeth. You are trying to bring your finger pads into contact with the upper molars.

    • You will need to pivot your body and elbows so that you can gently make the contact. Often this is best done in a standing position. It can be useful to make an additional contact on the frontal bone with your other hand.

- Ask your client to gently close their mouth around your fingers.

4. Negotiate space and orient to the primary respiration of the maxillae.

    - Spend time negotiating the space and listening for the health of the maxillae.

    - The maxillae may express internal and external rotation with a shape. Often there is a preference to one side and there may be patterns of restriction.

    - Acknowledge the detail of this and wait for states of balance to arise. Try to name the orientation of the maxillae with reference to its relationship to other structures around it: compression, sidebending or torsion.

    - Powerful responses can take place across the facial complex and in other parts of the body.

5. Negotiate ending.

Zygomatic bones

Zygoma comes from the Latin for yolk and you can see that the anatomists had a sense of the bones as yolked to the temporal bones through the zygomatic process. These bones are often referred to as 'the connectors' as they touch on so many other bones at the corner of the face. They are commonly called cheek bones and often take lots of blows from either falling, banging the head or being hit. Boxers must have serious zygomatic compression!

The zygoma directly contacts on to the sphenoid. In a craniosacral therapy session, the bones will often be involved in orbital patterns, or patterns of the jaw, as well as being strongly influenced by the temporals, so you can see how they may be pulled in all directions. It is interesting to make contact with your own zygomatic bones. You will notice one or both have strong expressions. Their typical craniosacral motion is internal/external motion around a vertical axis.

Orbits

The eye orbits are a miracle of body formational processes. They are composed of eight bones and a plethora of sutural joints, but always seem to form into a near-perfect ovoid shape. The orbits are a bit like the cheek bones in that they often take knocks from the outside world, which can lodge as compressions within bones or in sutures. Often one orbit is more expanded than the other. During treatments the orbits will commonly adjust and reorganize around their relationship to the face and the neurocranium, of which they are part of both. For more on orbits see Section 10.2 on the eyes.

Awareness Exercise: Following the diaphragm of the face

- Bring your attention to your mouth. Come into a sense of the size of the cavity of the mouth. Notice the roof of your mouth and the shape of it. Does it feel domed or flat? Does it feel comfortable? Does it feel spacious?

- If there is a sense of compression here it often comes from either the maxillae being medially compressed or from an inferior compression from the vomer above.

- Try to name how the body feels around your upper palate.

- Now tune into the craniosacral motion dynamics of the hard palate. How strong is the movement? This is a natural fulcrum for the face and ideally should have a doming and flattening motion similar to the respiratory diaphragm.

- As you deepen into these movements you may well get a sense of responses from other places within your body. Notice where these are; they may well be from other transverse diaphragms.

- Be open to states of balance occurring in the hard palate. Try to notice Becker's three-step healing process as it is literally happening right under your nose! As adjustments occur in the palate again notice responses across the body and the midline.

Midline of the face – ethmoid and vomer

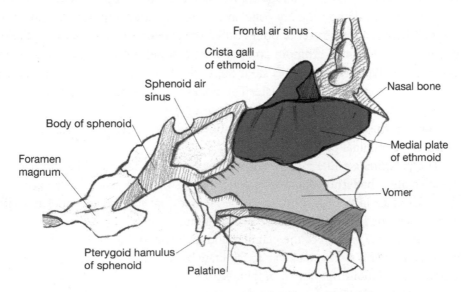

Figure 10.1.3 Mid sagittal section through the nasal cavity

At the centre of the face is a vertical arrangement between the ethmoid perpendicular plate and the vomer. These two structures lie on top of each other and form a centre line that bring the ethmoid, vomer and sphenoid into a strong relationship with each other.

The ethmoid sits at the centre of the eye orbits and is in strong relationship with the falx cerebri via the crista galli extending up through the ethmoid notch of the frontal bone. The vomer sits on top of the intermaxillary suture of the upper palate. This means the sphenoid is indirectly influenced by the dynamics of the mouth and eyes and cranial dura through these structures. Conversely, they are influenced by the sphenoid, so compression in the upper palate or between the eyes can be generated by SBJ patterns or intraosseous patterns in the sphenoid.

It is important to understand the array of connections between the face and the neurocranium. The ethmoid plate and the vomer can exhibit torsions along their length from torsion and sidebending forces in the maxillae and sphenoid.

Sometimes when there is strong compression in these bones, intraoral contact may be necessary to enable a more immediate connection to the structures involved. Therefore, bringing a cotted finger onto the upper palate can help enormously to resolve patterns in the vomer and ethmoid plate. Often resolution in this region is accompanied by a sense of the vomer and maxillae moving anteriorly and inferiorly.

The sphenoid and the face

At the back of the face sits the sphenoid. It is behind all the structures of the face. The lesser wings make up the back of the eye orbits, the body of the sphenoid is behind the vomer and the pterygoid plates are behind the upper molars.

The maxillae do not directly come into sutural relationship with the sphenoid. Instead there is a curious set of bones called the palatines that sit between the two bones (also the vomer, ethmoid and zygomatic bones are between the sphenoid and the maxillae). The palatines sit at the back of the upper palate and make up the back section of the hard palate. The bones are L-shaped and project up into the lower eye orbit contributing to the floor of the orbit. They are aligned along a groove in the pterygoid plates of the sphenoid. This section of the palatines is called the pyramidal process.

The palatines act like a spacer or washer between the sphenoid and maxillae. They create a buffering between the motions of the SBJ and the strong actions that take place in the functioning of the face, so that mastication does not affect and disturb the key motions in the neurocranium.

Allowing the motion of the maxillae and the sphenoid to come into synchrony with each other is a powerful way to facilitate harmony in the craniosacral system. Often this relationship can be impinged by the palatines holding compressive forces either from dental work or from impact injury. Direct blows to the front of the head can create a forcing of the palatines into the pterygoid plates. Often boxers have this in their system,[3] but it can equally occur from a fall or a crash.

The inherent treatment plan will reveal these patterns during the therapy session; making a contact to the exterior of the face can be quite sufficient to access these patterns and help the system adjust. Sometimes a direct contact to the back of the hard palate may be required in severe cases of compression.

Awareness Exercise: How the sphenoid interacts with the face

- Bring your awareness to your sphenoid. Create a very light awareness so the sphenoid shows its primary respiratory motion. Follow its movements for a while and then invite the facial complex into your perceptual field.

- Notice how the eye orbits are part of the movement of the sphenoid.

- Notice how the sphenoid and vomer interact with the maxillae and the ethmoid. The vomer moves forward from the body of the sphenoid.

- What is the sense of how the bones relate to each other in primary respiration?

- Be interested in the relationship between the pterygoid plates of the sphenoid and the palatines at the back of the upper palate.

- As the sphenoid moves in inhalation and exhalation what happens in the face as a whole? Stay with it for a while so you experience the movements as a combined holistic motion through the cranial base and face.

The neural face

Cranial nerves that supply the face

There are two main nerves to appreciate when orienting to the face: the trigeminal nerve (CN V: motor to the muscles of mastication and sensory to the face and most of the oral cavity) and the facial nerve (CN VII: motor to the muscles of facial expression and glands in the oral cavity). Both these cranial nerves fan out from the brainstem to innervate the structures in and around the oral cavity. The general facial hold is a great way of tuning into the nerve flow (see Figure 10.1.5).

Motor supply detail

The mandibular nerve, the third branch of the trigeminal nerve (CN V3), is the motor nerve supplying the muscles of mastication.

The muscles of the floor of the oral cavity have a complex nerve supply with contributions from the trigeminal nerve (CN V3), facial nerve and C1 spinal nerve via the hypoglossal nerve (CN XII).

The facial nerve (CN VII) carries the parasympathetic motor supply to the salivary glands. The fibres pass via the pterygopalatine ganglion between the sphenoid and the palatine bone/maxilla.[4] Disorders in this nerve are associated with disturbances in saliva, lacrimal glands, nasal mucosa and taste.

The muscles of facial expression are supplied by the facial nerve.

Sensory supply detail

The trigeminal nerve (CN V3) carries the parasympathetic sensory information from the glands and nasopharyngeal mucosa and tongue.

The TMJ joint capsule is innervated by the mandibular branch of the trigeminal nerve (CN V3).

The sensory nerves from the teeth are part of the trigeminal nerve (CN V3 for the lower jaw and CN V2 for the upper jaw).

Different branches of the trigeminal nerve carry the sensory supply from the dermatomes of the face.

The metabolic fluid fields of the face

Orienting to the embryology of the face offers a profound deepening of the contact. A very powerful way of working with stories that present through the face and jaw is to orient to the branchial arches and the fluid fields of the face (see Figure 10.1.4). They are formed as the early embryo folds. If you were to put a thick sock over your hand and bend your wrist the wrinkles that form on the underside would correspond to the branchial arches.

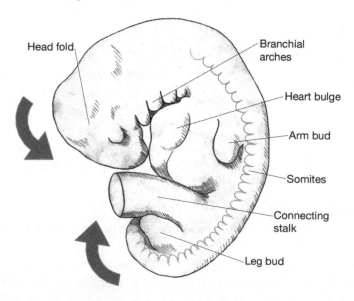

Figure 10.1.4 Branchial arches in a five-week-old embryo

The arrows show the curling of the embryo around the heart and early umbilicus in the first few weeks of life. The directions and actions of the biodynamic forces that shape the embryo are still present and perceptible in the adult

The structures form as densifications in the metabolic fluid fields of the embryo. Orienting to creating superior and inferior space between the horizontal fluid fields of the face is very powerful. It frequently means you can slide underneath many issues of activation, including issues dating from birth, from early attachment disorders, or from traumatic experiences or dental problems. Orienting to the fluid fields is a wonderful way of meeting the intelligence of the body and the deeper organizing forces.

Treatment Exercise: Orienting to the nerve flow and deepening into the fluid fields of the face

1. Start at the feet.

   - Take time to really establish resources, check in verbally, negotiate contact and wait for the holistic shift.

   - Orient to mid tide and the fluid body.

2. Make contact via the general facial hold.

   - Take your time to slow down and establish a safe holding field. The face and jaw can be a very charged area to contact.

3. Orient to nerve flow.

   - Try to get a sense of the information flow along the trigeminal and facial nerves to and from the brainstem.

   - What is the quality of the nervous system field? Frequently there can be a real sense of a hum or a buzz. Sometimes there is a sense of absence and a hidden quality to the jaw.

   - Support any settling and states of balance through the nervous system.

4. Orient to the fluid fields of the face and throat.

   - Deepen and widen your awareness. Allow the possibility of long tide and deeper states of stillness to emerge.

   - Can you go under any signs of activation and tissue patterning to an appreciation of the fluid metabolic fields of the early embryo?

5. Offer space.

   - Often there is a sense of compression top to bottom through the face – sometimes more pronounced on one side. Can you support a spreading and opening in the horizontally organized fluid fields?

   - The organizing forces inherently seek space and order. Can you be still enough to appreciate the intentions of the breath of life?

6. Negotiate ending.

7. Move to a different hold and slowly disengage.

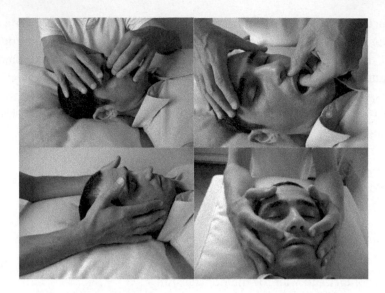

Figure 10.1.5 Facial holds
Clockwise from the top left: Ethmoid, midline of the face, general facial hold, angle of the mandible

10.2 THE EYES

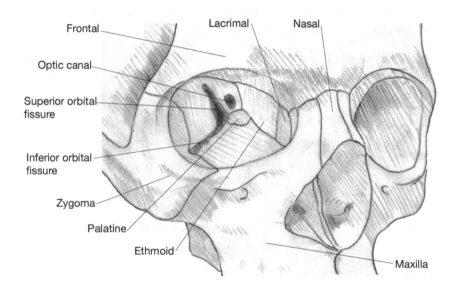

Figure 10.2.1 Bones of the orbit

Overview

> The visual system is made up of neurons and neurotransmitters, well-worn neural paths, associations and expectations. It is both hard-wired and soft, pliable and plastic. (Sewall 1999)

Vision is not a simple phenomenon. It often dominates the act of perception. Seventy per cent of the sensory receptors in the body are found in the eyes (Marieb 2006, p.272). To see things is to know them. Foucault charted an increase in medical power as the body was cut open and the inside was made available for sight (Jones and Porter 1998). The existentialists love the idea of the gaze; we become aware of ourselves through the gaze of the other.

As bodyworkers we are often striving to go beneath visual metaphors and come into a tactile, embodied way of perceiving. Sight is part of that, but is not allowed to dominate. Vision scientist and ecopsychologist Laura Sewall (quoted above) describes how visual perception is a whole body sense, particularly when sensing depth of field. She expands the definition of healthy vision to include a sense of embodiment and place. This all has implications for how our experiences might shape visual acuity.

Bates-related methods build on the conviction that eyesight is not just a mechanical process of acuity, but the body, mind, emotions, behaviour and environment are all interdependent factors in the act of seeing.[5] The beginning of a decrease in visual acuity is often attributed to an emotional stress.

According to Bates-related specialists, the external eye muscles are much stronger than would be necessary to simply move the eyeball. They have found that these muscles change the anterior–posterior length of the eyeball so that it functions with variable focal length, according to what the person is looking at and their thoughts and feelings about the object.

When the two oblique muscles tighten round the eyeball like a belt, they hold it in an elongated shape. Then the lens alone cannot focus the light rays onto the retina, resulting in myopia. This understanding forms the basis of treatment, essentially physical and imaginative exercises developed by Bates to restore the tone and flexibility of the external eye muscles, together with studying the principles of healthy vision.

Bates-related methods remain controversial in conventional medicine. The theory makes sense, but its application is beyond our experience. The notions that the shape of the eyeball and the process of vision are responsive to mechanical forces and our mental emotional framework provides many openings for treatment via craniosacral therapy. In this section we will orient to the shape of the eyeball and the orbit and we will also explore using the eyes as a route into the tone of the nervous system.

The sphenoid is essential in treating the eyes. It forms the back of the orbit; five of the six eye muscles attach to the sphenoid, and essential nerves for vision and controlling the eyeball pass through holes in the sphenoid.

Eyes and posture

Dealing with gravity is one of the biggest functions of the brain. Humans have a unique upright posture. Keeping balance involves integration of signals from the muscular skeletal system (proprioception), and the vestibular apparatus in the ear and the eye.

There are some simple tests you can use to demonstrate the link between the eyes and the musculoskeletal system. These links provide a theoretical framework for the importance of treating the sphenoid for any musculoskeletal issue.

- Try standing on one leg with your eyes closed; it is much harder without reference to the horizon.

- Contact the sub-occipital muscles, specifically the rectus capitus posterior minor (RCPM). You can feel the muscle twitch when you move your eyes, even when your head is still.

- Fix your eyes on a point in front of you. Now try turning your head, as far as it will go. With your eyes fixed ahead it is difficult. If you allow your eyes to point in the direction of the turn, you will suddenly be able to turn your head much further.

- Ask a friend with glasses to stand in their normal posture. Observe them again without their glasses. Frequently the whole attitude of the body will change (including the emotion you would choose to describe them; we can become very attached to our glasses).

- Standing behind a partner, make contact with the posterior superior iliac spines (PSIS). Ask your partner to open and close their eyes. Often you can notice a drop on one side of the pelvis via the PSIS contact.

Eyes and the nervous system

Eye muscles and movement and associated somatic nerves

There are six muscles that control the movement of the eye. Five of them originate on the sphenoid via a fibrous ring at the back of the orbit around the optic canal (see Figure 10.2.1 for the optic canal). The superior oblique has an attachment to the frontal bone, on the superior medial orbit, that acts like a pulley. The inferior oblique originates on the maxilla on the floor of the orbit. All six muscles cause rotation of the eye ball in various directions.

The six muscles are controlled by three different cranial nerves: the occulomotor nerve (CN III), the trochlea (CN IV) and the abducens (CN VI). The nuclei for these three cranial nerves are in the brainstem. CN IV and CN VI supply single eye muscles only, the superior oblique and the lateral rectus respectively. The occulomotor nerve has the widest influence; it controls four of the eye muscles, it opens the eyelids and it innervates the pupil via parasympathetic and some sympathetic fibres that pass along the occulomotor nerve.

There are two other cranial nerves that are relevant to the eye. The ophthalmic branch of the trigeminal nerve (CN V1) is involved in the corneal reflex (people who put in contact lenses learn to override this reflex closure of the eye). CN V1 also carries sensory information from the skin around the eyes. CN V1 enters the orbit through the superior orbital fissure.

The facial nerve (CN VII) supplies the lacrimal glands. This gland rests above the eyeball and produces tears which drain via the lacrimal duct into the nasal cavity. The facial nerve supply to the lacrimal gland passes through the inferior orbital fissure. The supply from the facial nerve is a mix of sympathetic and parasympathetic fibres that take complex routes to the orbit. The parasympathetic fibres synapse in the pterygopalatine ganglion between the palatine bone and the pterygoid processes of the sphenoid. This is a useful orientation for dry eyes.

The control of the eyes is quite a remarkable thing. There are many reflexes involved in tracking moving objects, accommodating for the movement of the head and coordinating the movements of the eyeballs. For example, the vestibulo-ocular reflex coordinates signals from the vestibular apparatus in the inner ear with eye movements. The processing of these signals involves brainstem nuclei and the cerebellum.

Optic nerve

The optic nerve is cranial nerve II (CN II). It carries the signals that are interpreted to create vision. The optic nerve is considered to be part of the central nervous system as it is derived from an outgrowth of the diencephalon during embryonic development. It passes from the back of the retina through the optic canal. The two optic nerves join and cross at the optic chiasma, anterior to the pituitary gland and superior to the body of the sphenoid. The first sign of a pituitary tumour can be vision issues due to swelling of the pituitary gland compressing the optic chiasma.

The signals from the optic nerve initially synapse in the thalamus (lateral geniculate nucleus) and then pass to the occipital lobe. The primary visual cortex, in the occipital lobe, is an important relay station in the processing of visual signals. There are 30 different areas involved in the perception of vision, including parts of the limbic system, an area better known for its role in processing emotion. Sight is an interpretation of incoming signals; meaning is at least as important as movement and shape. We see with our brain, not with our eyes.

Autonomic nervous system and the eyes

The pupils, the eye muscles and the eye lids are all strongly under the influence of the autonomic nervous system. The pupils expand under sympathetic stimulation. Allowing more light in is usually helpful for vision. One of the most common signs of sympathetic overactivation is getting headaches on a sunny day; the pupils are kept expanded by the increased sympathetic activity and fail to close adequately in bright light. The excess light coming into the retina is overwhelming and causes headaches.

Another sign of sympathetic activation is darting, rapidly moving eyes. The eye muscles are active (due to centrally acting sympathetic activity, not the pupil pathway described below). Rapidly moving the eyeball allows for constant scanning of the horizon for signs of danger.

The route the sympathetic nerves take to reach the pupil from the hypothalamus is unusual in that the nerves emerge from the base of the neck, pass through the superior cervical ganglia, then return to the head hitching a ride on the internal carotid artery. The sympathetic supply to the eye enters the skull via the carotid foramen and then some of the fibres join the occulomotor nerve and some join the ophthalmic division of the trigeminal nerve.

Parasympathetic supply, carried via the occulomotor nerve CN III, contracts the pupil in response to light hitting the retina: the pupillary light reflex. The Edinger–Westphal nucleus in the brainstem controls the pupillary light reflex.

The sphenoid and the orbit

'The prominent eyeball goes with the wide orbit (superomedial to inferolateral diameter) and the high great wing.' Sphenoid in flexion: 'Eyeballs equally prominent.' (Magoun 1951, pp.53 and 97)

Sutherland, as recorded by Magoun, noted that the sphenoid in torsion or sidebending/rotation would cause the eye to be more prominent and the orbit to be wider on the 'high side' in torsion or the 'concave side' in sidebending.

If you are looking at a face and notice the eyeball is more prominent or the orbit is larger on the right you might suspect, therefore, that there is a right-side bend (the right greater wing is closer to the front of the body) and/or that there is a right torsion (the right greater wing is closer to the top of the head) at the sphenobasilar junction (SBJ).

These clues should not be used to replace your palpation skills and do not become the focus of the session unless they emerge through the inherent treatment plan; however, they can be a useful starting point for an enquiry into the dynamics of the system. If you start observing faces, differences in the orbits and the eyes is one of the easiest shapes to spot.

Treatment Exercise: The eyes and the sphenoid

1. Start at the sacrum.

   • Establish resources, wait for the holistic shift and orient to mid tide.

2. Move to Becker's vault hold.

- Explore the dynamics of the SBJ.

- Allow any clues from the size of the orbit and the prominence of the eye to support, but not lead, your perception.

- Can you feel the sphenoid diving forward and widening on inhale? This is often a clear indication of health or that there has been a change in the system.

- For the purposes of this exercise just be aware of the shapes within the skull and the whole body.

3. Make contact with the eyeballs.

- Use an adapted frontal hold so that your middle finger rests on the eyeball.

- Take time to settle. Any pressure on the eyelid will be uncomfortable to receive; a featherlight touch is essential here. Make sure you have very strong elbow fulcrums.

- As you settle into the space it is acceptable to take your hands off and renegotiate the contact.

- Be careful not to narrow down your perceptual field.

4. Explore the eyeball, muscles and bones.

- Steps 4 and 5 are interchangeable depending on what presents. The system often quickly shows you either nervous system issues or structural issues.

- Can you get a sense of the shape of the eyeball? It is a fluid-filled ball. Sometimes it feels squashed and restricted. Is it elongated or short and wide?

- Often there is sense of soft tissue pulling through the muscles, or distortions through the orbit bones.

- Support Becker's three-stage process.

5. Orient to the optic nerves, the optic chiasma and the brain.

- Can you orient to the eyes as stalks sticking out from the brain? Sometimes you can get a real sense of being plugged into an active nervous system. Your awareness may be drawn to the optic chiasma, the brainstem, the occipital lobe or just a sense of the whole CNS.

- Notice any differences from side to side.

- Support Becker's three-stage process.

6. Return to Becker's vault hold.

- Notice any changes at the SBJ.

- Negotiate ending.

10.3 THE JAW AND THE TMJ

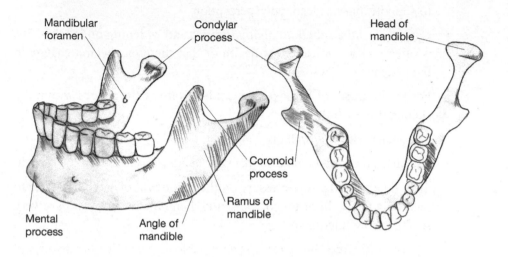

Figure 10.3.1 Lateral and superior views of mandible

The jaw is an incredibly common place for holding tension. During the case history it is very useful to ask about jaw tension, grinding (bruxism), mouth guards and dental problems. You may be surprised how often people will complain of jaw problems.

Consciously sitting with your jaw held tightly for any length of time quickly becomes an unpleasant experience. This exercise makes it clear how linked in the jaw is to fear, pain, love, grief, difficulty communicating and expressing ourselves, tension in our whole musculoskeletal system and holding right down into the heart, the guts and the pelvic floor. After clenching the jaw tight, releasing immediately gives a sense of relief, all the way down to the toes. The wide influence of the jaw is so obvious if you practise this on yourself.

Unfortunately the jaw is one of the areas where deep-rooted tension is often outside our immediate awareness. To soften and work with our own jaw dynamics is often very hard. As a practitioner, meeting that tension with skill, in the biodynamic paradigm, can have excellent results.

Clinical Highlight: TMJ self-test

Try the following self-assessment for the TMJ (downloaded September 2008 from www.wholebodymed.com/wbd.php).

Answer the following questions:

- Do you get frequent headaches or facial pain?

- Do you get frequent neck aches or shoulder aches?

- Do you find yourself clenching your teeth during the day?

- Do you grind your teeth at night?

- Do you wake up with your teeth clenched?

If you answered 'yes' to any of the above, especially two or more, there is a good chance you may have TMD (temporomandibular dysfunction).

Alignment of the jaw via the temporals

The anatomy of the temporal mandibular joint (TMJ) is complex. The literature (from dentistry and manipulative modalities such as chiropractic, osteopathy and physiotherapy) on aligning the jaw, and its significance for overall health, is frequently contradictory and unclear. Teeth removal, splints and braces to help relieve overcrowding and alignment issues are common, but are controversial.

The biomechanics of TMJ alignment are significant. Jaw tension is a frequent sign of stress. An alternative model of causation for jaw grinding is not over-activation but a continual reflex attempt by the muscles to adjust to misalignment of the biting surfaces.

The most effective way of supporting jaw alignment is to first work with the cranial base via the temporal bones. All the life events that impact the cranial base are relevant. The TMJ is such a dynamic area that just orienting to the position of the mandible is not always enough.

On inhale the mandible widens side to side, the two rami moving lateral, flaring out in relation to the old symphysis menti. Confusingly, classic biomechanics state that the coronoid processes move medially on inhale. This has not been our experience. If you are with the mid tide and the motility of the bone, it is much more useful to tune into a sense of the coronoid processes widening on inhale. Commonly you will feel one side of the mandible pulled superior and/or posterior. Resolution of inertial shapes often involves inferior and anterior space. The jaw thrusts down and out as it grows. Tight muscles often act to clamp the jaw upwards and backwards.

Treatment Exercise: Orienting to the temporal
bones and alignment of the jaw

1. Start at the innominate bones.

   - Take time to really establish resources, check in verbally, negotiate contact and wait for the holistic shift. Orient to mid tide.

   - The innominate bones often resonate with the temporals.

2. Explore the shapes in the whole skull.

- Using the vault or cradle holds move to the head. Differentiate between the neurocranium and the viscerocranium (facial complex).

- Do you notice any shapes through the bony facial complex? Does one side feel different to the other?

- Explore the muscles of the jaw. Can you orient to the sling made by the masseter and the medial pterygoid muscle? Can you get a sense of the tension in the lateral pterygoids?

- How is the mandible held in relationship to the cranial base?

3. Move to the temporal ear hold.

- Orient particularly to the dynamics of the temporal bones.

- Can you support a state of balance through the whole cranium through your contact at the temporals?

- Can you feel the temporal bones roll in and out evenly with phases of the tide?

4. Contact the angles of the mandible.

- Explore how inhale and exhale are expressed through the mandible. Can you feel the jaw widening on inhale?

- Is there still a sense of uneven movement? Often the work at temporals resolves many dynamics of the jaw. However, the additional intention of inferior and anterior space on the mandible can be useful.

5. Negotiate ending.

Development of the lower jaw

At birth the lower jaw is relatively much smaller, compared to the rest of the skull, than it is in the adult. As it grows it thrusts forwards and downwards. The developing teeth also change the shape and form of the jaw. The coronoid process also gets much bigger (see Figures 6.1.5 and 10.3.1).

The mandible is in two parts at birth. The joint is fibrous, and is called the symphysis menti. The joint surfaces are cartilage. (It is similar to the pubic symphysis but without a disc.) According to *Gray's Anatomy* the two halves of the mandible fuse between the ages of one and three (Standring 2005, p.483).

Muscles of the jaw

The muscles of mastication are very powerful. The temporalis and masseter are familiar to most people and easily palpated on the external surfaces of the skull.

On clenching the jaw you can feel the fibres of the temporalis contracting on the side of the head superior and anterior to the ear. The masseter is easily felt passing from the zygomatic arch to the angle of the mandible.

Harder to feel, and to visualize, are the very important pterygoid muscles. They are anchored on the pterygoid processes of the sphenoid. The medial pterygoid forms a sling with the masseter. The medial pterygoid, the temporalis and the masseter muscles all strongly close the jaw and are involved in chewing. Orienting to the sling of muscles is a very useful awareness.

The lateral pterygoid muscles open the jaw (along with gravity and some of the muscles connecting to the hyoid – not elaborated on here). What is interesting is that it attaches into the joint capsule of the TMJ and, even deeper, connects to the anterior part of the articular disc.

Ligaments and disc of the temporal mandibular joint

The TMJ is stabilized by three main ligaments. Biomechanically it is possible to orient to the alignment of the individual ligaments and offer space along the line of the ligament whilst contacting/stabilizing either the sphenoid or temporal bone as appropriate. The three ligaments:

- The lateral ligament from the zygomatic process to the condylar process (alignment inferior posterior).

- The stylomandibular ligament from the styloid process of the temporal bone to the medial surface of angle of the mandible (alignment inferior anterior).

- The sphenomandibular ligament from the underside of the sphenoid to the medial surface of the ramus of the mandible (alignment inferior).

The TMJ is a very unusual joint. The two sides have to move together or, at the very least, accommodate to movement initiated at the other side. The condyle of the jaw has two movements on jaw opening – it rotates and slides anteriorly. It is a very mobile joint. On opening, often there is a lateral shift that can be felt at the TMJ, from one side back to the other. This side-to-side wobble and uneven movement of the condyles is not an optimal situation.

There is an articular disc that should move with the condyle as it rotates and slides forward. It should follow the curves of the mandibular fossa and articular tubercle on the underside of the zygomatic process of the temporal bone. *Gray's Anatomy* likens the disc to a banana skin that permits movement of the joint. There are two synovial cavities, one above and one below the disc, that lubricate the joint.

To help the disc move and stay in place, between the moving condyle and the fossa, the lateral pterygoid muscle acts to pull it forward and the posterior elastic material acts to pull it backwards.

Often problems occur when the disc gets out of sync with the condyle. There are different classifications of misalignment. Most frequently the disc is pulled too far forward. On jaw opening and closing, as the condyle partially engages and disengages with the misaligned disc, there is often a clicking sound. Sometimes there is a complete dislocation of the disc and this contributes to locking of the jaw.

10.4 THE THROAT
The hyoid

The hyoid is an unusual and interesting bone. It floats in an arrangement of muscles, ligaments and fascia, suspended in front of the throat. Typically it is at the level of the third cervical vertebra. You can palpate it on yourself in the space underneath the jaw and above the Adam's apple (thyroid cartilage). If you swallow you can feel it move. You should also be able to feel it as a dense lump that moves side to side when you push.

There are a host of muscles that hold the hyoid in place. Suprahyoid muscles attach superiorly to the mandible and the temporal bone, notably the diagastric muscle. Infrahyoid muscles attach inferiorly to the sternum, the clavicle and the scapula. There are also some muscles that connect the hyoid posteriorly to the tube of tissues that form the pharanyx. One of the authors' most surprising sessions receiving cranial work was to feel their shoulder tweaking as the therapist contacted the hyoid. It was not until the author looked up the omohyoid muscle, going from the hyoid to the upper border of the scapula, that they understood the anatomy behind the experience.

There is a strong ligamentous attachment inferiorly to the thyroid cartilage. The hyoid is an integral part of the deep cervical fascia that connects the cranial base, the inferior maxilla, the mandible, the structures of the throat (the pharynx, hyoid, thyroid and cricoid cartilages), the thyroid organ and the carotid sheaths, going all the way down to the sternum and the pericardium (Tufts 2009). That is a huge potential zone of direct influence if we can begin to engage with the hyoid in biodynamic craniosacral therapy.

Awareness Exercise: Posture and the throat

- Try finding a neutral upright standing posture. Look for strong feet, your weight not forwards or backwards or on the left or the right. Try engaging your pelvic floor and feeling strong in your core muscles. Let the tube of your neck lengthen and your shoulders spread. Try a lift though your heart and a smile on your face. Enjoy the feeling of balance and openness for a few minutes.

- Let your heart sink, your head jut forward and your belly go slack. Become a sack of potatoes. Keep holding this posture and notice what happens. Not pleasant, but if you walk down the street and look at people it is a very common posture.

- Keep holding the shape. Particularly notice your throat. Can you feel a sense of tightness or compression? Often this posture is coupled with a blocked throat, an ache in the lower back, weight going forward and a clawing of the toes.

- From this exercise it is possible to see that shifts in the space and connections in the throat could help with toe pain and low back pain. Some osteopaths link together big toe problems, low back pain and sore throats. It is all connected. We love exercises like this; they endlessly demonstrate that the whole body works as a unit.

The facial complex and the social nervous system are essential to expressing emotion

One of the most successful ways of working with the face, jaw and throat (the facial complex) is to appreciate the importance of the neurology. The jaw and throat often act like a weather vane indicating problems of activation in the brainstem. The jaw and throat frequently hum with nervous tension. The cranial nerve nuclei that control the facial complex are all located in the brainstem – very close to the autonomic centres that control our responses to stress and overwhelm.

Porges (2003) is clear that whole subsets of cranial nerves fire together in a phased response to stress. In humans the first responses are about communication and orientation. Porges' classification of the social nervous system links together cranial nerves V, VII, IX, X and XI. They control sucking, swallowing, voice, breathing, middle ear muscles, heart rate, ingesting, facial expression and head movements. Neurologically there can be no doubt that the face, jaw and throat can hold deep imprints and patterning in response to our experiences.

A tight throat, feeling choked, crying, having a plum in your throat and feeling unable to speak are very common experiences. The ability to express emotion, to articulate our needs and communicate all depend on space and openness within a fully functioning face, jaw and throat area. Being in practice will quickly demonstrate that many people frequently feel blocked and stuck in the throat and have very tight jaws.

Treatment Exercise: The hyoid

1. Start at feet.

   - Establish resources, wait for holistic shift and orient to mid tide.

2. Make contact with the hyoid via an adapted jaw hold.

- To contact the hyoid, keep the general face hold, but move your hands slightly towards the feet so that you can place your middle finger on the lateral parts of the bone. You will need to sense through the soft tissues. Maintain a delicate contact.

- Allow a tissue awareness and support Becker's three-stage process.

- Facilitate a state of balance in relationship to a fulcrum.

- Classic intention is of inferior/anterior space.

- Can the hyoid float in the tissue field?

3. Options to explore.

- Use a different hold – one hand on the hyoid and the other hand below neck or on the sternum or on the head or shoulder.

- The throat is a powerful, intimate place; it may be important to resource and pace the treatment as required.

- CNS facilitation may be present.

4. Orient to branchial arches.

- Use the state of balance as a gateway to a deeper state.

- Orient to fluid field and embryological intentions.

- Clues that might tell you you are in touch with formative forces: fluid-membranous field rather than bones, wide field awareness, sense of a small being in your hands, big head relative to the body, clear sense of midline, non-tidal growth patterns become present.

5. Negotiate ending – via cradle or return to feet.

Summary of Chapter 10

Appreciating how powerful a place the face is in the body and how its state of health has global effects is an important feature of the work. The face meets the world in many ways from the moment of birth onwards. So learning to be confident and sensitive in your approach to working with specific patterns that commonly arise within the facial complex will produce great results.

Here are some of the skills that can develop from the chapter material:

- Recognizing birth patterns in the facial complex, including vertical and horizontal shapes, distortions of the cranial base and their relevance to the face, appreciating the midline of face, and the palate as a transverse diaphragm.

- Orienting to the eyes. Common possible stories that emerge around the eyes are the dynamics of the orbit and the sphenoid, the shape of the eyeballs and appreciating the eyes as outgrowths of the brain.

- Understanding the ramifications of chronic jaw tension and its effect on all the systems of the body including the neuroendocrine–immune responses, digestion, posture and emotions.

- Working with the hyoid as a natural fulcrum for the structural and emotional health of the throat.

Notes

1. We strongly associate poor dental work as the one of the main factors adversely affecting the body. Dentistry is a very complex area. We have had long conversations with a number of dentists over the years. We always come away stimulated, but rarely with a consistent, clear approach. If your client does not seem to respond we would strongly recommend looking in their mouth. *Whole Body Dentistry* (Breiner 1999) is an interesting exploration of dentistry that discusses toxicity and much else.

   Metal irritation also seems to be a problem. A few years ago we realized that the majority of our long-term clients with hard-to-treat issues had significant amounts of metal dental work in their mouth. We find change happens much more slowly with people with large amounts of amalgam fillings, gold teeth, metal crowns, metal braces, poor-fitting bridges and plates. (Also tongue and lip piercings – the problem is not just toxicity but metal irritation in a sensitive environment.) A neurological explanation is that metal acts as an irritant to the sensitive membranes and structures of the mouth (King 2008), a bit like walking around with a pebble in your shoe. The irritation causes a whole spinal cord response called the flexor withdrawal response. This upsets the proprioceptive mechanisms of the body and leads to aberrant musculoskeletal output throughout the whole body. Our very strong experience is that a whole host of chronic disorders including knee pain, low back pain, shoulder pain, neck pain and tiredness will clear much more quickly when the metal in the mouth is removed. As we get more experienced we are increasingly aware of a particular quality of nervous activity in the facial complex that indicates metal irritation.

2. The work of Price offers another insight into the cause of problems in the facial complex. He was a dentist who travelled the world in the 1930s documenting the effects of nutritional changes as people moved away from traditional foods to more processed foods. He discovered huge increases in the amount of cavitations in younger generations and quite radical changes in the shapes of faces (narrow, poorly formed dental arches, crowded teeth, narrow nostrils). He has many photos from different indigenous cultures showing significant narrowing of the facial complex following the change from traditional food. You can view his book *Nutrition and Physical Degeneration* online via http://gutenberg.net.au/ebooks02/0200251h.html.

3. One of the authors had a phase of treating people from a boxing club.

4. Working to create space around the pterygopalatine ganglion, by working with the palatines between the maxilla and the pterygoid processes of the sphenoid, is a classic piece of biomechanics that may be helpful for sinus issues and irritated nasal mucous membranes.

5. For this discussion of the Bates method and the complexity of the visual process we are very grateful to Viola Sampson (2005).

Joints

11.1 INTRODUCTION TO JOINTS

In the East, longevity has been understood for a long time to be intimately linked to the mobility of the joints. You are as old as your joints. Therefore, yoga and chi kung emphasize stretching and opening joints to create supple bodies and only then can prana or chi move through their channels properly.

Without stable, mobile joints your posture will not be optimal and there will not be a smooth transition of weight through the joints, resulting in increased wear and tear. It is as if the body has a dynamic between suppleness and postural alignment versus poor posture, wear and tear, joint compensations, tension, lack of suppleness and rigidity. Along with that comes a decrease in energy, emotional contractions, mental rigidity and narrowing of perceptions.

Broad mind/postural balance/spacious synovium all work together and are part of a whole reality. Sustainability of stress for the joints is different for every individual; some people's constitutions are so strong they can work down a coal mine and smoke 30 cigarettes a day and still maintain health. The power of potency and the right DNA are significant.

Clinically this therapy can produce tremendous results with joints. This is a prime area for research. Some joint conditions are amongst the most painful of physical conditions, so any relief is a positive result. This therapy can affect joint conditions powerfully and it can easily be used for joint rehabilitation, recovery from joint operations, supporting hip/knee replacement, knee injury, and joint diseases.

Can joints recover from physical deterioration? Yes; bone is constantly being remodelled in line with the forces present. All joints will be conducive to aligning back to the original blueprint of health if the conditional forces affecting the joint are resolved. Even someone with chronic osteoarthritis or rheumatoid arthritis will try to make the right moves back to health. It does not matter how chronic the condition is, the body can move towards greater health. The possibility of health is never lost, it is the imperative of life. Shut down, low potency, physical restriction, pain, degeneration – all of these phenomena may be the healthiest options available at a given point in time. The body has no choice but to respond to a deeper interaction with the breath of life; however, the degree of response is down to the individual's overall health, constitution and internal awareness.

Synovial joints

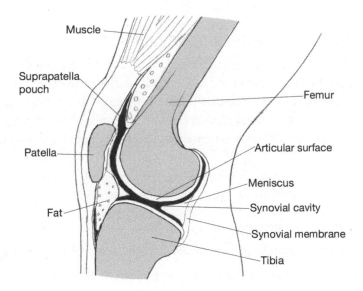

Figure 11.1.1 Sagittal section of the knee joint showing the synovial cavity

The most common and the most moveable type of joint in the human body are synovial joints. The joints of the limbs and facet joints of the spine are synovial joints with great freedom of movement, necessary for allowing the full mobility of the arms and legs and the back and neck. There is a balance struck between stability and large ranges of movement. Often the joints need lots of support to continue to function at their optimum throughout life. Clinically this means you will spend lots of time orienting to overloaded and misaligned synovial joints in your practice.

All synovial joints are hydraulic systems. The ends of the bone are lined with shiny hyaline cartilage. Ligaments and the joint capsule bind the joint together. The ends of the bones do not actually touch; there is fluid space bounded by a synovial membrane. This membrane secretes synovial fluid. In health the fluid causes the joint surfaces to glide over each other; think of a glass sliding on a table covered in oil. Synovial joints are an engineering wonder. Despite injury and misuse these joints will go on working even with mechanical issues. Look at professional soccer players and how often they damage their knees; they still manage to continue with the help of physiotherapy, surgery and painkillers. The body can almost fully recuperate from dramatic injuries; often soccer players are back and in full training within the same season from something as dramatic as cruciate ligament damage. This not only says lots about modern medical and therapeutic care but how powerful the body is. It helps greatly that the individuals are athletes in peak physical condition, it shows how the potency of the whole system is a critical factor in recovery.

Fibrous joints and cartilaginous joints

The other common kind of joints are fibrous joints and cartilaginous joints which are mostly in the head and between the vertebral bodies of the spine. The sutures in the head are fibrous joints. The disc joints of the spine are typical examples of cartilaginous joints with a strong fibrous ring of cartilage and a soft pulpy nucleus pulposus in the middle. These joints have less mobility than synovial joints.

Awareness Exercise: Global joint exercise

- Bring your awareness to your right knee.

- Let your awareness deepen so you find the sense of fluid in the joint.

- Stay with that and open out to the potency field around the body. See what happens.

- Your joint should start to charge up and as the fluids infuse with potency notice how the surrounding tissue adjusts.

- Fluids, potency and tissues are in relationship and the structure is able to optimize.

11.2 TREATING JOINTS

Treating joints is treating the body. All elements of the body meet at joints:

- Synovial fluid.
- Connective tissue/ligament.
- Muscle/tendon.
- Synovial membrane/epithelial secreting tissues.
- Bone/cartilage.
- Nervous system/mechanoreceptors/pain receptors.
- Hormone/immune system.

A spinal vertebral joint also has a visceral relationship.

Of course, in a way everything is a joint, including synapses, cell membranes, ion gates, lymph nodes, Bowman's capsules, etc. A joint is a meeting place and a junction, a transition from one place to another.

As a therapist the most common condition to come through your clinic space is joint dysfunction. It is so common for people to have joint injuries, congenital defects, whiplash, lower back problems, hip/knee replacement, and arthritis. The list is endless and the better you understand joints the more successful you will become as a therapist. Know this:

- When you hold a joint you are in contact with the whole body.

- One joint changes and they all start to change as if joints talk to each other.

- The body is a series of tissue and fluid fields oriented around joints.

- Joints are reservoirs of potency. Synovial fluid has some similarities with CSF, so you've got a whole network of ventricles.

- One adjustment at a joint has a knock-on effect through the whole body connective tissue framework.

General principles for working with joints

The site of the pain is rarely the cause of the problem. Never just treat a joint locally. Fulcrums in the spine, the cranium and organs are at least as important as any local joint dynamics. Remember to trust the inherent treatment plan. However, if someone comes with a painful joint, it is useful to acknowledge the joint and make contact there during session work, if only to satisfy a surface need of the client that you are working on their presenting issue.

Under-resourced and overwhelmed clients will take longer to heal. Even with acute presenting issues, creating safety and resources and helping clear dissociative processes and/or over-activation are often the essential first steps. Many chronic joint issues will resolve by paying attention to the whole person. Often these are cases that have been treated unsuccessfully by other bodyworkers who have focused on the local dynamics and structural issues. The embodied skills to work with overwhelm are particularly clear in biodynamic craniosacral therapy.

Pain and emotion always go together; joint pain is no different. Do not fall into the trap of assigning particular themes to particular parts of the body. For example, knee problems are because 'you cannot get over things' or left-sided issues are about 'issues with your mother or not integrating your femininity'. The human experience is way too complex for simplistic maps of that kind. Allow individual stories to emerge using your verbal skills during your hands-on clinic work.

Useful orientations are: Can you help the structure you are drawn to work with come back into relationship to the whole? Can the joint and limb express primary respiration orienting to the midline and to its natural fulcrums on the midline? L5 is often mentioned as the natural fulcrum for the legs and C7 the natural fulcrum for the arms.

Given the above, specific orientations, based on a clear knowledge of the anatomy of individual joints, will enormously speed up the process of healing. Some introductory thoughts for individual joints are given below.

It is possible, with skilled palpatory awareness, to feel and treat the quality of nerve flow between the centre and periphery. Treatment that appreciates nerve flow can break the cycle of flexor withdrawal, facilitation and nociceptive loops. You can use a two-handed contact between the peripheral structure and the spine (see Figure 2.3.5).

Treating limbs

Often one limb will feel and move quite differently to another limb. It is extremely effective in practice to be aware of this. Figure 11.2.1 shows some common bilateral holds that will enable you directly to compare primary respiration in each side. Remember on inhale the legs and arms externally rotate. On inhale each joint will naturally seek space; the joints will express motility as a sense of expansion and opening.

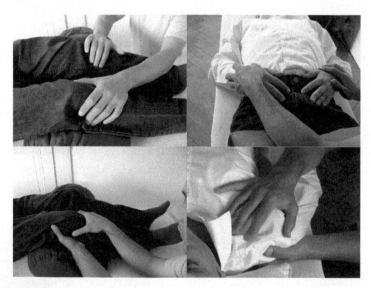

Figure 11.2.1 Contacting limbs and joints
Top row: Bilateral contacts can be very useful to compare how one side is expressing primary respiration compared to the other. Bottom row: Making contact around the joints

Develop the skill of trying to feel the whole outline of the body, from wherever you make contact. Often it feels as though one limb is missing or is smaller or is just very hard to contact. If this is the case, see if you can expand your awareness to invite the missing part back into relationship with the whole. Use verbal skills to invite the client to explore how their brain is mapping out their body. 'How does x compare to y?' 'Does the outline of your body feel in proportion? For example, are your hands or feet too big, too small, too close, or too far away?' What cannot be felt is often the fulcrum, rather than the busy noisy part that is tight and complaining.

Allow the possibility of an embryological awareness. Orient to how the limbs budded out from the body in the early embryo (see Figure 10.1.4). Allow the limbs to balance, like a delicate see-saw, in relationship to the midline.

Clinical Highlight: Nerve flow

There are three ways of orienting to the flow of information between the spine and the periphery. Nerve flow is easiest to feel either via the nerve roots or via the spinal cord segments:

- *Nerve roots.* Orient to where the nerve root leaves the spine through the intervertebral foramen and feel the flow along the nerve to the structure it supplies. The somatic nerve roots from C5 to T1 innervate the arm and shoulder, forming the brachial plexus. The sympathetic nerves exiting from T1 and L2 supply the viscera. The somatic nerves exiting from the lower lumbar vertebrae supply the structures of the lower back and legs. For example, the nerve roots L4 to L5 (and S1 and S2) form the sciatic nerve and innervate the back of the leg and foot. The femoral nerve roots emerge from L2 to L3 and innervate the front of the thigh and hip flexors.

- *Spinal cord segments.* Orient to the spinal cord segment where the nerve originates. Orient to the nociceptive (pain) loops between a painful structure and the relevant spinal cord segment. The important anatomical piece here is that the spinal cord ends at around L1 and that the lower spinal cord segments are at a different level to the similarly named vertebrae. For the lower legs and back, facilitated spinal cord segments can therefore be felt at the thoracic lumbar junction. For the cervical region the spinal cord will be facilitated at the level of the similarly named vertebrae.

- *Embryological segments.* Orient to the nucleus pulposus in the intervertebral disc. This is the natural fulcrum for two adjacent vertebrae and the natural fulcrum for all the tissues that grew in the embryo from the somite that developed at the level of the nucleus pulposus. This awareness has a slower quality than nerve flow; it is about embryological intentions. Orientation to the limbs budding out from the somites can be very useful.

11.3 KEY JOINTS: AXIAL SKELETON
Occipital atlantal junction

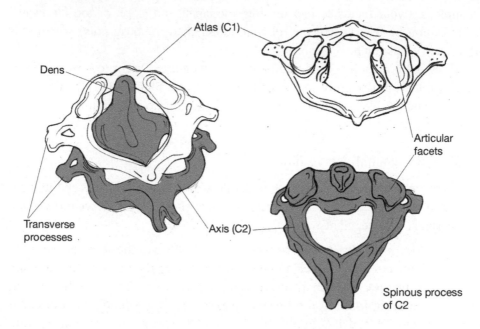

Figure 11.3.1 Atlas and axis

The whole weight of the skull and its movements of rotation, nodding and sidebending is supported by a relatively small set of joints comprising three bones: the occiput, the atlas (the first cervical vertebra or C1) and the axis (the second cervical vertebra or C2). The joint complex is unique in the body. It is sometimes called the occipital triad, the upper cervical complex or the occipitoatlantal axis/ complex as well as the occipital atlantal junction (OAJ).

The articulation of the atlas with the axis is complicated, comprising four distinct joints:

- There is a pivot articulation between the dens of the axis and the ring formed by the anterior arch and the transverse ligament of the atlas. Here there are two joints: one between the posterior surface of the anterior arch of the atlas and the front of the dens; the other between the anterior surface of the ligament and the back of the process.

- There are also bilateral gliding synovial joints between the articular processes on the superior surface of the axis and inferior surface of the atlas.

There are many layers of ligaments between the bones of the occipital triad. The alar, apical (or odontoid), transverse and cruciform ligaments are an unusual network of small ligaments around the dens. There are also the facet joint capsules, ligaments that bind to the arches of the vertebrae, and continuations of the longitudinal ligaments running the length of the spine that connect into the inferior parts of the occiput and sphenoid.

As if this is not complex enough there are a whole series of suboccipital muscles (rectus and oblique capitis muscles) that help maintain stability and control of this area of the body, plus a complex cervical nerve plexus to deal with the fine adjustments and movements needed to keep the head and neck in balance.

The amazing thing is this doesn't go wrong that often. It mostly goes right and there is enough movement and balance to allow the head and spine to co-relate. However, the most common musculoskeletal dysfunction after lower back pain is neck pain. This can lead to headaches, poor mobility and a general stagnation of potency in the head.

Upper body tensions frequently start from the upper cervical complex, so don't be surprised if you are often drawn into this area. Many people become tight and compressed at the OAJ when they are stressed and activated. Contact at the atlas is particularly powerful as it is at the centre of the complex. Often you will feel many small adjustments in the suboccipitals and then the atlas will feel like it is floating anterior and widening. Relief to the whole body comes from this adjustment along with a reduction in nervous tone.

Treatment Exercise: The occipital atlantal junction

1. Start at the atlas.

   - Establish resources, wait for the holistic shift and orient to mid tide.

   - The atlas hold is an adaptation of the cradle hold, with a little more precision in the finger contact. You may need to move your hands slightly inferior so that your finger tips or pads can be in contact with the posterior arch of the atlas. There is no spinous process on the atlas so the first midline bump you feel, moving inferiorly from the occipital inion, will be the C2 spinous. Your finger pads should make contact laterally to the hollow between the inion and C2.

   - It is possible to be even more precise. Keep your second fingers in contact with the atlas but allow your first/index fingers to extend to contact the transverse processes of the axis. With this hold you will be in contact with all three bones of the occipital triad. It takes a little practice to get the landmarks.

2. Orient to the atlas floating between the occiput and axis.

   - The atlas is often relatively posterior on the occipital condyles. Tight neck muscles and arching of the head during birth both tend to create this pattern. The atlas really seems to enjoy the intention of anterior space. It is a wonderful feeling to experience the atlas floating in the fluid of its synovial joints between the axis and the occiput.

3. Orient to superior and inferior space between the axis and the occiput.

    •   There is frequently compression within the occipital triad. This 'telescoping' can feed in all the way to the SBJ and often originates in birth. Detailed awareness of the ligaments and tissue relationships is particularly helpful in this orientation, as is also being clear in your contact on the occiput and axis.

4. Orient to intraosseous patterns within the occiput.

    •   The occiput was in four parts at birth. Often there is a sense of narrowing across the condyles or rotation between the squama and the condyles. Birth and intraosseous issues are often the key with the OAJ.

5. Negotiate ending, maybe at feet or the pelvis.

Lumbosacral junction

This is a place of critical health for the whole body. When it is working well there is an ease and balance in the joint and all of the surrounding ligaments and muscles. The spine is able to curve with ease as the body moves and the whole weight of the body is smoothly translated through the joint. When it is not working there is lower back pain, muscles are over-contracted and there is compensation through the legs and pelvis that can create whole body patterns. The spine loses its flexibility and there is uneven translation of weight through the area so that the hips become out of balance and strains develop through the pelvis and spine.

The strains are commonly in the erector spinae muscles and the iliolumbar and lumbosacral ligaments that attach onto the transverse processes of L5 and L4 and the anterior longitudinal ligament is often under a great deal of stress. All of this in time will affect the viability of the L5 disc joint which may often bulge or in extreme cases rupture. The most common cause of days off work is lower back pain and it's not hard to see why this is such a global problem with people having such poor posture and weak body tone. Over time this will affect breathing and walking, and energy levels will decrease.

As a practitioner your client may commonly present with low energy or headaches but as the sessions proceed the underlying pattern of lumbosacral restriction will show itself. This is one of the most common muscular skeletal issues in the body. L4, L5 and S1 is a reflection of the C2, C1 and occiput relationship and the potency of the ligaments are critical for health and balance. Spend time getting to know the ligaments at the lumbosacral junction (LSJ) and the pivotal roles of the psoas, quadratus lumborum and lower erector spinae muscles. All of these muscles contribute to lumbar stability.

Sacroiliac joints

The key joints of the pelvis take the weight of the body from the lumbar spine and split it into the innominate bones before moving through the hips down the legs. These joints have large articular surfaces that can cope with the upper body weight. The joints are ideally mobile and even; however, that rarely is the case and often the sacrum is oriented to the left or the right in a sidebending shape or rotated/torsioned left or right.

Inevitably these patterns affect the spine so that it takes on C curving and torsion patterns or at its worst scoliosis. Of course, the spine can affect the sacroiliac (SI) joints so that rotations in the spine cause the sacrum to orient in a similar way. You will notice as a practitioner that there is commonly compression into one of the SI joints which can create a whole set of strains in the legs, hips and pelvis.

A powerful way to contact the SI joints is to bring one hand to the sacrum and by craning your arm across the front of the pelvis rest your palm and fleshy part of your forearm on the anterior iliac crests. This contact will allow you to get a 3D perception of the pelvis in relationship to the SI joints. This perception will facilitate states of balance to arise across the whole pelvis.

11.4 KEY JOINTS: LOWER LIMB

Hip joints

The hip joints are huge joints surrounded by some very strong muscles. It is a common joint to be painful and to experience wear and tear.

Hip anatomy

Bones: The head of the femur angles in to articulate with the innominate bone, via the acetabulum. The hip socket is deep in the groin; most people will point to the greater trochanter when asked about the hip joint.

Hip muscles: The main muscles to know about are the psoas, the gluteals and the piriformis. The psoas originates from the front of the transverse processes and lateral vertebral bodies of T12 to L4; it inserts into the lesser trochanter. It is a strong hip flexor. A tight psoas, pulling the lumbar arch into lordosis, or a long and weak psoas are common patterns. It is a wonderful muscle to make friends with, linking the spine to the legs.

The three gluteal muscles strongly extend the hip. They form the bulk of the buttocks and are important postural muscles and hip stabilizers.

The piriformis is the main external rotator, extending from the front of the sacrum to the greater trochanter. It is an interesting muscle as the sciatic nerve passes beneath it. Because of this anatomical closeness it is suggested that piriformis tightness is implicated in sciatica.

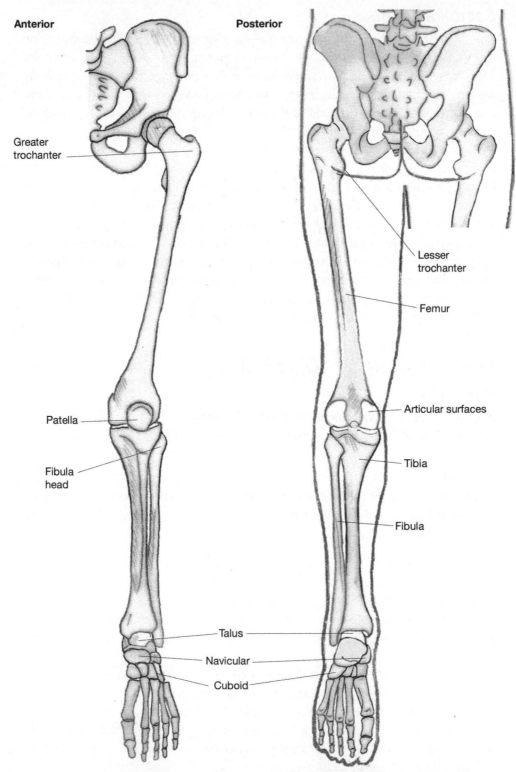

Anterior

Posterior

Greater
trochanter

Lesser
trochanter

Femur

Patella

Articular surfaces

Fibula
head

Tibia

Fibula

Talus

Navicular

Cuboid

Figure 11.4.1 Left leg bones and joints: anterior and posterior views

Connective tissues: The joint capsule surrounds the joint.

Clinical focus: The dynamics of the hip joint are so tied into the lumbosacral junction and the sacroiliac joints that often treatment of those areas resolves pain presenting in the hip. In health the hip joint will feel fluid and will express a smooth internal and external rotation.

Knee joints

The knee is a particularly vulnerable joint. It is one of the most common joints to be injured in sport; it will not be long in your practice before you meet someone who has injured their knee playing football or skiing or from overdoing the lotus position in yoga. There is a common 'terrible triad' of a torn anterior cruciate ligament (ACL), damaged medial collateral ligament and damaged medial meniscus. In acute injuries there is often a sequence of 'pop, pain and can't straighten'.

The knee also is one of the most common places for people to experience osteoarthritis.

> Almost one in three Americans older than age 45 reports some type of knee pain, and it's a common reason that people visit their doctors or the emergency room. (MayoClinic.com 2009)

Arthritis simply means 'wear and tear'. The term frequently generates anxiety for people and joint pain is seen as an inevitable consequence of getting old. This is just not true; even with some wear and tear in the joints there is not an absolute correlation to pain. By improving the alignment of the joint, the proprioceptive control and the potency resources of the whole system, our experience is that even chronic joint pain of many years can be significantly relieved.

Osteoarthritis (OA) often affects single joints, typically knees, hips and thumbs, but it can be any freely moveable joint, including spinal joints. OA is quite different from rheumatoid arthritis (RA). RA is often a systemic disease of excessive immune activity that can target joints. In RA many joints, often smaller joints, are involved. It can happen quite suddenly. The over-active immune response can lead to destruction of the joint.

In OA, persistent wear and tear, due to poor joint mechanics and poor proprioceptive feedback and control, causes damage to the cartilage that protects the joint surfaces. There will be inflammation, swelling, pain and loss of function. Over time, if untreated, the body starts laying down more bone to protect the surfaces, leading to osteophytes and joint thickening that restrict the range of movement.

The good news is that cranial work can be fantastic in helping recovery from acute knee injuries and in treating chronic knee pain. All the general principles of working with joints apply. Some highly effective, specific explorations are given in the clinical highlight below.

Knee anatomy

Bones: The knee joint is primarily the tibia hinging on the femur. The distal end of the femur has two large, shiny and smooth-sliding surfaces/condyles. Between the femur and the tibia are two unique crescent-shaped pads of fibrocartilage: the medial and lateral menisci.

Two other bones form parts of the knee: the patella is a sesamoid bone in the tendon of the quadriceps muscles; laterally the fibula head attaches to some important muscles and ligaments.

Knee muscles: Anteriorly the insertion of the quadriceps group crosses the knee joint, attaching to the tibial plateaux. The quads straighten/extend the knee. A frequent pattern is for the vastus medialis of the quads to be too weak and the lateral ilio tibial band (ITB) to be too tight. This causes tracking problems of the patella and can cause inflammation of the joint. It is a common intervention of soft tissue practitioners to recommend loosening the ITB (often painfully) and strengthening the vastus medialis (partial squats, often hard work).

Posteriorly the hamstring group insert onto the tibia and fibula and the calf muscles attach to the femur; both groups cross the joint. Often the hamstrings are relatively weak compared to the quads. The calf muscles are often very tight. The popliteus is a muscle crossing the back of the knee that unlocks the knee after straightening.

Connective tissues: There are two sets of ligaments that are essential to the stability of the knee. The two lateral ligaments (medial collateral and lateral collateral) stop the knee wobbling from side to side. The two cruciate ligaments cross over inside the joint; they are extensions of the joint capsule. They attach the tibia to the femur and prevent forwards or backwards movements of the tibia on the femur.

Clinical focus: See the clinical highlight below.

Clinical Highlight: Common patterns in the misalignment of the knee according to Dr Mark Charrette DC (2005)

The alignment of the tibia to the femur is the essential relationship in knee issues. There are three possible patterns at the knee joint:

- The whole tibia is relatively posterior to the femur.
- The lateral part of the tibia is posterior; the tibia is externally rotated in relationship to the femur.
- The medial part of the tibia is posterior; the tibia is internally rotated in relationship to the femur.

From being someone who generally got mediocre results with knee issues, one of the authors started getting radically better results after learning to feel the above patterns. We highly recommend exploring the alignment of the tibia on the femur with the possibility of the tibia moving anteriorly.

Ankle and foot joints

Over-pronation of the feet is the pattern in more than nine out of ten people (Charrette 2005). As the arches flatten and roll in, the feet, due to the nature of the arches, will also flare outwards (think Charlie Chaplin). This tends to happen more on one side than the other; it is a very easy pattern to spot if you start looking at feet. The pelvis on the side of the more-turned-out (over-pronated) foot will tend to rotate anteriorly and drop inferiorly. The alignment of the feet is therefore essential for the whole posture.

Ankle and foot anatomy

Bones: The tibia and fibula and the tarsal bones are the interesting bones of the lower leg. There are seven tarsals; of these it is worth getting to know the talus, the navicular, the cuboid and the calcaneus (heel bone). The talus articulates with the distal tibia and fibula.

Muscles: The gastrocnemius and the soleus are big flexor muscles that lift the heel; they are often very tight. A study on cats, quoted in King (2008), showed that activation of the calf muscles stimulates the adrenal glands.

The anterior tibialis, running down the front of the shin, is often spectacularly tight. It draws the foot towards the head (extension or dorsiflexion of the foot). There is a bunch of smaller muscles that move the toes and control lateral movements of the foot.

Connective tissues: The arches of the feet are maintained by ligaments. According to Charrette (2005) muscles only provide 25 per cent of the support to maintain the arches of the feet. Most of the work is done by ligaments. A pessimistic belief about the recovery capabilities of ligaments (the plastic deformation model argues that once overstretched it is very hard to get elastic tone back in a ligament) states that once we have dropped arches then they will always be dropped.

Clinical focus: Painful inflammatory foot conditions are surprisingly common. The general points about treating joints all apply.

A specific intention is to explore the position of the cuboid bone; the lateral border is often superiorly rotated, particularly in inversion strains of the ankle (rolling over the outside of the ankle). The connective tissues over the cuboid will often feel puffy and swollen in this case.

Exploring space in the relationships between the talus and the tibia and fibula and between the talus and the navicular can be very helpful.

11.5 KEY JOINTS: UPPER LIMB

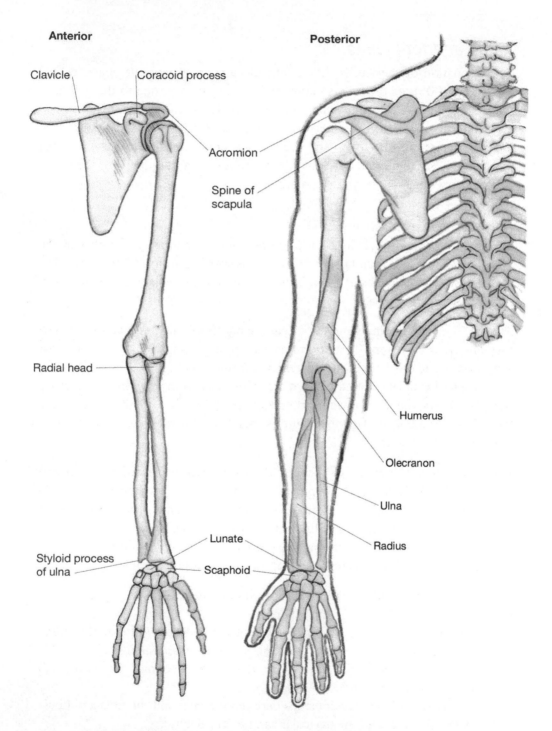

Figure 11.5.1 Left arm bones and joints: anterior and posterior views

Shoulder

The shoulder is an incredible joint. The range of movement permitted is astounding. There is a complex arrangement of muscles and bones to bind the humerus to the scapula and the scapula to the skeleton. It can be a tricky joint to treat as there is so much going on (Broome 2000).

Shoulder anatomy

Bones: The shoulder joint involves three bones: the scapula, the clavicle and the humerus. The coracoid process of the scapula is an anterior projection from the scapula. There are four articulations that make up the shoulder complex: the sternoclavicular joint; the acromioclavicular joint; relationship of the scapula to the ribs; and the glenohumeral joint. The scapula is attached to the ribs by muscles. The glenohumeral joint is the ultimate ball and socket joint.

Shoulder muscles: The rotator cuff often dominates the dynamics of the shoulder. It's composed of the tendonous sheath of four muscles that attach to the head of the humerus from the scapula: the subscapularis, teres minor, infraspinatus and supraspinatus. The subscapularis and supraspinatus are often weak, leading to difficulties stabilizing the shoulder blade and abducting the shoulder. The rotator cuff can commonly become aggravated by the strains running through it; ideally there should be a smooth biotensegrity. Via the trapezius and the latissimus dorsi the shoulder complex is directly attached to the whole of the spine. The big pectoral muscles on the front are often very tight, pulling the shoulders forward. Many of us struggle to engage the serratus anterior muscles that draw the scapula inferior and onto the ribs. The deltoid, biceps and triceps are very powerful muscles that cross the shoulder joint. There is even a muscle that attaches from the scapula to the hyoid – the omohyoid.

Connective tissues: The joint capsule has to accommodate all the shoulder movements. It is relatively weak in terms of binding the joint; it primarily secretes and contains synovial fluid. One theory around the cause of frozen shoulder (rarely a simple condition to treat) is that the capsule becomes inflamed and sticks to itself limiting movement, causing adhesive capsulitis.

Clinical focus: The relationship of the shoulder to the neck is of paramount importance. The nerve flow through the brachial plexus can be compromised. Shoulder muscles will be inhibited due to cervical spinal subluxations.

The alignment of the clavicle between the sternum and the acromion is often neglected; this can be very important in shoulder dysfunction.

The upper and mid thoracic vertebrae and ribs will often hold stories in hard-to-treat shoulder issues.

Elbow, wrist and hand

Elbow and wrist pain are common. Carpal tunnel issues arise from impingement of the nerves that supply the hand on the anterior surface of the wrist.

Elbow, wrist and hand anatomy

Bones: The radius and ulna and the carpal bones are the interesting bones of the lower arm. There are eight carpal bones; of these it is worth getting to know the scaphoid (it often fractures when people try and break their fall with a straight arm) and the lunate.

Muscles: Wrist extensors are on the posterior surface of the forearm. Wrist flexors are often very tight (lots of typing, holding on and clenching). They attach on the anterior forearm on the medial epicondyle of the humerus. This area is often very sore on palpation.

Connective tissues: The carpal tunnel is formed by the natural arch of the two rows of the carpal bones and the transverse carpal ligament. The lunate acts like a keystone (Charrette 2005).

Clinical focus: The lunate often moves anteriorly, collapsing the arch and compressing the nerves and tendons of the carpal tunnel. This is frequently associated with tight forearm flexors. The intention of supporting the arch and the lunate moving posteriorly is very helpful for all sorts of wrist issues.

Orienting to the alignment of the radius, especially at the elbow, can be helpful.

Summary of Chapter 11

Joint issues are so ubiquitous that becoming skilful in treating them is a must. Being confident to work with a whole range of joint conditions will help your practice immensely. Recognizing how the health of a joint can affect the health of the whole system will create a powerful relationship to the whole that is often the very thing that is missing when joints become dysfunctional. The important phenomena stressed in this chapter were how to relate to joints as places of natural vitality and crossroads in the tissue, fluid and potency fields.

Key skills from this chapter:

- Being able to differentiate the tissues at a joint: fluids, ligaments, bone, cartilage, tendon, muscle, nerve.

- Feeling the health at a joint and the potency in the fluid synovial cavity.

- Feeling nerve flow between the centre and peripheral structures.

- Facilitating the reorganization of a limb through tuning into its primary respiratory motion and allowing embryonic movements to emerge. Letting the body balance between the limbs and the midline.

Practice Development

12.1 WHY DO YOU WANT TO BECOME A CRANIOSACRAL THERAPIST?

Know your purpose

Being clear on why you are or why you want to be a craniosacral therapist is vital. This is a question you will ask yourself on many occasions. Working in the therapeutic field is not for everyone. It can be both exciting and illuminating, but it can also be hard work and often very demanding of you at many levels. Helping to resource someone's system and supporting the processing of trauma can be exacting, plus a great responsibility. However, the upside is that you are constantly engaging with the deeper aspects of life. What a wonderful job to be paid to listen to the breath of life! Most of the time the work is uplifting and makes you feel great.

Passion is the defining attribute of most successful therapists. To build a successful abundant practice you need to be hungry; it will not just fall into your lap. Being a skilful practitioner unfortunately does not mean being a busy practitioner. You can trust what you have been taught – biodynamic craniosacral therapy is profound work that can facilitate deep, lasting change in people's suffering. The breath of life is the mover of the universe, so you are in relationship with tremendous power. Your clients do not know that. To build a thriving practice means taking on the identity of a small business person; this includes skills such as marketing, business planning, selling your version of health and self-motivation and reflection. As a biodynamic therapist you are taught to wait and to facilitate the conditions for change; the shift to a more active way of being to promote yourself and your work is often confusing. The authors remember many painful hours waiting for the universe to send us clients. It doesn't work like that in the competitive world of private healthcare. If you are clear about your belief systems, and do not impose them, it is fine to shout them from the roof tops and you can sell yourself and your model with integrity. Biodynamic craniosacral therapy can be a hard thing to understand for many people. The name is unhelpful for one thing, and the art of doing nothing is counter-intuitive for most people.

At some stage in your career there will come a moment when you really learn to trust your skills and to trust the unique qualities that you bring to the therapeutic relationship. You realize the amount of suffering you can be with in another person and you will begin to realize just how profound the biodynamic cranial model is. We hope it happens to you sooner rather than later. It is a wonderful moment and becomes a touch point for your own growth and future session work. When you are learning and starting out as a practitioner it can be helpful to be in touch with similar peak experiences from your life, those experiences that taught you what it is to be alive. These form the bedrock from which you can be present to create a safe holding field for someone else. There is a wonderful model of the wounded healer;[1] from the depth of your own suffering you know what is required to meet another human being in pain.

12.2 HOW TO EARN A LIVING AS A CRANIOSACRAL THERAPIST: SOME THOUGHTS ON BEING IN PRACTICE

An overview of creating a practice

Be energetic

- Put it out there that you want to treat.

- No one is going to come to you if you do not believe in your skills.

- It takes commitment and drive to build a practice.

- This work is hard – it is a process of continual development.

- Keep working at your boundaries.

- Establish yourself by being there for people. Don't even think of cancelling clients unless there is a very good reason.

- When joining a new centre, one shift a week gives very few options to clients who want to see you. Consider a minimum of two shifts at different times of the week; it shows much more commitment.

Make connections

- Build a BCST support network (peers, mentor, supervisor).

- Work in pairs with clients who are not responding deeply to one-to-one treatment – it can really shift the whole agenda.

- Work alongside other health practitioners (prescribing modalities such as Western herbs, TCM, homeopathy and nutrition can all really support the breath of life).

- Reception staff in a new clinic can make or break your practice – give them free sessions, give free sessions to their partners/friends, give their granny a free session.

- Marketing and leaflets are fine, but word of mouth is where it really happens.

Word of mouth

- Word of mouth is the most effective way of building a practice.

- Every successful client is a gateway to a whole community of people. Two or three clients who are good networkers will probably make your practice.

- As a minimum get the client to take away some of your cards or leaflets; ask them to tell their friends and family.

- Use your social connections.

- Get your diary out before the clients leave. People nearly always forget to rebook as soon as they intend.

Sell yourself and cranial work

- Clients are seeing you for a reason – there is not a better practitioner just round the corner.

- There can be negative reinforcement – the clients who get better quickly leave; the ones with chronic, hard-to-shift problems stay in your practice.

- Be clear on your belief systems around health and learn to articulate them.

- Target the message to the individual. (Two extremes might be one: a very expansive breath of life explanation and a short and sharp biomechanical explanation.) Golfers want to swing better, mums want to be less tired, everybody wants more energy, better sleep, less pain… How do you think BCST achieves these goals?

- Specifically address the need the client presented with. The inherent treatment plan can meander a bit, so some short first-aid work during the session is nearly always useful.

- Charge decent money. It is much easier to drop your price for a fixed number of sessions rather than try and raise it after a few sessions.

Short sessions and a course of treatments

- Little and often is much better than long, everything-in-one-go sessions.

- Most people have chronic health problems and would benefit from a course of treatments.

- Two treatments a week may be necessary for clients in acute situations.

- Do not be afraid of recommending long-term treatment plans (Sills: 'I recommend a minimum of 10'; Ukleja: 'I often recommend two years of treatment').

- Do you really need an hour to treat? We would advise 45-minute sessions. The breath of life doesn't hang around if you don't.

- Having regular breaks built into your schedule means you can occasionally run over if there is a client who needs time to settle.

- Work at building your stamina – practise treating people back to back. Develop a rhythm of moving towards, engaging and moving back out of contact.

Make good decisions at the start

- This work is not that portable; when you find a good clinic or set up it is hard to move on and develop a whole new client group.

- Make a business plan.

- Review your business plan and audit your work.

- Do the simple stuff – insurance, first aid, keep records, get an accountant.

What kind of therapist do you want to be?

Working with particular client groups can be a very attractive way of making a successful practice and creating variety, plus taking the work into new areas. BCST often has success around conditions other therapies don't do too well with. These include: low energy states (chronic fatigue, ME, depression); autoimmune issues (ME, rheumatoid arthritis, MS); and persistent states (fibromyalgia, colitis, psoriasis). Specializing in some of these areas makes a lot of sense. Why not run a migraine clinic? Or a clinic for cerebral palsy? Or a stress clinic? Or a lower back clinic?[2]

It makes sense to become confident with basic issues that many people are suffering from: back pain, neck pain, headaches, emotional overwhelm, stress, and the autonomic nervous system.[3] Most of any therapist's day is spent meeting these kinds of conditions. Becoming competent at knowing what you are in relationship to is very important in the biodynamic approach. This means being able to name what you are in relationship to: how does neck pain feel; what's the sense of emotional flux in the body; what does it feel like when someone's sympathetic nervous system is aroused? Self-reflect on what you are good at, and target continuous professional development courses in the areas you need support.

You may feel strongly about working with different sections of society. Many practitioners are drawn to working with pregnant women, some practitioners to babies or infants, some to teenagers and some to working with people later in life by offering treatments in aged care facilities or hospices. It's useful to know what group of people attracts you and making an effort in establishing the work in that field. Other possibilities are: health professionals, women, chronic pain, trauma, mental health, sports injuries, and cancer.

The other decision to make is whether you treat from home or a clinic. There are many advantages to both. Working from home is very common in certain countries but not in others, so that might be a factor about where you work from. Working from home means you can establish your own unique practice environment. It's also very convenient and low cost. However, you are working alone without colleagues or other kinds of therapists around you. This is a big factor in the work: keeping in touch with others in the healing profession, receiving stimulation and support and not feeling isolated. It can also help to boost your practice through referrals and the efforts of the clinic to advertise its therapists. For some therapists working from their own space is very desirable, but for others it may feel too vulnerable and unsafe having members of the public coming into their home.

Making a living out of it

Have a good look at the way you relate to money. It's vital that you understand your worth as a trained therapist and as a person. You are dedicating your time and energy to someone else's health and bringing a professional aptitude to it. Confidence and ability apart, you are offering your time and commitment to another individual and this is worth something. The easiest way to avoid confusion is to simply set your clinic fee to the going rate in your area; then your fee is neither too low nor too high. Don't bother thinking about whether you are worth it because you have just qualified. For people who are much more experienced and have a reputation, they may decide to set a higher fee, which is very common practice.

Work out how much money you want to make from your practice. Then work backwards to how many clients you need at the going fee rate; you now have your goal set for your practice. Be sensible and practical about how much income you want to make. Being a therapist is not about having a hobby, it's about having a career and making a living from something you believe in and enjoy.

Creating a BCST introduction talk

In order to ignite your practice you will have to engage with the public in advertising your services. One powerful way of doing this is to hold free or low-cost talks on the therapy. These talks will give interested people a more direct experience of what the therapy is about and its benefits; rather than simply picking up a leaflet and reading it, it will take them a step further. For some people this might be just what they need to come along for a treatment.

You can become skilled at presenting these talks and helping people to obtain a more direct experience of what the therapy is. It is important to get the elements of the talk right from the start so that you are clear about what you are trying to achieve and convey. Here's a suggested format for a talk:

- Use images, especially anatomy images. BCST has a very exciting view into the body's anatomy and physiology and is based on medical science. It also means you are using a scientific way of explaining the therapy. One of the major features of BCST is its orientation to felt sense and body awareness through anatomy.

- Keep the language simple. Avoid 'cranio speak'. Use words that everyone will understand. Rather than trying to explain the grand theory of the work, try to explain a few of the interesting features of the therapy. For instance, biotensegrity, relating to the whole, reciprocal tension, the properties of water, the relational field.

- Try to bring in as many guided awareness exercises as you can. For every bit of theory you present, try to ground it with an exploration of the body. Come into body awareness in different ways, exploring perception and exploring presence.

- Try to be interactive with your audience. Make sure there is time for questions and answers. These can often lead to interesting discussions, but you always need to be prepared to bring things back to your main themes rather than digressing too much. Sometimes demonstrating a treatment can be a powerful way for people to understand the therapy. You can talk as much as you like about it, but describing a live treatment is more interesting. Keep it short; it doesn't need to be too long.

Creating a brochure and a website

Ultimately your practice will grow through word of mouth. However, producing an impressive and well-designed brochure and website is an important tool in attracting clients and making a statement about who you are, and how you practise and run your business. Invest some money in a creative designer and spend time creating a look that reflects you and what you feel about the therapy you are offering. Members of the public like to see that someone is offering a professional service and creating a brochure and website is part of that in the modern world. Make sure your website is search-engine optimized so that it appears high in the rankings when people are searching for local therapists. Just a few medium-term clients who book with you through your advertising will mean it has paid for itself. The important thing is how you describe the work. Look around at other definitions of the therapy and write your own so that it represents your beliefs and what you think are the important features of it as practised by you. Bring your energy into it; that's what will attract people to come to you for treatments.

A simple model for change: 'Take the loads off the back of the donkey'

There is no one way to approach pain. The causes of pain are multifactorial and complex. A simple idea is to 'take the loads off the back of the donkey'. If we pile weight on the back of a donkey it will become an unhappy donkey. It will be tired, slow, in pain and be prone to getting ill. We could whip it, feed it donkey stimulants (sugar? carrots?) or try and make it stronger. If we keep piling on loads, however strong it is, at some stage the donkey will collapse. The smart treatment option is not to treat the overwhelmed legs or the painful back. The best choice is to remove as many loads as possible.

Loading a donkey also illustrates some other principles around pain. Predicting which leg will collapse first is very hard; it is a complex donkey with unique stresses and strains. Also, there is no sense in saying that the cause of the problem was the last load applied. How often have you heard something similar to 'My back went when I bent down to tie my shoelaces'? You dig deeper and your client tells you that they are under pressure at work, their relationship is not going well, they have an old sports injury, they slouch at the computer and who knows what else. Which is the cause? They all are.

There are some very common things that load our systems, interfere with the control mechanisms and energy economy of the body and prevent us from working to our optimum. You will get great results in treating all types of pain by working to remove these loads from your clients' systems:

- Structural dysfunction: any joints being out of line (especially the spine and cranial bones) cause interference.

- Visceral issues: musculoskeletal pain frequently involves clearing interference to the functioning of the nervous system that originates in organs.

- Poor nutrition and environmental toxicity.

- Stress and unprocessed overwhelming experiences, especially dissociation.

- Poor dental work and piercings: metal can really inhibit essential reflexes.

- Inflexible beliefs and life statements: these are often tied into birth and early experiences.

12.3 PROFESSIONAL CONSIDERATIONS

Ongoing training and support

The important thing is to exemplify being a health practitioner. Ultimately you are an advert for your practice and a representative of the therapy. The essence of this body therapy is to manifest the breath of life. In order to do this you will need to have a personal health practice that addresses what you eat and drink, how you move and how you relate with others. As a client, I am going to be very impressed with a health practitioner who looks healthy, who has a clarity of mind and is sensitive. Receiving regular treatment is an essential aspect of ongoing support that can be forgotten by many therapists. You are coming into contact with trauma through the practice of this therapy and you will always need therapeutic support to help your system deal with this, along with anything that is arising in your personal life. Find a practitioner whose approach works for you so you have a place of support and resource. Create a daily practice around internal awareness through meditation, yoga, chi kung or some form of regular activity and bring about a strength and stamina to your system.

Belonging to a CST association is an important statement of your intention around the work. Associations create standards in practice and education and stand for quality assurance. All professional associations insist on continual professional development or education and for good reason, as it is vital to keep involved in the honing of your skills and in touch with the cutting edge of the work. This is especially true of biodynamic CST, as it's such an evolving science. Here are some of the major CST associations:

- CSTA – UK (www.craniosacral.co.uk).

- BCTA – North America (www.craniosacraltherapy.org).

- Cranio Suisse – Switzerland (www.craniosuisse.ch).

- PACT – Australasia (www.biodynamic-craniosacral.com).

In addition, there is an international affiliation of BCST training colleges that have created minimum standards in the BCST approach to education: IABT (International Affiliation of Biodynamic Trainings). See www.biodynamic-craniosacral.org.

Legal considerations

Huge changes have taken place in the alternative and complementary therapy fields over the past few decades. One of the major shifts has been a move towards greater regulation. Much of this has been driven by a legislative atmosphere that has made it imperative to take out personal indemnity insurance as a private practitioner. This varies depending on which country you live in. In many countries it is mandatory to have insurance in order to practise. Often part of joining an association is to gain access to low-cost block insurance schemes.

Local associations will also have a code of ethics. Cranial work consists of intense personal relationships involving touch. There is plenty of potential for confusion for both the therapist and the client. There is an excellent sample code of profession conduct available from the IABT website. We strongly recommend reading the code and getting supervision. See www.biodynamic-craniosacral.org/standards/code_of_conduct.

12.4 TAKING CASE HISTORIES

Treatment records

Finding your own way of taking a case history and how you want to approach your client on the first visit is important. It is a primary event as you are gauging their health, their expectations, and what they want from the treatment, that is, what they want treated and what their desired outcome is. Professionally you need to be diligent and know what your client is coming for and whether they are suitable for treatment. Sometimes it can be unclear why people come for treatment and you need to spend time creating clarity around this for both yourself and your client. Otherwise how can you measure success? It might be that you don't feel qualified to treat what your client is coming with; then you should consider referring them on to another professional health practitioner you feel is more appropriate. Knowing practitioners in allied fields whose competence you trust is a very useful resource. It may be that you feel you don't want to treat the client for personal reasons. You don't feel safe with them perhaps, or their trauma is something you don't feel confident or able to meet or cope with. This is fine. You are quite within your rights to not proceed with further treatments and under no obligation to do so. You are also honouring your own health and abilities.

Being relaxed, natural and empathetic will create a warm and open ambience that puts your client at ease and allows them to be open and honest. This is such a big feature of being a successful body therapist. Most people will be naturally anxious about coming along for a touch therapy and disclosing personal information and history. An ability to allow people to settle will greatly enhance the therapeutic effects. That means you as the practitioner are calm, present and open.

It's important to record your treatments, especially the first one, as this will act as a reminder of how your client's health was at the start of the therapeutic relationship. Practitioners do this in many different ways, often by using a form with prompts on certain aspects of your client's health and general details. Some practitioners are not so formal in their approach, and they are more interested in recording how the client presented their description of themselves rather than creating a format or series of questions. The important thing is to gain a sense of how the client is and why they have come and to be able to record that on a client record. Don't forget that they can have access to this at any time and it might be best to write as if you wouldn't mind your client seeing it. That way the record is in simple, easily understood language, non-judgemental and consistent with what has been disclosed in the sessions.

Clinical Highlight: Some guidance on taking a case history

Useful information – short version
Two good useful opening questions are the following.

What brought you to the session today?
This is about their presenting condition or conditions. As a minimum you need to ask how long it has been there, has it happened before, known causes, how it affects their life and, if it is a chronic condition, what is the longest pain-free period they have had in the last few months.

Are there any major things in the past you would like to tell me about?
This is where they can tell you about significant life events. You may need to prompt by asking: Have you had any big operations, dental work, falls, accidents, broken bones, major illnesses or long periods of taking medication?[4]

A good set of follow-up questions are the case history questions discussed in Chapter 3 under Dissociation (see p.90). They are suitable for getting an idea of the overwhelm in someone's system: Do you get cold hands and feet? Do you bump into things? Are you sensitive to loud noises or bright lights? Do you ever have a sense of being detached? Are you more anxious than you would like?

Finally, another good set of follow up-questions are: Are there any major life events going on for you at the moment? Is there anything going on for you in your family, your relationship, around your home or your job? (Our experience in clinical practice is that the vast majority of people who present with acute pains will have an unresolved issue in some major part of their life.)

Useful information – long version

How are they?
Let the client lead. Give them space to do this just as you would in a hands-on session. Be in a state of balanced attention. The way they describe how they are feeling is very informative.

How is their health?
Facilitate your client to describe their health, not just their pathology. The way they describe their concept of their health is revealing.

Are they resourced?
- What are their resources?

- How resourced do they feel they are?
- In their life and within themselves?

How is their vitality?

- Level of energy.
- Full of life?
- Fatigue/exhaustion.
- Concentration and memory.
- Will and direction of life.

Do they have support?

- Friends, family, relationships.

Do they experience pain or discomfort in themselves and their body?

- Places of pain.
- Difficult feelings or experiences.
- Combination of both.

How do they physically function?
Breathing, eating, moving, sensing (seeing, hearing, tasting, smelling), sleeping, libido.

Detailed questions about their major systems
Digestive, uro-genital, menstrual cycle, liver, CNS, endocrine, cardiovascular, respiratory, muscular, skeletal.

Traumatization
Any traumatic event that they feel had a strong effect on their lives, for example, birth, death, break-ups, injury, illness, abuse.

Medication

- Are they on medication now or have they been in the past?
- Long-term or short-term?
- What kind of medication?

12.5 ASSESSING YOUR CLIENT'S HEALTH

Skills of obtaining a clear picture of someone's health are vital to the success of the treatments, not only in terms of the body response but also so that you can give your client meaningful feedback. Creating baselines to assess change is part of any therapist's skill. Below is an attempt to keep it simple. The basic assessment uses words and ideas that are not craniosacral therapy terms. In many ways you are listening to just these qualities within your client's system. This assessment can create a baseline of health for you to compare with future states of health. This is good for your client who will receive your feedback of treatment progress and notice the improvements within their system.

Clinical Highlight: Basic assessment – how to form a clear picture of someone from a touch perspective

Motion

- Is there any?
- How much?
- How fluid is it?
- Direction and quality?

Space

- Does their system feel spacious?
- Is there a lack of space?

Aliveness

- How alive do they feel?
- Do they feel vibrant or tired?
- What is their tissue quality like?

Communication

- Does the client's system come to meet you?
- How readily does it 'engage'?
- How easily is there a 'conversation' with the breath of life?
- How responsive are they?

Presence

- How present does the client seem visually?
- Does their system feel present?

Emotional state

- Is there an emotional tone that comes to you?
- What part of the body does it come from?

Clinical Highlight: Craniosacral assessment – how to form a
clear picture of someone from a craniosacral perspective

Here's a list of questions to help you with identifying the health and
responsiveness of your client's system using craniosacral therapy terminology.

Motility

- Do you notice movement within structures?
- Breath of life in the cells?

Potency

- Is there strength/vitality/vibrancy?
- Does your client's system feel resourced?
- What's the amount of potency?

Tide

- Is there a tide?
- What are the nuances of the tide: amplitude, unfoldment of the tide, symmetry and transition of phases?

Stillness

- Can your client be still?
- Can their system rest and access a stillpoint?
- Is there a sense of spaciousness?

Places of organization

- How well does the breath of life express around the natural fulcrums of the body?
- Is it having to orient around a place or area of tension or hyperactivity?
- Is there an inner/inherent response?

Relationships

- How much mobility is there between structures?
- Is there an interplay of tissue, fluid and potency?
- Is there a sense of connectivity and reciprocal tension?

Language for touch

Developing a language for touch (written and verbal) is a crucial skill in biodynamic
craniosacral therapy. How to explain the work and to whom helps the client

understand the process of the work and helps you to become clearer about what you are perceiving. The easiest approach is to make your language understandable for everyone, so avoid any craniosacral therapy jargon and keep to common terms. It's very effective to describe the biodynamic body process so that your clients can hear how the treatment has unfolded.

Words for change

Relaxing, softening, unified, fluid-like, adjustment, reorganization, harmonious, realignment, balancing, resolving, transitioning, transforming, processing, lengthening, expanding, widening, spacious, integration, remembering, unwinding, letting go, releasing, reconnecting, unravelling, rewired.

Words for difficulty

Restricted, contracted, compressed, static, dense, inert, lack of movement/flow, dissociated, resistant, congested, stagnated, constricted, sluggish, low energy, protected, stuck, blocked, patterned, shut down, non-responsive, cut off/separated, intransigent, hyper/hyposensitive, disorganized, activated/charged, numb.

Words for health

Motion, movement, flow, fluid, ease of motion, deepening, glide, engaging, responsive, body intelligent, communicative, continuity, tensegrity, connectivity, vibrant, lively, potent, responsive, still, quiescent, balanced, midline, organized, healthy, expressive, alive, resourced, effervescent, tingling, shimmering, sparky/electric, integrated.

Words for process

Process, trauma expressions, shock effect, somato-emotional release, emotional release/clearing, emotional process, tissue memory, early patterning, accessing patterns, dissolving, reworking, activating, resolving, transforming, shifting, surge, build-up, expressing.

'How many sessions do I need?'

This is the question all therapists are asked. It's understandable that your client will want to know the extent of the treatment plan so that they can have a sense of their level of commitment and when they may practically be alleviated from their condition. However, the nature of the body is complex and the movement back to health can be quite circuitous. Healing is rarely in a straight line. The important thing is that you will not know how well someone's system responds until you have treated them a few times. This is a good thing to tell your client. You can tell something about someone's level of health and responsiveness from the first session, though, and that is something you can base your ideas on about how well someone might do, but it is only a snapshot. What you don't know is how well they will maintain the changes that occur in the sessions and how deep the changes will go. People's deeper resources can only be known after observing their systems over a number of sessions, so it's reasonable to say, 'Come back for a few sessions, in order to monitor progress.' An important thing to understand is that nobody can resolve their system in just one session. Our bodies need reminding of the deeper health.

Often therapists divide conditions up into two categories: acute and chronic. This makes a lot of sense and knowing which category your client is in will help with how you deal with them and your expectations of recovery. Chronic conditions have taken time to manifest and have become embedded within the body. They will clearly need time to resolve. Commonly low energy states go along with chronic conditions and so the lack of available potency will mean the body can only do so much. As a rule of thumb chronic states will take a medium- to long-term treatment plan, so upwards of ten sessions and perhaps as much as a whole year of treatment. The beauty of this therapy is that it rapidly enables the body to harness its deeper health and optimize on all levels, so you notice that people become healthier quickly. However, it's important to be pragmatic as a therapist. The body has remarkable properties of recovery and reorganization, so it's crucial that you do not limit this by your attitude around someone's health. Being open to the possibility of remarkable change is a powerful thing to offer in your relational field. The pragmatic side of you however knows that people can take time to change and increase their health, so there may be no dramatic changes or huge leaps in health, more a slow progress to better health. There again there may only be so much your client's system can do and their health level plateaus. You need to be accepting of this. The outcome is not always what you would like to see, so being equanimous about your client's outcome is a very helpful state of mind.

Acute conditions are quite different. This is something that is active now in the body and the body's defences are attempting to deal with it. The body's energies are already activated and a BCST practitioner can help enormously with recovery from the trauma. As a minimum, helping the body to deal with shock is a vital contribution to the body's deeper healing. Allowing the autonomic nervous system to settle and balance, along with accessing the midline health and creating a whole body awareness, will quickly bring the body into a greater physiological health. The efficacy of BCST in balancing shock effects is breath-taking and the application to recovery from trauma such as injury to the body, emotional distress and medical intervention is what you will notice regularly as a practitioner. The field is well known for its application to babies and mothers around the birth event.

Biodynamic craniosacral therapy is unusual in that it can hold the spectrum of healing from very effective and quick pain relief in both acute and chronic conditions in a few sessions, to a deep enquiry of what it means to exist in a body over a number of years. Some people see it as silent psychotherapy. Other people use it as a gentle form of physiotherapy, osteopathy or chiropractic. Many of our clients have been diagnosed with life-threatening illnesses such as cancer and find BCST a source of ongoing support. Part of the fun in practice is the wide variety of conditions that you will work with. Another rule of thumb is a practice that is made up of a third of short-term clients (up to ten sessions), a third of medium-term clients (three to nine months) and a third of long-term clients (more than a year). If you are only seeing short-term clients it may be good to explore the messages you are giving out about how cranial work can support ongoing change. Some practitioners see more like 75 per cent long-term clients; it depends on your style of practice and what you focus on. Initially it is good to review the progress between three to six sessions and around ten to twelve sessions; life events happen and the goals of the sessions need to be constantly negotiated.

12.6 HOW TO BE A PRACTITIONER OF EXCELLENCE

Safety in practice

Boundaries with clients are a vital part of a body therapy that has a very intimate and empathic touch.[5] As a safe practitioner you need to be clear who you are as an individual, what your intentions are as a therapist and where your body ends and your client's begins. The power of presence and detached observation is everything in this therapy. The more you observe yourself and your arising feelings the more you know yourself at the conscious and the unconscious levels. Orientations towards power and control do not belong in the therapy space. The ideal attitude is more about humility and graciousness and excitement about the unfolding of health right in front of you. When traumatic expressions arise in the therapy these qualities of a practitioner become very important and allow for a clean, undisturbed process that does not involve any elements from your internal state. That's true safety in practice.

Being resourced is essential. It is one of the key things you offer, your own health and abundance as a model for your client's system to be inspired by, so you need to look after yourself. Receive regular treatments yourself, keep fit and healthy in your body, feed your body what it truly needs and create order in your life. The breath of life is the ordering principle of the body and its emergence in a treatment session brings the body to a higher state of order. Exemplify this through your internal order and your relationship with the breath of life within you; you then become a representative of order. Be careful about over-extending yourself. Try to work within your capacity. At first, this therapy takes a lot of stamina to become accustomed to, and you need to move into this slowly and in a paced way. Being with people's trauma in a very intimate way takes some getting used to. The more you sink into your midline the more you will feel resourced. The more you can introduce your client's system to their breath of life the easier it gets for you. The first year in practice is about integrating what you have learned and experienced during the training and building up stamina. Most people can earn a decent living treating between 20–30 clients a week. You need to build your stamina to be able to get to treat that many people for at least 40 weeks a year.

Supervision is such a useful support, especially during the first few years of practice when you will be dealing with clients and events that you are not familiar with. Having an experienced supervisor to turn to for advice and support is vital and is a cost that you should build into your business plan. Make sure your supervisor is the person for you by meeting a few supervisors and forming a connection. Many BCST associations make supervision a mandatory requirement during the first year of practice.

Cleanliness and health go hand in hand. Your personal hygiene is part of the safety of your client. Making sure you keep your hands and nails clean during your practice day is a pre-requisite for a professional therapist. Most therapists wash their hands after and/or before a treatment session to maintain hygiene and to have a ritual of starting or finishing the session. Look at how you present yourself. The clothes you wear, the way you hold yourself and how well kempt you are is part of what people respond to. It is the same with your practice space; this too needs to be clean and have a good feel.

Structure of a treatment session

A treatment is in many ways quite simple; there's a beginning, a middle and an end, just like everything else. There's certainly a unique moment when you first touch someone's system. Then the whole landscape of the body shows itself to you for a minute or two before the inherent treatment plan starts to move the body into its priorities. That's when you can tell how things are, what has changed and what is the lie of the whole land. It's like a view of the terrain from the hill top before you start to walk through the land. The first part of the session is often associated with CRI expressions that include tissue shapes, local fluid fluctuations and the body accessing more superficial patterns, often connective tissue/muscle oriented. These settle down over a period of ten minutes and there is a sense of balance of left and right. The body may have moved through several states of balance before it comes into a deepening into the midline and a holistic shift towards a deeper, more whole body, fluid state. This is where the breath of life can really show itself in its fuller glory and where much deeper shifts take place that involve the whole body state. This is typically the middle of the session where deeper process and resolution is being accessed and where potency is emerging much more dynamically. This commonly emerges after a stillness and ends in an even deeper stillness. The last part of the session is about rest and connecting to wider fields of relationship.

If there are traumatic expressions they are often expressed when the system shifts into the second phase of the treatment. More authentic and engrained patterns of experience express themselves in this phase and quite often this can be traumatic. The relational field creates such a containment and access to deeper potency that often the trauma has moved through a whole shift to resolution before the final phase of the treatment. All of this of course depends on the level of health of the client and it may take many sessions before the trauma is accessed and there is some processing of it.

Being skilled

This is everything. You know how it is when someone who is skilful puts their hands on you. It makes a huge difference to how the body responds and to how confident a client feels with you. There is an air of knowing and presence around an experienced and skilful practitioner. How can you become this person? Experience is something that unavoidably only comes through hundreds of sessions and hundreds of clients. This can't be reproduced in any other way. However, what you can do is hone your skills through being diligent, putting your hands on as many people as you can, and working at creating a greater acuity, an ability to differentiate and know what you are in relationship with. That's the key to success, to know what the body is telling you, to be able to feel the arising forms. You can do this by working hard at studying anatomy, and making it real by relating it to felt sense. Spend time exploring your own system and become familiar with how your tissues feel, all the different varieties, your fluid states, biodynamic health expressions and how the body reorganizes itself. The more sensitive you are to your system the more sensitive you will be to others.

Developing trust in deeper intelligence

'Trust the tide' or 'Trust the breath of life' are common phrases in the craniosacral field. It is an acknowledgement of the underlying force of health in the body; the more you surrender to its force the more powerfully your treatments will go. Notice how deeply and quickly your clients change as you adopt the biodynamic approach to craniosacral therapy. The modality has developed through practitioners noticing more efficacious changes by becoming neutral and allowing the body to change in relationship to its natural health and not through practitioner intentions. To truly embrace this approach you must see for yourself the power of being a knowing presence and of accessing the body's intelligence. You must also de-programme yourself of years of education which has taught you to do and to act in order to bring about change. You are letting go into the power of life, the power that makes things grow. We can help plants grow by offering them the right conditions, but in the end it's the plant that does the growing, we don't do that for them. It is the same in a treatment. The relational field is the optimal growing environment that stimulates the potential for growth and reorganization.

A lot of the art of this therapy is to be able to let go of your intentions to 'do', intentions which reduce the body's options and create a lesser vehicle for allowing the matrix of life to shine through. There are exciting and challenging shifts that are needed within your bodymind that allow you to personally grow to a greater state of attunement with our intrinsic nature. We see biodynamic craniosacral therapy as an endless dance between you and your clients. It can be constantly refined and you will be constantly challenged to develop your skills to work with a wider range of people and their conditions. Just when you think you have got it, the next client who walks through the door will show you something new.

Notes

1.   Cheiron is the Greek version.

2.   Ged Sumner set up and ran the Health Living Centre (www.thehealthylivingcentre.co.uk) in North London. Craniosacral clinics that have been on offer there for a number of years are: ME Clinic, Pregnancy, Mothers and Babies Clinic, Performers Clinic, Children, Teenagers and Parents Clinic as well a low-cost Teaching Clinic (in conjunction with the Craniosacral Therapy Educational Trust).

3.   'Osteopathy…had the skill to directly interpret and influence autonomic activity using perceptual and palpatory skills. The level of awareness that can be developed in this regard is much greater than any scientific instrument… *Perhaps 80 percent or more of disease is directly traceable to ANS imbalance*' (Jealous 1999).

4.   It is incredible what people can miss out when you take a case history. Keep returning to these questions over the first few sessions. Apart from forgetting, people disclose more as they learn to trust the space. One of the authors once had a client who presented with neck pain but who omitted to disclose that he had had an operation for decompression of his foramen magnum due to prolapse of his brainstem. This is important for a craniosacral therapist! It only came to light after the author noticed the scar on the back of his neck.

5.   Su Fox (2007) is a craniosacral therapist and psychotherapist who has written an excellent book on the therapeutic relationship. Egan (1997) is very good on being a reflective practitioner. Mitchell and Cormack (1998) is also a good book on being a complementary therapist.

Glossary

Becker's three-stage process Seeking, Settling and Reorganization. The state of balance occurs in the settling phase. Derivation: Becker, Sills.

Biodynamic In craniosacral therapy biodynamic designates an attempt to always work in relationship to the whole. The starting point is orienting to slower tides than CRI, being aware of midline function and embryological forces and letting the breath of life do the work. Derivation: Bleschchmidt, Jealous, Sills.

Biodynamic forces Forces of health; act to centre conditional forces. Interaction with conditional forces gives rise to patterns of experiences. Derivation: Becker.

Biosphere Energetic or potency field around the body; Jealous talks of a distance of 18 inches. A zone of influence, a personal space, where the heat of the body may extend out to; can be the same as the space that is crossed when someone is too close to you. 'The biosphere is the body and the field of potency and environmental exchange around it' (Sills 2001, p.423). Derivation: Becker.

Breath of life The animating creative force of life. Derivation: Sutherland.

Conditional forces Forces of experience, for example knocks, falls, toxins, life events, birth, trauma. (Also called biokinetic forces by Becker.)

CRI Cranial rhythmic impulse – quickest palpable tidal unfoldment of breath of life. Variable rate but usually 8 to 12 cycles/min or approximately 6 seconds to complete a cycle. Derivation: Osteopaths Rachel and John Woods in 1961, according to McPartland and Skinner (2005).

Dynamic stillness The stillness that underpins everything. The potent void from which activity spontaneously emerges. A cranial cosmology might be: There is a transmutation from void to movement to energy to fluids to form. Derivation: Becker, Sills.

Exhale Sinking, narrowing side to side, contracting phase of primary respiration.

Field Describes a fabric or matrix or energetic space that we all exist in. The relational space that we can perceive. A zone of influence. Merleau Ponty talks of an extended phenomenological 'flesh' (Abram 1996). Derivation: A term used in physics.

Fluids The water-based, non-solid parts of the body. Within cells, around cells and in vessels. We are 65 per cent water.

Fulcrum A fulcrum is something that organizes or influences. Frequently it can be considered to be the thing that organizes motion. All motion has a fulcrum. A natural fulcrum is the optimum fulcrum for the creation of form and movement laid down in the embryo. Natural fulcrums are often centres of potency on the midline and can move, or automatically shift, with the tide. Inertial fulcrums arise due to conditional forces and have a fixed, static quality, they give rise to a sense of fragmentation and loss of relationship to the midline. Derivation: Sutherland.

Holistic shift A settling of the system where a felt sense of wholeness emerges and the fluid tide clarifies. From Becker we can add that the will of the client (and the practitioner) lets go into the will of the breath of life. Derivation: Sills.

Ignition A permeation of order and coherence through the potency field. The spark or initiation of potency transmuted into the fluids of the body. Derivation: Sutherland.

Inhale Widening side to side, rising, expanding phase of primary respiration.

Inherent treatment plan Describes the natural order of the healing process. At any one time, given the resources of the client and the quality of the relational field held by the practitioner, there will be a primary issue that can begin to resolve. The inherent treatment plan is a decision made by the breath of life and emerges during the session; it is not a sequence imposed by the client or the practitioner. Derivation: Becker, Sills.

Long tide Slowest, most stable tidal expression of primary respiration. Considered to express as 100-second cycles of inhale and exhale, in a wide field of action. Derivation: Becker.

Midline Organizing central axis of the body.

Mid tide Term developed at the Karuna Institute to designate middle tidal unfoldment of the breath of life; used to be called potency tide. Generally described as 2.5 cycles/min or approximately 24 seconds to complete a cycle of inhale and exhale. Derivation: Sills.

Original health Same as original matrix.

Original matrix An epigenetic knowing that emerges from the activity of the body. A blueprint for form. Derivation: Jealous (but not this definition).

Patterns of experience The shapes that arise in the body due to the interaction of conditional forces and biodynamic forces. There is an organizing centre to a pattern of experience that is also called a fulcrum. At the heart of the pattern of experience there is a core of biodynamic potency centring the shape.

Perceptual field The area that your sensing body is in direct relationship to. The phenomena you are aware of that make up your perceptual reality/field. 'The beyond-the-horizon, by withholding its presence, holds open the perceived landscape, while the under-the-ground, by refusing its presence, supports the perceived landscape' (Abram 1996, p.214). So by widening your perceptual field you increase your perception to what is withheld, over the horizon. You are in effect going into the future. And by deepening your perceptual field you increase your perception to what is refused, under the ground. You are in effect going into the past. Think of being in a room; the person who has the sharpest hearing knows when someone is about to approach the door. Their present time includes the future of the colleague who is not yet aware the door is about to open. As a craniosacral therapist, deepening and widening our perceptual field allows us to feel what is hidden in the other's body; it allows us to have some relationship to their past and their future by increasing the possibilities of the present moment.

Potency Liquid light or fluid within the fluid. The cranial word for energy. An ordering force that has the potential to organize and do work. It manifests through the fluids and transmutes with every cycle of primary respiration. Derivation: Sutherland. (Last two sentences are from Sills.)

Potency field See *Biosphere.*

Practitioner See *State of balanced awareness.* Derivation: Jealous.

Primal midline The notochord remnant passing through the vertebral bodies and body of the sphenoid and ethmoid. Also called the anterior midline.

Primary respiration Subtle rhythmic expressions of the breath of life. Can be felt at different rates or as different perceptual states. Sometimes used to denote the action of long tide only (for example, Shea 2007). Derivation: Sutherland.

Relational field 'The conjoined fields of interplay between practitioner and client' (Ukleja 2009a). Derivation: Sills.

Resources Anything that supports health. Useful to orient to the sensations that resources generate in the body.

Ritual of contact A consistent approach to making contact that supports the required relational field for biodynamic craniosacral therapy. We use 'Self, Other, Field' as a simple way to remember a ritual of creating a state of balanced awareness in our selves, negotiating physical contact with the other and orienting to a wide perceptual field and primary respiration. Derivation: Sills.

State of balance Systemic settling around the organizing centre of a pattern of experience. Also called state of balanced tension. Derivation: Sills.

State of balanced awareness A place where your attention is neither coming nor going. Your awareness is balanced between your own internal space and the space around you, including the client. It is equivalent to a practitioner being neutral.

Stillness A quality that emerges in session work that we strongly associate with health. Sutherland was clear that the power of the tide is in the stillness. A universal quality in nature that allows a reconnection to the breath of life.

Stillpoint A temporary cessation of the expression of primary respiration in the body. Sutherland emphasized the importance of a stillpoint as a fulcrum for the fluctuation of cerebrospinal fluid. A stillpoint is a state where the potency of the system recharges. To be clear, the long tide does not ever go still, nor is it ever in shock; it is a very stable tide. Even though the long tide is still happening, in deep stillpoints the sense of stillness is the pervasive perception.

Systemic neutral As healing deepens the systemic neutral is 'the dynamic equilibrium between universal and conditional forces that becomes a gateway to long tide and dynamic stillness, and even to the breath of life itself' (Ukleja 2009a). Derivation: Sutherland, Becker, Jealous.

The tide Used interchangeably with primary respiration. Derivation: Sutherland.

Tissues The material, more solid, structures of the body: bones, muscles, connective tissues. Can also include nerve tissues and organs.

Transmutation 'It is a change into another nature, substance, form or condition' (Sutherland 1998, p.291). He goes on to relate this to a 'potential in the center; the function, a different condition' (p.292). It is about the interchangeability of energy and matter. Derivation: Sutherland.

References

Abram, D. (1996) *The Spell of the Sensuous*. London: Vintage Books.

Acland, R.D. (2004) *Acland's DVD Atlas of Human Anatomy*. London: Lippincott Williams and Wilkins.

Ainsworth, M. and Bowlby, J. (1965) *Child Care and the Growth of Love*. London: Penguin Books.

Al-Khalili, J. (2003) *Quantum – A Guide for the Perplexed*. London: Weidenfeld and Nicolson.

Armour, J. (2008) *How Does the Heart Display Emotional Intelligence?* Unpublished lecture notes from The Relational Heart Conference run by Confer, London.

Attenborough, D. (2002) *Life of Mammals*. DVD from the BBC.

Barral, J.P. and Mercier, P. (1988) *Visceral Manipulation*. Vista, CA: Eastland Press.

Becker, R. (1997) *Life in Motion*. Portland, OR: Rudra.

Becker, R. (2000) *The Stillness of Life*. Portland, OR: Rudra.

Blake, W. (1803) *Auguries of Innocence*. Available at www.online-literature.com/poe/612, accessed June 2010.

Blechschmidt, E. (2005) *The Ontogenetic Basis of Human Anatomy: The Biodynamic Approach to Development from Conception to Birth*. Berkeley, CA: North Atlantic Books.

Bolte Taylor, J. (2009) *A Stroke of Insight*. Available at www.ted.com/talks/lang/eng/jill_bolte_taylor_s_powerful_stroke_of_insight.html, accessed Oct 2009.

Breiner, A. (1999) *Whole Body Dentistry*. Fairfield, CT: Quantum Health Press.

Broome, R.T. (ed.) (2000) *Chiropractic Peripheral Joint Technique*. Oxford: Butterworth-Heinemann.

Brown, D. (2006) *Tricks of the Mind*. London: Channel 4 Books.

Buckminster Fuller, R. (1961) 'Tensegrity.' *Portfolio and Art News Annual 4*, 112–127, 144, 148.

Capra, F. (1992) *The Tao of Physics*, 3rd edn. Fort Lauderdale, FL: Flamingo Press.

Carrick, F.R. (1997) 'Changes in brain function after manipulation of the cervical spine.' *Journal of Manipulative and Physiological Therapeutics 20*, 529–545.

Castilho, S.M., Oda, Y.J. and Santana, M. (2006) 'Metopism in adult skulls from southern Brazil.' *International Journal of Morphology 24*, 1, 61–66.

Chaitow, L. (1999) *Cranial Manipulation – Theory and Practice: Osseous and Soft Tissue Approaches*. Edinburgh: Churchill Livingstone.

Charrette, M. (2005) *Charrette Extremity Adjusting Protocols*. Lecture notes from Dr Mark Charrette DC.

Damasio, A. (2000) *The Feeling of What Happens – Body, Emotion and the Making of Consciousness*. London: Vintage Books.

Damasio, A. (2006) *Descartes' Error*, revised edn. London: Vintage Books.

Dawkins, R. (2009) *The Greatest Show on Earth – The Evidence for Evolution*. London: Bantam Press.

Dean, N.A. and Mitchell, B.S. (2002) 'Anatomic relation between the nuchal ligament (ligamentum nuchae) and the spinal dura mater in the craniocervical region.' *Clinical Anatomy 15*, 182–185.

Diamond, J. (2005) *Guns, Germs and Steel – A Short History of Everybody for the Last 13,000 Years*. London: Vintage Books.

Egan, G. (1997) *The Skilled Helper: A Problem-Management Approach to Helping (Counseling): A Systematic Approach to Effective Helping*, 6th edn. Pacific Grove, CA: Brooks Cole.

Emerson, W. (2009) *2009 Workshop Schedule*. Available at www.emersonbirthrx.com, accessed Oct 2009.

Encyclopedia Britannica (2009) *P'u (Daoism)*. Available at www.britannica.com, accessed May 2009.

Feynman, R.P. (1998) *Six Easy Pieces: Fundamentals of Physics Explained*. London: Penguin.

Fox, S. (2007) *Relating to Clients: The Therapeutic Relationship for Complementary Therapists*. London: Jessica Kingsley Publishers.

Frith, C. (2007) *Making Up the Mind – How the Brain Creates Our Mental World*. Oxford: Blackwell Publishing.

Gendlin, E. (1981) *Focusing*, revised edn. London: Bantam New Age Books.

Gilman, S. and Newman, S.W. (1996) *Manter and Gatz's Essentials of Clinical Neuroanatomy and Neurophysiology*, 9th edn. Philadelphia: F.A. Davis Company.

Gintis, B. (2007) *Engaging the Movement of Life: Exploring Health and Embodiment Through Osteopathy and Continuum.* Berkeley, CA: North Atlantic.

Goldacre, B. (2008) *Bad Science.* London: Fourth Estate.

Guyton, A.C. and Hall, J.E. (2000) *Textbook of Medical Physiology*, 10th edn. London: Saunders.

Held, L.I. Jr (2009) *Quirks of Anatomy – An Evo-Devo Look at the Human Body.* Cambridge: Cambridge University Press.

Herrigel, E. (1953) *Zen in the Art of Archery.* London: Vintage Books.

Holmes, J. (1993) *John Bowlby and Attachment Theory.* London: Routledge.

Ingber, D.E. (2008) 'Tensegrity and mechanotransduction.' *Journal of Bodywork and Movement Therapies 12*, 198–200.

Jackson, M. (2002) *Pain – The Science and Culture of Why We Hurt.* London: Bloomsbury PBK Original.

James, W. (1902/2008) *The Varieties of Religious Experience.* London: Routledge.

Jealous, J. (1994) *Around the Edges.* Bradford on Avon: The UK Sutherland Society.

Jealous, J. (1999) *Accepting the Death of Osteopathy: A New Beginning Winter.* Thomas L. Northup Lecture, AOA Convention, 1999 AAO Journal.

Jealous, J. (2004) *The Biodynamics of Osteopathy.* CD series.

Johnson, S. (2001) *Emergence.* London: Penguin Books.

Jones, C. and Proter, R. (1998) *Reassessing Foucault: Power, Medicine and the Body.* Routledge Studies in the Social History of Medicine. London: Routledge.

Juhan, D. (2003) *Job's Body: A Handbook for Bodywork*, 3rd edn. Barrytown, NY: Barrytown Ltd.

Kandel, E. (2007) *In Search of Memory.* London: W.W. Norton and Co.

Kandel, E., Schwartz, J. and Jessell, T. (2000) *Principles of Neural Science*, 4th edn. Columbus, OH: McGraw-Hill Education.

Kern, M. (2006) *Wisdom in the Body*, 2nd edn. Berkeley, CA: North Atlantic Books.

King, S. (2008) *Live Without Pain.* Cheltenham: Naturality Press.

Lane, N. (2005) *Power, Sex, Suicide – Mitochondria and the Meaning of Life.* Oxford: Oxford University Press.

Lao Tzu (1993) *Tao Te Ching.* Translated by S. Addiss and S. Lombardo. Cambridge, MA: Hackett Publishing.

Levin, S. (2009) *Biotensegrity.* www.biotensegrity.com, accessed November 2009.

Levine, P. (1997) *Waking the Tiger – Healing Trauma.* Berkeley, CA: North Atlantic Books.

Lindley, S.E., Carlson, E.B. and Benoit, M. (2004) 'Basal and dexamethasone suppressed salivary cortisol concentrations in a community sample of patients with posttraumatic stress disorder.' *Biological Psychiatry 55*, 9, 940–945.

Mae Wan Ho (1999) *Coherent Energy, Liquid Crystallinity and Acupuncture.* Talk presented to British Acupuncture Society, 2 Oct. Available at www.i-sis.org.uk/lcm.php, accessed May 2010.

Magoun, H. (1951) *Osteopathy in the Cranial Field*, 1st edn reprint. Fort Worth, TX: The Sutherland Cranial Teaching Foundation.

Maitland, J. (2008) *How Two Biodynamic Theories Masquerade as One.* Unpublished article.

Marieb, E. (2006) *Essentials of Human Anatomy and Physiology*, 8th edn. London: Pearson.

Martini, F. (1998) *Fundamentals of Anatomy and Physiology*, 4th edn. London: Prentice Hall.

Mason, J.W., Giller, E.L., Kosten, T.R. and Harkness, L. (1988) 'Elevation of urinary norepinephrine/cortisol ratio in posttraumatic stress disorder.' *Journal of Nervous and Mental Diseases 176*, 8, 498–502.

MayoClinic.com (2009) *Knee Pain.* www.mayoclinic.com, accessed May 2009.

McBratney-Owen, B., Iseki, S., Bamforth, S.D., Olsen, B.R. and Morriss-Kay, G.M. (2008) Development and tissue origins of the mammalian cranial base. *Developmental Biology 322*, 121–132.

McPartland, J.M. and Skinner, E. (2005) 'The biodynamic model of osteopathy in the cranial field.' *Explore 1*, 1, 21–32.

Melzack, R. and Wall, P. (1996) *The Challenge of Pain*, updated 2nd edn. London: Penguin.

Mental Health America (2008) *Factsheet: Stress: Know the Signs.* Available at www.nmha.org/go/mental-health-month/stress-know-the-signs, accessed Sept 2008. Copyright © Mental Health America.

Milne, H. (1995) *The Heart of Listening*, Vol. 2. Berkeley, CA: North Atlantic Books.

Mitchell, A. and Cormack, M. (1998) *The Therapeutic Relationship in Complementary Health Care.* Edinburgh: Churchill Livingstone.

Moussavi, S., Chatterji, S., Verdes, E., Tandon, A., Patel, V. and Ustun, B. (2007) 'Depression, chronic diseases, and decrements in health: results from the World Health Surveys.' *Lancet 370*, 851–858.

Myers, T.W. (2001) *Anatomy Trains – Myofascial Meridians for Manual and Movement Therapists.* Edinburgh: Churchill Livingstone.

Neira, S.C., Elliott, R. and Isbell, B. (2006) 'Can craniosacral treatment improve the general well-being of patients?' *The Fulcrum 38.* Available at www.craniosacral.co.uk, accessed May 2010.

Nelson, K.E., Sergueef, N. and Glonek, T. (2006) 'The effect of an alternative medical procedure upon low-frequency oscillations in cutaneous blood flow velocity.' *Journal of Manipulative and Physiological Therapeutics 29,* 626–636.

Newell, D. (2003) 'Concepts in the study of complexity and their possible relation to chiropractic health care: a scientific rationale for a holistic approach.' *Clinical Chiropractic 6,* 15–33.

Oschman, J. (2000) *Energy Medicine: The Scientific Basis.* Edinburgh: Churchill Livingstone.

Perrow, C. (2005) *CTET Practitioner Training.* Unpublished lecture.

Pert, C. (1999) *Molecules of Emotion.* London: Simon & Schuster.

Petkova, V.I. and Ehrsson, H.H. (2008) *If I Were You: Perceptual Illusion of Body Swapping.* www.plosone.org, accessed May 2010.

Pinker, S. (2002) *The Blank Slate.* London: Penguin.

Porges, S. (2003) 'The Polyvagal Theory: phylogenetic contributions to social behavior.' *Physiology and Behavior 79,* 503–513.

Porges, S. (2008) *The Polyvagal Theory: Neurophysiological Bases, Phylogenetic Origins, and Clinical Implications.* Unpublished lecture notes from The Relational Heart Conference run by Confer, London.

Price, W. (2008) *Nutrition and Physical Degeneration,* 8th edn. Lemon Grove, CA: Price Pottenger Nutrition.

Ramachandran, V.S. (2004) *A Brief Tour of Human Consciousness.* New York, NY: PI Press.

Redwood, D. and Cleveland, C.S. (eds) (2003) *Fundamentals of Chiropractic.* Edinburgh: Mosby.

Roth, H.D. (2004) *Original Tao, Inward Training (Nei Yeh) and the Foundations of Taoist Mysticism.* New York, NY: Columbia University Press.

Rothschild, B. (2000) *The Body Remembers – The Psychophysiology of Trauma and Trauma Treatment.* London: W.W. Norton.

Sampson, V. (2005) *CST and Myopia.* CTET undergraduate project.

Sapolsky, R. (2004) *Why Zebras Don't Get Ulcers,* 3rd edn. New York, NY: Owl Books.

Scarr, G. (2008) 'A model of the cranial vault as a tensegrity structure, and its significance to normal and abnormal cranial development: research report.' *International Journal of Osteopathic Medicine 11,* 80–89.

Scarr, G. (2009) Personal Communication.

Schleip, R. (2003a) 'Fascial plasticity – a new neurobiological explanation. Part 1.' *Journal of Movement and Bodywork Therapies 7,* 1, 11–19.

Schleip, R. (2003b) 'Fascial plasticity – a new neurobiological explanation. Part 2.' *Journal of Movement and Bodywork Therapies 7,* 2, 104–116.

Schore, A. (1999) *Affect Regulation and the Origin of the Self.* Lawrence Erlbaum.

Schultz, R.L. and Feitiss, R. (1996) *The Endless Web: Fascial Anatomy and Physical Reality.* Berkeley, CA: North Atlantic Books.

Seaman, D. and Winterstein, J. (1998) 'Dysafferentation: a novel term to describe the neuropatho-physiological effects of joint complex dysfunction. A look at likely mechanisms of symptom generation.' *Journal of Manipulative and Physiological Therapeutics 21,* 267–280.

Sewall, L. (1999) *Sight and Sensibility – The Ecopsychology of Perception.* London: Tarcher Putnam.

Shapiro, F. (2001) *Eye Movement Desensitization and Processing – Basic Principles, Protocols and Procedures,* 2nd edn. London: The Guilford Press.

Shea, M. (2007) *Biodynamic Craniosacral Therapy,* Vol. 1. Berkeley, CA: North Atlantic Books.

Shea, M. (2008) *Biodynamic Craniosacral Therapy,* Vol. 2. Berkeley, CA: North Atlantic Books.

Sheldrake, R. (2009) *A New Science of Life: The Hypothesis of Formative Causation.* London: Icon Books.

Sills, F. (2001) *Craniosacral Biodynamics,* Vol. 1 – *The Breath of Life, Biodynamics, and Fundamental Skills.* Berkeley, CA: North Atlantic Books.

Sills, F. (2004) *Craniosacral Biodynamics,* Vol. 2 – *The Primal Midline and Organization of the Body.* Berkeley, CA: North Atlantic Books.

Sills, F. (2009a) *Being and Becoming – Psychodynamics, Buddhism, and the Origins of Selfhood.* Berkeley, CA: North Atlantic Books.

Sills, F. (2009b) Personal communication on organ dynamics.

Simeon, D., Knutelska, M., Yehuda, R., Putnam, F., Schmeidler, J. and Smith, L.M. (2007) 'Hypothalamic-pituitary-adrenal axis function in dissociative disorders, post-traumatic stress disorder, and healthy volunteers.' *Biological Psychiatry 61,* 8, 966–973.

Singh, S. and Ernst, E. (2008) *Trick or Treatment? Alternative Medicine on Trial.* London: Bantam Press.

Soho, T. (1987) *The Unfettered Mind.* Translated by W.S. Wilson. Tokyo: Kodansha International.

Standring, S. (2005) (ed.) *Gray's Anatomy,* 39th edn. Edinburgh: Elsevier.

Stearns, S. (2008) 'Bush pressures US Congress to boost AIDS funding for Africa.' *Voice of America.* Available at www.aegis.com/news/voa/2008/VA080212.html, accessed Mar 2010.

Stone, C. (1999) *Science in the Art of Osteopathy.* Cheltenham: Nelson Thornes.

Stone, C. (2007) *Visceral and Obstetric Osteopathy.* Edinburgh: Churchill Livingstone Elsevier.

Stone, R. (2009) *UK Polarity Therapy Association.* Available at www.ukpta.org.uk/Dr_Stone.htm, accessed Oct 2009.

Strous, D., Maayan, R. and Weizman, A. (2006) 'Review: the relevance of neurosteroids to clinical psychiatry. From the laboratory to the bedside.' *European Neuropsychopharmacology 16,* 155–169.

Sutherland, W.G. (1990) *Teachings in the Science of Osteopathy.* Portland, OR: Rudra Press.

Sutherland, W.G. (1998) *Contributions of Thought,* 2nd edn. Fort Worth, TX: The Sutherland Cranial Teaching Foundation, Inc.

Suzuki, S. (1970) *Zen Mind, Beginner's Mind.* Boston, MA: Weatherhill.

Taleb, N.N. (2007) *The Black Swan – The Impact of the Highly Improbable.* London: Penguin.

Taylor, J.G. (2001) *The Race for Consciousness.* A Bradford Book. Cambridge, MA: The MIT Press.

Terry, K. (2009) *Working at the Level of the Soul.* Available at www.karltonterry.com/index.php/page/181, accessed Oct 2009.

Thayer, J. and Lane, R. (2000) 'A model of neurovisceral integration in emotion regulation and dysregulation.' *Journal of Affective Disorders 61,* 201–216.

Tufts (2009) *Cervical Fascia.* University Department of Anatomy and Cellular Biology Medical and Dental Gross Anatomy. Available at http://iris3.med.tufts.edu/headneck/Index.htm, accessed Mar 2009.

Ukleja, K. (2005) *Karuna Practitioner Training.* Unpublished lecture.

Ukleja, K. (2007) *The Fluid Brain.* Unpublished lecture notes, Da Sein Institute.

Ukleja, K. (2009a) 'Biodynamic: what's in a name?' *The Fulcrum,* letter, Sept. Available at www.craniosacral.co.uk, accessed May 2010.

Ukleja, K. (2009b) *Craniosacral Biodynamic Approaches to the Viscera.* Unpublished lecture notes, Da Sein Institute.

Upledger, J. (2009) *Upledger Institute UK.* Available at www.upledger.co.uk, accessed Oct 2009.

Van der Kolk, B., McFarlane, A. and Weisaeth, L. (eds) (1996) *Traumatic Stress: The Effects of Overwhelming Experience on Mind, Body and Society.* New York, NY: The Guilford Press.

Vu, H.L., Panchal, J., Parker, E.E., Levine, N.S. and Francel, P. (2001) 'The timing of physiologic closure of the metopic suture: a review of 159 patients using reconstructed 3D CT scans of the craniofacial region.' *Journal of Craniofacial Surgery 12,* 6, 527–532.

Wade, A. (1997) 'Small Acts of Living: everyday resistance to violence and other forms of oppression.' *Contemporary Family Therapy 19,* 1. New York, NY: Human Sciences Press Inc.

Watkins, A. (2008) *Heart Rate Variability and Its Implications.* Unpublished lecture notes from The Relational Heart Conference run by Confer, London.

Wilkinson, R. and Pickett, K. (2009) *The Spirit Level: Why More Equal Societies Almost Always Do Better.* London: Allen Lane.

Winfree, A. (1987) *When Time Breaks Down – The Three-Dimensional Dynamics of Electrochemical Waves and Cardiac Arrhythmias.* Princeton, NJ: Princeton University Press.

Yuasa, Y. (1987) *The Body – Toward an Eastern Mind–Body Theory.* New York, NY: State University of New York Press.

Subject Index

Author Index